Medicine and Body Image

Resource Planning for the Poor

Terence Ryan

IAD
Institute of Applied Dermatology
Effective Care through Integrative Medicine

WORDS by DESIGN

Produced in association with

WORDS by DESIGN

www.wordsbydesign.co.uk

ISBN: 978-1-909075-56-6

This edition published by
Institute of Applied Dermatology
Centre for Integrated Medicine & Public Health
IAD junction, Uliyathadka, Madhur Road
Kasaragod, Kerala, India PIN: 671124
Phone: +914994-240862, 240863 Mobile: +918137022233
email: iadorg@gmail.com
website: www.iad.org.in

This book reprint is for free distribution in South Asia Association of Regional Cooperation (SAARC) countries

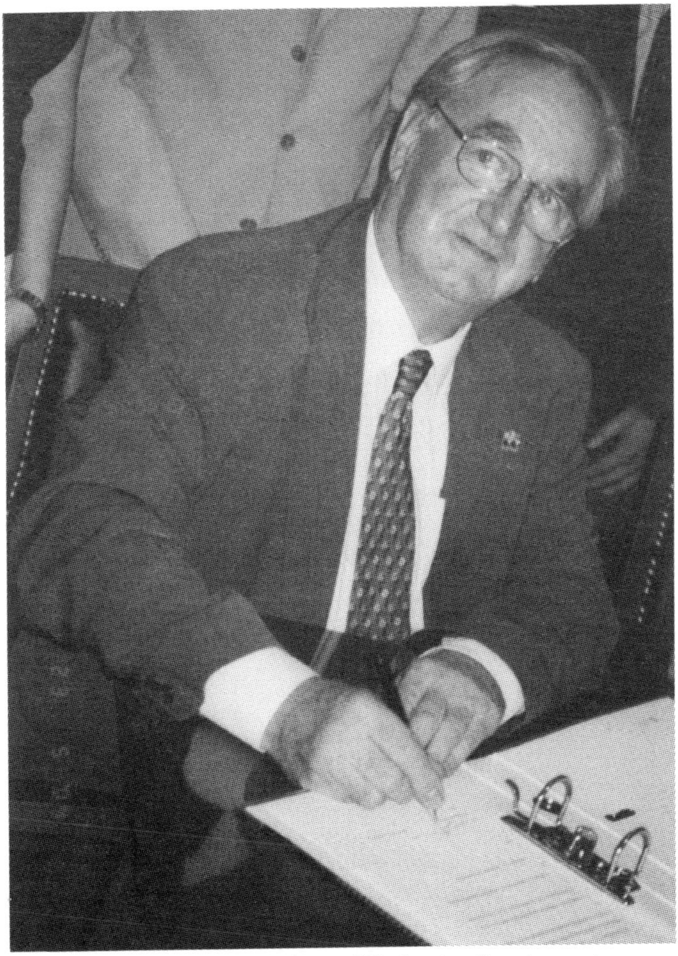

Signing a Memorandum of Understanding to create a system for training village health workers.

To Anne my wife,
my daughter Josephine and son James,
son-in-law James Del Mar,
and grandchildren Cosmo and Adelaide,
with thanks for their encouragement
and support over many years.

CONTENTS

Acknowledgements

The writing of this autobiography was enormously helped by the reading through and detailed commentary of the first six chapters by the late Max Blythe whose comments, following his own experience of writing biographies, gave me the confidence to complete this story of my experiences.

I describe the building up of Oxford Dermatology which would not have been possible without the encouragement of Dr Renwick Vickers and my initial collaborators Rodney Dawber and Fenella Wojnarowska. George and Christine Cherry, by adding much under the heading of The Oxford International Wound Healing Foundation, brought much glory to the department's international reputation.

The later Global Planning had Darrell Wilkinson as my initial stimulator and Al Kopf, Stuart Maddin, Francisco Kerdal Vegas and Henning Grossmann as my first collaborators on the International Foundation of Dermatology, who tackled all the problems, showing both wisdom and passion. From the earliest moments of discussions I recognised Roderick Hay as an essential source of knowledge and negotiating skills worth recruiting as soon as possible.

I have been generously awarded and must especially thank Stephen Ersser for initiating my Professorship at Brookes University and Honorary Degree at the University of Hull, and Wolfgang Marsch for a very grand inauguration at Martin Luther University, Germany.

Terence J Ryan

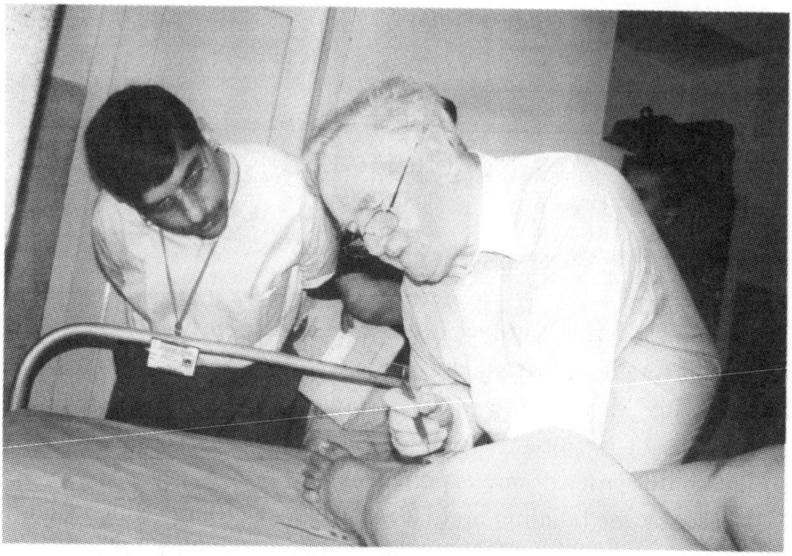

Terence Ryan after retirement from Oxford, as Mentor at the Institute of Applied Dermatology, Kerala, India, with the Director of the Institute Dr S.R. Narahari

1: FAMILY BACKGROUND

My mother always told everyone that father was a descendant of Irish kings ruling the territory of Owney on the borders of Tipperary and Limerick. This is very possible as most Irish descend from tribal leaders. The name Ryan was anglicised from other names such as O'Mulryan at the turn of the nineteenth century. By tradition I was given, at the age of 21, a signet ring with the family crest of a griffin and a motto: 'Rather death than disgrace'. My father, Gerald John Ryan, was born in 1902 in the comfortable home *Melrose* of an aunt in cool Ootacamund[1] in the Nilgiri Hills of South India. Eighty years later it is little changed, painted with a pink wash and overlooking a field of arum lilies. He spent much of his childhood in Burma, near Shwegu in the north and Moulmein in the south, where his family were in the teak business – his father being a Conservator of Forests.[2] My father's brightest memories at Shwegu were of his pony and climbing into the Mingun Bell, the second largest in the world. His younger sister, Shelagh, remembered, as a ten-year-old, travelling to the family in an oxcart from Rangoon, taking several weeks.

The relevant Ryan tribe is based in Scarteen near Limerick and Tipperary. It is famed for its *Black and Tan* hounds on which the family spends its money earned by arranging hunts for Americans.[3] Rather less is spent on a decaying family home. A family tree was revealed on which there was a Hugh Ryan of 1799 with a scribble: 'No legitimate heir.' It is thought that Hugh Ryan might have sired two children, including John Ryan who boarded the *Repulse* in 1823 to sail with the Irish Army to Madras, and who was to sire the Ryan family in India. The family in Ireland is Catholic but the family in India was strongly Protestant. John was one of the first soldiers to find his way in the hot summer of 1840 to the Nilgiri Hills, and after leaving the Army after a few years, making a little money in Australia, he returned to India to build houses on the Nilgiri hillsides at Ootacamund. He and his many descendants are buried, the majority after a very early death from childhood infections, in the Protestant church of St Stephen's. There are many sources of knowledge of the family in Ootacamund, including a local history text[1,3] and the records of the Masonic lodge, while in a famous public library one can see attractive drawings of early Ootacamund on which houses are labelled 'Ryan'. While mostly in the business of forestry and growing Cinchona for quinine as a treatment for malaria, at one stage they went a little to the west and lost money looking for gold. It was the forestry interests that took the family to Burma where my father spent his childhood.

My father's mother developed tropical sprue and was brought home to the London School of Tropical Medicine where she died in 1910. His father, Cecil, then married a missionary schoolmistress. In 1913, my father was sent home to school from Burma to live with an aunt in Sutton from the age of twelve. He went to Ellesmere School with his brother where he excelled in boxing and field sports. He then studied engineering at the Crystal Palace School of Engineering and joined the Glasgow firm of Sir Willam Arrol which built the Forth Bridge. He played hockey for the Cartha Athletic Club, the leading Glasgow sports club, and worked on the Tay Bridge. Immediately after the war there was the Depression, money was short, and in 1922 he was made redundant.

As a result of playing tennis with friends in the south of England, one of whom was Deputy Secretary in the Automobile Association's head office, he was offered a patrol job on a bicycle at the Polegate roundabout between the London highway and the coast route to Lewes and Winchester. He was responsible for an AA telephone box at the roundabout.[4]

He was lonely and lodged in Polegate – and, in search of company, went to a local dance in Polegate Village Hall, close to where Kathleen May Knight lived.

Kathleen May Knight was born on 25th May 1900. She saw herself as a fitting contemporary for Queen Elizabeth the Queen

Mother, and was pleased to have Gemini as her sign of the Zodiac. Exactly who were her twin personalities is difficult to define, but one was certainly larger than life. My mother later claimed that Bob fell instantly in love with the sound of her voice which my mother claimed was notable for her elocution, and also that she only used 300 words of basic English, which was apparently in vogue at the time. Being the centre of attraction was linked with her capacity to make everyone laugh, and the stories she told were always well embellished, so that in due course she could never tell one anything without exaggeration. She loved laughter, and it was first recorded at the age of four, at a village concert when – dressed as a large rose to recite a poem – she was so consumed with giggles that it was never recited, but the entire audience collapsed in laughter.

The family history of mostly Sussex farming stock included several who were nineteenth-century mayors of Lewes but also some who had residence in the debtors' prison in Lewes Castle. The story of her family, her two elder brothers and elder sister, is described by her brother Cecil Knight in 'Memoirs of an Eventful Life'.[5] Cecil, who was a snob, did not mention that they were poor. Indeed, bankruptcies affected the family in the nineteenth century, and her grandmother kept a diary recording this terrible development. Her father, Clement Knight, was a corn merchant. A legacy of £9,000 from Grand-uncle Weller allowed the purchase of a fine house and garden, *Heatherwood* in Buxted. As the youngest and perhaps most attractive of the Knight children, my mother received a great deal of attention, and throughout her life thereafter she aimed to be at the centre of it. She had a happy childhood except for some life-threatening events. The first of these was when she fell down a well, and was missing for several hours. Her brother Cecil in his memoirs attributes her survival to his having taught her to float. The second near miss was when she fell on a scythe, cut her hand badly and developed tetanus – from which, at that time, it was unusual to survive. The wound was exposed to the air and incised frequently: these were kitchen table operations while she was anaesthetised with chloroform.

Throughout her life she treated her pets as preferable or equal to humans, and in early childhood, her greatest friend, kept at an uncle's

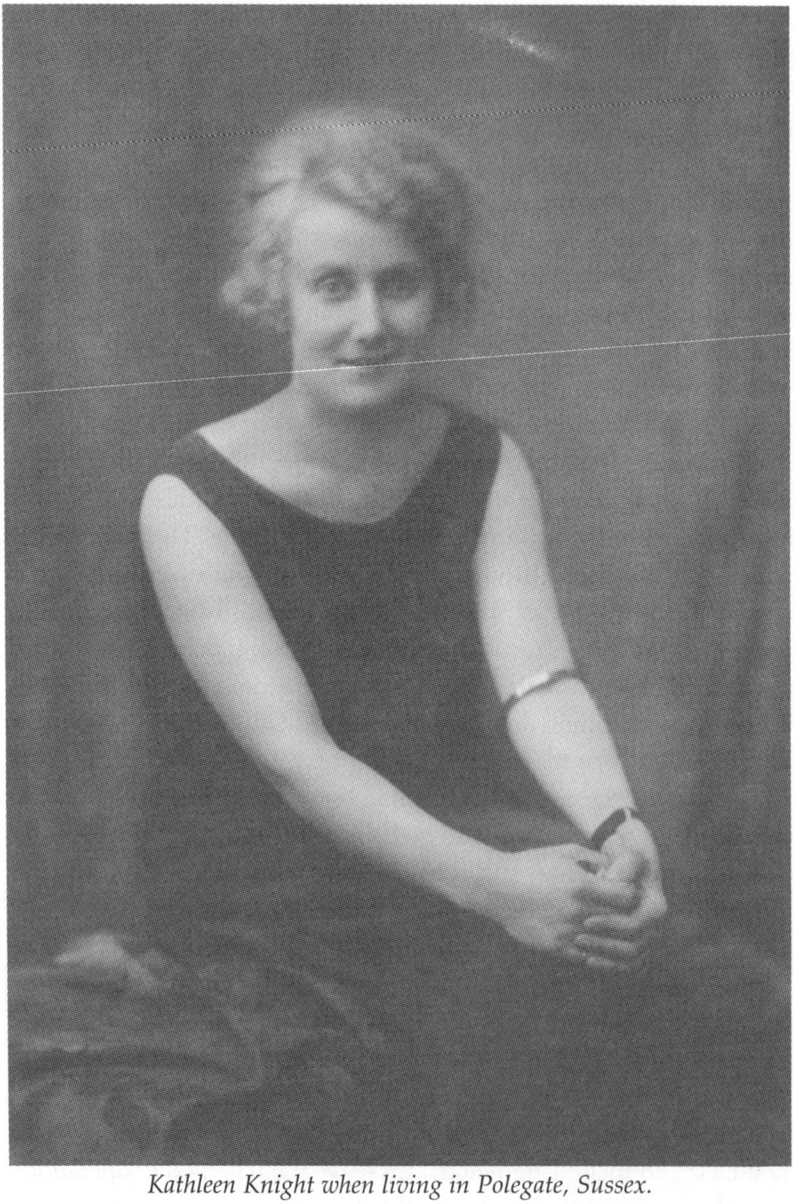

Kathleen Knight when living in Polegate, Sussex.
An attractive teenager, engaged three times, having spent two years in France and Belgium driving ambulances, cars and motobikes

farm two miles away, was her donkey which accompanied her everywhere – including, on one occasion, up the stairs to her bedroom, where it refused to move either forwards or backwards, and eventually had to be carried downstairs backwards by the farm-hands.

At about the age of twelve, a happy childhood came to an end when her mother died of cancer. Her mother had survived a mastectomy for cancer of one breast when Kathleen was aged six. Both mastectomies were performed at St Bartholomew's Hospital, London. For a year, dressed in black, Kathleen had to stay with a strict and gloomy aunt, where amongst other things she became sick and despairing over two tasks – the making of a black rug, and the learning of the *Gypsy Rondo* for the piano by Haydn. Only a small black dog gave her any happiness during that period. When her father married again, she was never able to accept her new stepmother; she was sent to boarding schools and expelled from three of them. The first time was, when in quarantine with mumps, she escaped to play with the doctor's sons next door and gave them mumps. On the second occasion, in a dormitory, one of the girls requested that she must always say 'please' when passing her bed, for which she received a broken nose from Kathleen's hairbrush. The teachers at one school gave her prizes for punctuality and truthfulness. This she never forgot and always arrived too early, and always reminded one about her truthfulness when it was clear that her latest tale was unbelievable.

In 1914 war broke out, and in its third year, at the age of sixteen, she claimed to be older and was recruited into the Armed Forces. Photographs show her as an attractive blonde. She was proud that her 'dimensions' were the same as the Venus de Milo, ignoring the fact that she was five inches shorter! She dropped the name of Kathleen and was variously known as Patricia, Patrick, Pat or Patsy. During the war, she spent at least a year in France as a dispatch rider and an ambulance driver, and for a short period helped to train the horses of the Canadian cavalry. At the time of the battle of the Somme, she was a chauffeur of senior officers between HQs and hospitals.[6] At one stage, she fell into a trench with the dead, and remembered the stench thereafter. At the end of the war, Pat did

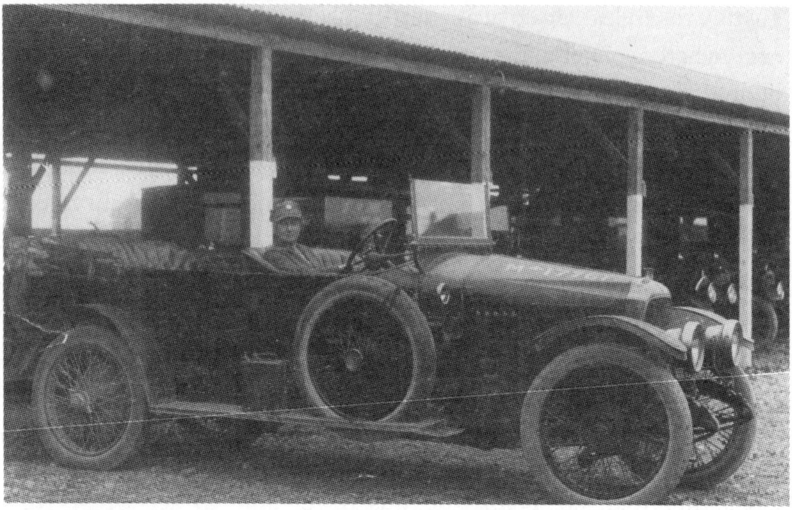

Kathleen Knight driving senior officers between headquarters and hospital

mostly a chauffeuring job of medical specialists and she drove a very large staff car. Pat noticed that one of the medical officers, Ned White, was looking yellow. A diagnosis of jaundice was made, and he was saved from going to the front and thereafter claimed that Pat had saved his life. He remained her family doctor until his death, 40 years or so later.

Her discharge from the Army was 25th November 1919. Several letters of appreciation were sent from the Quartermaster-General which would have relevance to her subsequent career in the next war (see note 4 in Chapter 2).

Kathleen Ryan had been engaged twice, once to a doctor, who became Westminster Hospital's chief pathologist, and then to a London diamond merchant. That was shortly after the end of the war. The main event in this period was the meeting with Gerald John Ryan, known as Bob Ryan, in 1923, after which she ditched the diamond merchant pretty quickly. Bob was not yet 21 and his parents in India would not give permission for him to get married. A letter to Pat, from Bob Ryan's father, dated April 1923, actually states that he had no objection to their being engaged saying, 'I know now you won't be foolish and marry in a hurry. Young Bob is a wonderful fellow. Make him set to make good in his profession. He must not chuck it now.' But not heeding his parents' wishes, immediately after reaching 21, the banns were read at Polegate church – by which time his parents were hurrying back by boat from India to stop the wedding, arriving a day too late.

Cecil Ryan was right in predicting that they would have financial difficulties, and five days before the wedding Bob Ryan wrote of 'more money worries' – having only £1 on the day of the wedding, for buying scraps for Pat's dog Bonzo!

On the first visit to the new in-laws from India, Pat borrowed a Bentley and a large empty trunk in order to hide their poverty. Later, father-in-law Cecil Ryan was successfully taught to drive by her. They saw Cecil and his wife rarely during their retirement in England. After the wedding, Pat advertised as a valet with driving skills, and she also drove lorry chassis from Dover to London.

Immediately after the marriage, Pat Ryan was chauffeuring in Clapton, and when she had time off, my father, as an AA patrol, might bicycle into Eastbourne when she would catch a glimpse of him 'for two short minutes'. Otherwise they met only on Sundays. They wrote daily and my mother, who was anxious he would meet other girls, valued this daily contact for reassurance. Bob Ryan frequently visited her father Clement Knight, who had long given up control of his daughter and must have been grateful for such a pleasant young man to take over his ill-disciplined daughter.

Later, when in the summer Bob was drafted to help at the harbour at Newhaven, he had a motor-cycle combination and repair equipment. He lived in digs with other harbour staff and played hockey for Newhaven, and while there was selected to play for the Sussex County as outside right.

Bob was soon promoted to being the AA Port Officer at Newhaven. Members of the AA had documents to be checked and cars were driven onto platforms and lifted onto the ships. In rough weather, vehicles could be lost overboard. It was clear from letters kept by my mother until her death that both before and after the wedding they saw each other only at weekends until Bob became the AA Harbour Superintendant at Folkestone and Dover, 1924-26, and they began living together. Later, when Bob took charge of the AA Sussex County Office in Brighton, they felt much better off and had a comfortable first-floor flat.[7]

These were mostly happy times. Pat was determined to have fun, and took up riding. Many of her long-term friends stemmed from that time and their circle of hockey friends included several members of the Sussex team. These were days when they enjoyed camping on the Sussex Downs and going to dances and concerts.

Pat looked for ways to boost their finances. Her piano skills provided extra money as an accompanist at a ballet school and she made decorative matchboxes for a Brighton store. Elsie Thompson was a girlfriend with whom my mother had most laughs. Her husband, Percy, had a good tenor voice. Shortly after the death of the first-born of the Thompsons they attended a musical evening. Percy was singing Coleridge Taylor's *Hiawatha* which has a line including the words 'leaped to meet me'. Percy's false teeth dropped out at that point; Elsie and Pat became hysterical with laughter. The audience thought that Elsie was suffering from grief due to the death of her child, and was crying not from laughter. Elsie left, and could be seen from the window clinging to the railings, consumed with laughter.

Many of the stories were about making the most of their money. At one stage, when the Charleston was all the rage in Paris, they decided to spend all their money on going to Paris to learn this new dance. Trips to the Continent were possible and affordable because Bob Ryan was in charge of the shipping of cars for the AA from Folkestone. When they came back, they were the Charleston King and Queen of the Folkestone dance halls. They visited the Folies Bergère when the famous cabaret star Josephine Baker descended from the ceiling dressed in bananas and sat on Bob's knee. Pat's love of animals meant that she always had to have an exotic beast or two. They were probably one reason for delaying having a family and they featured both in her camera and her storytelling. Her favourite animal was a large harlequin Great Dane known as Bill – a very handsome animal, with which she used to walk down the front at Brighton. On one occasion she met Edward, Prince of Wales, who asked whether the dog was for sale.

One of Pat Ryan's trips overseas without Bob was for a first experience of skiing at Zermatt. This was the occasion of a famous avalanche which left them stranded for several weeks. On another visit, she tried to out-ski everyone by taking a dangerous short cut and broke her leg.

The 1920s were noted both for the financial difficulties of the population but also for the partying. My mother was a great one for joining movements and I have a collection of her badges and emblems. One day she would be a Methodist, another a Catholic. For periods she had joined the Fascists and admired Oswald Mosley, then it was the Black and Tans in the wars of Southern Ireland, and then there was Hitler who did not immediately repel her – but she was always on the lookout for a laugh. My father focused on doing his job and playing hockey as well as possible. Against this background there was no question of having a family until well into their thirties, which was unusual at that time.

Notes on Chapter 1

1) Price, Frederick (1908), *Ootacamund: A History*. Rupa & Co., Dakshin, Bangalore, India, purchasable at Higginbottom's, an ancient and well-known bookstore chain found throughout South India.

2) In 1987, on a visit to Burma and Sri Lanka on behalf of the University of Oxford (organised by Drs John Ledingham and David Warrell, to celebrate the 150th anniversary of Sri Lanka's Medical School), I was given by the Burmese forestry department some mid-nineteenth-century records of the family. They included details of holidays, children's schooling and much else. Sadly, my father died of lung cancer while I was there.

By an odd coincidence, an Australian colleague, Gerry Bodeker, with whom I closely collaborated from 1990, was told by his elder sister that our families had collaborated in Burma in the teak industry. When his elder sister was aged two, the family had a visit from a bald-headed Mr Ryan. He sat in a low-lying chair up to which the child crept and, fascinated by a bald head which she had not seen before, tickled it with a feather. Mr Ryan unknowingly brushed it away as with a fly. Happily, the child left the room without there being any comment, only to return with a small toy train engine which she ran over the visitor's head.

3) The New Zealander Thady Ryan, an Olympic medallist of Equestrian sport, headed the Ryan clan and died in 2014. His biography is mostly about his being Master of the Hounds. Ryan, Thady, MFH, (2002), *My Privileged Life with Scarteen Black and Tan Hounds*, Derrydale Press, Lanham, New York.

My extensive Ryan family records are much indebted to my cousin Vanya Orr and are held by cousin Fay Ross-Magenty, Lockeridge, near Marlborough.

4) A key to the AA telephone boxes was a popular item, strictly for members. There was a well-known AA piece of advice to members, and in the early days a main function of AA patrols: 'If a patrol does not salute, stop and ask him why.' Usually it was to report a police trap! Barty-King, Hugh (1980), *The AA: A History of the First 75 Years of the Automobile Association 1905-1980*. Published by the Automobile Association, Fanum House, Basingstoke, Hants.

5) The story of the Knight family is described in *Memoirs of an Eventful Life* by Kathleen's brother Cecil Knight (Lavenham Press, Lavenham, Suffolk, 1980). Cecil married the daughter of a burgomaster whose first husband fathered Audrey Hepburn.

6) It is possible that my mother may have driven the American surgeon Harvey Cushing, the biographer of Oxford's most famous Dr Sir William Osler. She was on duty, driving doctors near the battlefield hospital when Revere Osler, the son of the Regius Professor of Medicine at Oxford, was severely injured and this famous American surgeon, Harvey Cushing, was called in to attend to him. In *With the British Medical Corps in France*, in *Consecratio Medici and Other Papers* (Little, Brown and Co., Boston, 1928), he describes hundreds of vehicles and only mentions male drivers. He visited countless crowded field stations and hospitals with British and French soldiers with terrible wounds.

7) They lived in an upstairs flat with their Great Danes and other species of dogs at 68 New Church Street, Hove, Sussex.

2: A Pre-World War II Childhood and an Eventful War

Eventually, after ten years of marriage, Pat and Bob decided they would have children, and in 1932, aged 32, my mother became pregnant. Eventually, in July, her family practitioner, Ned White, arranged for her to be induced by a Queen Charlotte inflatable bag method of induction, which had recently been introduced. After a long period in labour at home in which it seemed not to work, in a small first-floor flat in Hove, Ned performed a Caesarean, delivering her a son. She remained extremely ill after that for several weeks. It was a bad experience which she frequently talked about, especially to her son. Ned wrote a poem about the event to be given to me at the age of twelve. It was not thought safe for my mother to have a second child, and one further pregnancy in 1938 was followed by an abortion.

On the advice of Grandfather, I was named Terence John, since in Ireland they distribute a card which states that Terence means 'He is hard-working and doesn't give up'.

I was brought up by a succession of helpers including a young German girl called Jenny Vogel, the daughter of a Viennese Poet Laureate. Having been brought up to believe that the English were tall and wore formal dress, she never quite got used to the informalities of being an *au pair* girl in the family of Pat and Bob.[1] She was surprised to be met at Brighton station by Pat Ryan, dressed in her nightdress and slippers.

My earliest memories are when still in Hove. A single step, carpeted in green, had to be climbed into the parents' bedroom. Unhappy memories were unloved meal times. There was *Milk of Magnesia*, synthetic orange juice and small cartoons of cream. Labelled as having 'acidosis' meant being the topic of conversation, displayed and looked upon with sadness by all visitors. Lunch was

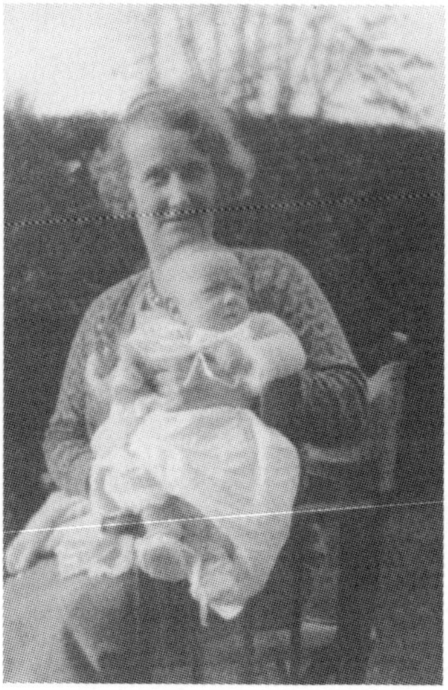

The first photograph to be taken of Terence with his mother at the home of her father in Buxted, Sussex

always a slow business, being fed spoonful by spoonful to some 20 or more squirrels in my stomach, all with identifiable names.

The attention from my parents was not generous. Although there are lots of photos of me on my mother's lap or being wheeled in a pram, in later years my mother told me I did not strike any chord with her until at about the age of four when she saw me looking out of a window crying as she departed, and she then knew that she was cared for. My father said she could have me as an infant but he would take over when he could teach me cricket. Such an event never occurred and anything like it was not greeted with joy by a very shy child.

Contacts were maintained with Mother's family: with my grandfather Clement Knight, walking downhill in Buxted, Sussex, a short distance to see the trains. But I kept clear of Step-Grandma who had a hairstyle like an Alice in Wonderland queen and illustrations in her Mother Goose's Nursery Rhymes frightened me.

My mother's Great Danes were good friends, allowing me to ride them, pulling a sledge in the snow or allowing me to paint them with whitewash, but the harlequin Dane killed my pet white rabbit and a bull terrier terrifyingly killed neighbours' dogs.

In 1935, my father was promoted to take up control of the AA's North of England office in Nottingham. On leaving Sussex, the *Sussex Daily News* described him as having unfailing tact and a comprehensive understanding of the difficulties of the motoring public and the trade – and hard to replace as a hockey player.

My parents looked at a few houses together but eventually my mother chose to rent *The Elms* at Bottesford, near Nottingham, a

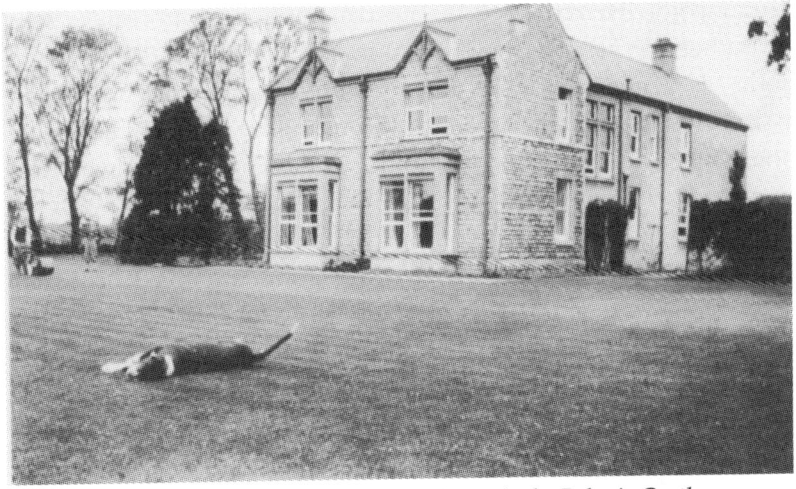

The Elms, Nottinghamshire, which overlooks Belvoir Castle. Bill the Great Dane in the foreground.

house that was rather too grand to be affordable. It was a late Victorian house that had a long drive with daffodils and a lawn with a ha-ha that looked out on a windmill across fields, at the back of which was Belvoir Castle. *The Elms* was owned by Mr Marsh and son Alec, the starters of the Derby. It had stables and was surrounded by fields. I was nervous when placed on horses and worried when watching my mother break them in. A horse named Goldilocks threw her and nearly broke her back.

My father began his immaculate gardening with a perfect lawn for tennis and a kitchen garden. He was always alone – neither I nor my mother were expected to help, and this was to remain so throughout my life. The house had a drawing room and dining room with large low-lying windows which the dogs and all of us used as exits into the garden. There was a nursery and a kitchen in which frilly-hatted maids lived.

Shortage of money to pay for all this was a problem. My mother's close riding friend Rex Remington solved this by every now and again turning up, having sold some of his parents' silver – and eventually he moved into the house as a companion and gardener, saving the expense of a gardener and bringing useful extra income. He remained for 3½ years until the outbreak of war. My father was at work in an office in Nottingham, and Rex was at home as a companion to my mother, enjoying the riding and assisting with the parties she loved arranging and holding. The house was cold, and wood had to be sawn each day, mainly by Rex, to provide enough fuel.

In 1936, it was thought appropriate for me to have a governess, and a Miss Leaf arrived and stayed for a few months. I heard my mother state that Miss Leaf had 'BO' and wondered what possession that might be. For the 1936 Coronation, Miss Leaf made a red, white and blue suit for my golliwog and helped me read *Black Sambo*, a popular child's book of the time. There was very little social contact with children. There are memories of people dressing up for a village fête, a first visit of a circus and visiting the poor, whose names were all surnames. The grander neighbours were more reverentially addressed. There was a Miss Middlemass, a garden snob, who gave us a rare flower called 'Mysotis' which my mother denied all knowledge of – a little blue flower which we discovered was forget-me-not which already grew abundantly in our garden.

I heard my first ghost stories from one of the kitchen maids, who was dismissed for telling them to me. Not much time was spent with my parents nor with Rex, but I felt left behind when they went off anywhere. They visited the local 'movies'. I thought this was someone taking the pictures of the wall of the house and moving them round. Why did they have to leave our house to do that? My first movie was not until about the age of eight, partly because Cedric Greenep, one of my father's hockey friends, said *Snow White* was too frightening for me.

Miss Leaf did not last long and briefly there was a share of another governess in the village.

Cedric Greenep, who had acted as proxy godfather when the proper one did not turn up, visited regularly over 30 years and allowed the four-year-old to repetitively act as a snake to kill him and then to wave a magic wand to bring him back to life. Cedric was accused of borrowing and not returning money, for which he was chased round the garden naked, with Pat Ryan thrashing him with a horse-whip.

There has never been a record of my father's views on my mother's boyfriends that went with the house or the horses. It is apparent from photographs that he enjoyed tennis parties, ferreting and organising shooting parties, and also poaching, using sultanas to attract pheasants into the beam of his car headlights on the Belvoir estate.[2]

To be in the presence of my father alone invoked severe shyness which was not enjoyable for either of us. He tried teaching me cricket, took me for drives in his car and attempted to interest me in shooting, but these sessions with my father were uncomfortable as I was very shy in his presence. Not being a courageous child, I disappointed both parents at children's parties when I would not jump out of a tree on a suspended rope, or would not leap with glee into a swimming pool. My mother's noisy and ribald humour also worried me. In my case, the only child syndrome was a lack of friends and shyness when visiting others.

In 1937, after two years at *The Elms* at Bottesford, probably for reasons of affordability, there was a move closer to Nottingham – to Bingham and a red brick house on the main road close to the church. The rooms were not large but here too there were maids – most of them were homesick, and there are memories of them in tears while having to be kitted out with specially-made clothing and frilly caps. The Bingham house had a long garden where my father could usually be found, beyond which was a railway. I claimed that every train driver was my best friend and spent much time waving to them. Rex, who was with us at both houses, used to look after vegetables, sheds and stables – now without horses. My mother's much younger stepbrother, Uncle Eric, helped to make a concrete path with all our palm marks and initials. Grandfather Clement Knight taught me to ride my first bicycle there. Whereas all my mother's family were well-known to us, the Ryan family were not, and my father lacked any inclination to see them.

When eventually I started at a private school, in a neighbouring village, it was my father's job to take me there with one or two other pick-ups on his way to work. At the age of five-and-a-half, the new school required social adaptation. It was wrong to kiss little girls, but dancing with them to the tunes of nursery rhymes, such as *Ring a Ring a Roses* and *London Bridge is Burning Down*, was enjoyably acceptable. I vividly remember the pictures illustrating my first reading books and began to take an interest in drawing.

Termly reports showed reasonable achievement but a very great number of absences, perhaps on days that Father could not get me there. There was a two-week period boarding, with much enjoyment because of evening games, while my mother had an abortion.

After about the age of five, there were early morning visits to my mother in bed after the departure of my father to work. They were often times for visits of her boyfriends with morning tea and practical jokes with raucous laughter. I would join in the laughter but actually felt quite frightened by the jokes played and their ribald humour.[3] On one occasion, there was a water-fight throughout the house with increasingly large containers of water. Finally, a large aluminium bath used for bathing the Great Danes was filled with water and thrown at my mother on the stairs. On another occasion, there was the throwing by Rex and Pat of each other's belongings out of the front windows onto the main street until all clothes cupboards were bare and there were heaps of clothing in the road outside.

There are happier memories of staying in a cosseted stress-free environment without meal enforcement, in a disused train carriage at the beach at West Wittering, with my mother's elder sister Aunt Lil. Travel there was in an old *Austin* driven by 70-year-old Uncle Charles who prided himself at not changing gear even once between London and the coast. Sometimes my parents stayed nearby with lots of friends in a local pub. On one occasion, my father assisted with sand castles.

In 1937, all was to change. A war began to threaten. My mother, at the age of 37, was a sought-after young woman who had had experience of World War I.[4] World War II did not burst upon us as my mother, at the age of 37, was recruited as a part of preparations from 1937. With experience as a driver in the previous war she was appointed as a volunteer section leader of the Women's Legion Mechanical Transport (WLMT) Section. But she also received a letter from Lady Londonderry of Londonderry House in London, who wrote that her help and interest would be deeply appreciated to discuss the formation of a Women's Defence Association, and in September 1938 it seemed that the WLMT would be responsible for all Royal Air Force requirements, and all the clerical and general duties of all forces. However, it was a thorough muddle with the War Office issuing instructions but with the three Armed Forces remaining uncertain as to whether they were responsible for either a single women's organisation or up to three separate Auxiliary Territorial Services. My mother was given responsibility for recruitment in the north of England for a new organisation to support the RAF, in a letter adding, 'I am sure we can give the RAF a fair deal but training should be on RAF lines and not on Military lines.' She was recruiting volunteer drivers, clerks, equipment managers, supervisors, cooks, orderlies and fabric workers.

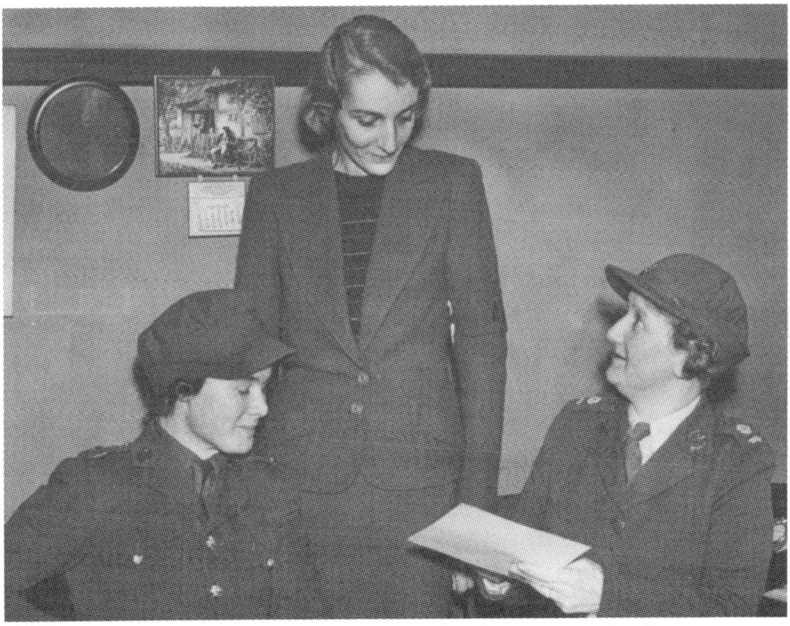

Pat Ryan (far right) recruiting for the Women's Legion Mechanical Transport in 1938 based in Nottingham

There were numerous points of contention, such as who should pay, and how much for what badges or uniforms. The Air Ministry, by now planning their own branch of a women's auxiliary service, wrote that all candidates must be British Subjects of pure European descent, and that the WAAF (Women's Auxiliary Air Force) was 'not to register upholsterers, photographers, tracers and draughtsman. However, teleprinters must be intelligent and able to type 30 words a minute.' The HQ was said to be in existence but no buildings had been purchased. My mother worked from home, juggling service commitments and domestic responsibilities. It was still an age in which titles determined who was in charge but now only a year was to pass and that age was to vanish. In December 1938, a new Drill Hall was opened for my mother in Nottingham by the Duke of Portland. She was now writing to and receiving letters to both Lady Londonderry and Lady Belper – the latter, for example, about the purchase of gas masks for her company. My mother enjoyed the company of the Ladies Londonderry and Belper. By April 1939, she was Nottinghamshire's County Commandant for what was to become the WAAF, but the Women's Legion wrote: 'You are not County Commandant for us and it is not possible for you to continue duties with us.'

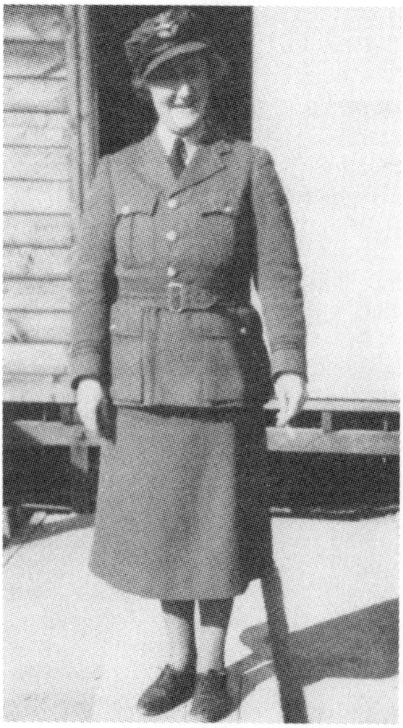

Pat Ryan in her first WAAF uniform outside her newly opened office at Hucknall, Nottingham, at the outbreak of war

By June 1939, Pat was addressing the language to be used for drill, and details of the tests that recruits would be expected to pass. On 28th June, the King approved the new Women's Auxiliary Air Force and the blue colour of their uniform. On 12th July, the Air Ministry was instructing her 'to only approve Women's Legion instructions if deemed suitable by herself, and any rejection of their recruits should be managed tactfully'. Lady Belper advised her to keep the Air Ministry quiet 'for three or four weeks until we know what we want'. A letter from the Naval and Military Club[5] informed Pat that the War Office thought their recruitment was 'another snob show'. It became well-known that the Women's Legion's nose was out of joint. There seems also to have been an Auxiliary Territorial Service in Nottinghamshire, headed by Lady Belper.

There was correspondence about emoluments of 50 shillings per week for other ranks and three guineas for officers, and although the King had said they should be blue, there was correspondence about the khaki uniforms which were actually issued.

It was now only two days before the outbreak of war. On 2nd September, my mother wrote to Lady Belper, saying,

> *I arrived on Tuesday to report to Hucknall to see if I could do anything, and interviewed the Air Vice-Marshal, who gave me authority – acting on an Air Ministry letter – to call up the 15th WAAF Company. They reported for duty immediately. We took possession of an office, dressed in our new uniforms, and transport was obtained to and from Nottingham until yesterday, 1st September, when quarters were fitted and they are confined to barracks here. Please forgive me for neglecting my duty to you in notifying you of all this, but we have been working 24 hours a day and are very proud to be the first WAAF Company called up. The Air Vice-Marshal and whole staff at Hucknall were treating us extraordinarily well, looking after our comfort and helping us in every way that is possible. Their one concern is that we are working too hard. Our orders are now not to try and do the impossible, and to get our administrative side going. My strength is about 60 and has to be increased to 187 immediately.*

And they were soon to be much involved in plotting and decoding.

On reading the official list of the WAAF in 1940, my mother is listed just as another Flight Lieutenant and none of the above volunteer work with its various senior titles is listed.

I have no memories of any of this story of the WAAF except its ending, sitting in front of the radio with my mother and Rex on 3rd September, listening to the famous 'We are at War!' announcement. In mid-1939, blackout had to be made and there was the first wearing of gas marks. My mother used to tell people that she had asked me whether I would like to go to Canada, and having heard of a boat of British evacuees being torpedoed, I said, "No!"

When the war came, all the contents of the house were packed up by Rex and put in store. It was a foul winter but, still short of money, we managed to make £7.10.0 (£7.50) on the apples from the garden that had been stored away.

And so it seems my mother played her part in history, for at least one year as a volunteer, by being one of the first to be recruited and to command the Women's Auxiliary Air Force. Maybe, too, hers was the first WAAF Company to be called up. If so, this is the first time this has been recorded apart from very frequent reports in the Nottinghamshire newspapers.

Two days before war was declared, my father joined the Sherwood Foresters regiment.

Once war was declared, my mother found a WAAF to drive me in an *Austin* 8 down to Worcester to stay with my step-grandmother Minnie Ryan, who had a very small seventeenth-century cottage overlooking the churchyard at Hanley Castle near Upton-on-Seven. Water was obtained from a hand pump and the weekly bath was a copper tub squeezed in against the walnut family dining table. It was in the tiny garden of this seventeenth-century cottage that I came to know the behaviour of every inhabitant. There were no children to play with, so spiders and slugs were important interests and even companions to talk to.

Grandma had been a Protestant missionary school teacher. She had not had children of her own, and the experience was like being at boarding school. During the day, one went to classes in the local village school – which were not memorable – but in the evening and on Saturday morning, one had intensive tutorials, the best of which were nature walks. There was tuition in astronomy and the identification of trees. There was a polishing of prayer books in the adjacent church, and some very long church services. The three-hour service on Good Friday is remembered as a barely tolerable experience. There were also table manners to develop, and brushing one's own shoes. It was an intense period without any of the wild gaiety or stresses that had characterised home life. At the age of seven, I was ready to learn and was grateful for any reading matter – which included a newsletter of the University Mission to Central Africa, written for the young which described finding solutions for the problems of the peoples of the British Empire. In February 1940, following commendation while with a unit in Britain, my father was promoted to Lieutenant and sent with the British Expeditionary Force to France, adding to worries inflamed by bad war news.

I was largely unaware of the war, and what was happening to my parents, one of them setting up WAAFs at various aerodromes, and the other fighting in France and then retreating to Dunkirk. Rare half-day meetings with my mother would always end in tears, because saying goodbye was grim.

Having established the WAAFs in Hucknall, my mother moved some six months later to Aston Down in Gloucestershire to start up the WAAFs there.

In the early summer of 1940, I was billeted within a few miles of Aston Down aerodrome and my mother was able to see me about every three weeks. The house, later demolished, was *The Vicarage* of Amberley, near Stroud. It had stairs under which we would take cover when there were air raids. We would listen each night to the sounds of aircraft and try to identify them as British or German. I shared a bedroom with three East End evacuees, which should have been playmates, but I spent more time with the Vicar's teenage family who were home before taking up war work. The East Enders were rough companions, and one had to compete for the few kind words and friendships. We often had to sleep in air-raid shelters. The vicar's sermons seemed very long on Sundays,

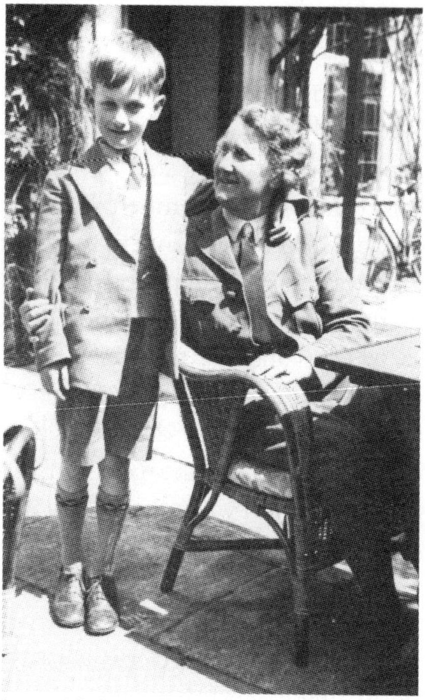

Terence staying with his mother one weekend at the requisitioned headquarters at Aston Down near Cirencester

and the rest of the week he completely ignored the children in the house.

Initially I went to a small kindergarten run by a middle-aged lady with plaits circling her head, who taught French, but after one term it was followed by a prep school called St George's, which was oppressive. It was my most unhappy period. There was always the fear of the cane, although not experienced. There was 'rugger' and cross country runs, Latin and Greek, bread and dripping for tea, and no pleasure. Eventually, I found a solution to my feelings of oppression, and encouraged a small fat boy to walk home with me along a rather solitary path and then attacked him. At the age of eight, it was probably the worst thing I have ever done.

There was a long silence following my father's transfer to France and my mother eventually heard from him only on his return on 30th May when he wrote from Aldershot:

Well! Well! Here I am back in England. I landed at Dover yesterday morning from Dunkirk and the first thing I did was to dash on the platform to send you a wire. I sent it to the Adjutant at Harwell and asked him to tell you I was home because I did not want you to receive the shock of a telegram direct [as these usually reported a death], especially at this particular time, and I do hope he passed it on to you.

'Well, darling, a great deal has happened during the last few weeks. When we left Rennes about three weeks ago, we were rushed up into Belgium, near Brussels, and from that time we have been all over that awful triangular bit of country. We never stayed more than one night in one place and rarely had more than two hours sleep in one night. Anyway, the day before yesterday we were near Cassel but had orders to return to Dunkirk. Off we started – hog-frogging with our quite inadequate transport – some marching, some riding, turn and turn about. Eventually I got a company and a half on the dunes near Dunkirk and returned to pick up more. I got so far, only to find that there was no hope of getting transport through and I was ordered to destroy all our trucks. We kept one and with the driver got nearer to Dunkirk when that one had to be ditched and rendered useless. My small party then began to march and we soon contacted the battalion who had been ordered to hold a bridge over the canal south of Dunkirk. At this point, our CO ordered me to get back to Dunkirk, to try to 'win' some transport and bring back the 1½ companies which I had already left there. So off we trudged again. ten miles of most unpleasant walking. Halfway there, we met the Brigadier of our Brigade who told me there was no hope of my getting the run back and that I was to continue to Dunkirk and wait there with them. Well, off we went dead tired and eventually arrived on the racecourse at Malo-les-Bains where the one-and-a-half companies had been left – but no sign of them. I made enquiries and found they had already embarked – it was now 11.00pm and raining hard. We marched on another two miles along the sands towards Dunkirk Quay where eventually I found an officer controlling embarkation. He told me to get on board as

> *it was essential to get all British troops off as soon as possible. So I and my little band of eight drivers finally got on board at 4.ooam and set sail for Dover where we landed at 9.00pm. I don't know what has happened to the rest of the battalion and am rather worried about them. I do hope they got through safely.*

Towards the end of 1940, my mother was moved to Harwell aerodrome. Her rank at this time was Flight Lieutenant, and she was due to be promoted to Group Captain. In 1941, I lived on a farm nearby. The Germans bombed Harwell every day, at midday and midnight. Harwell had no guns, and the planes flew over so low that one could see the pilot very easily. One was always running to the shelter, but it was a fine summer, and I enjoyed some friends of my own age. There was a worrying session following being given piggy-backs by a pilot who was absent without leave, and there was a session involving me in identification, and his court martial. There were feelings of insecurity, and episodes of bad behaviour, losing my temper and throwing cabbage stalks at my mother.

I was treated very kindly at the aerodrome, and explored Wellingtons, Lancasters, Spitfires and other planes, as well as once or twice in a Link Trainer. I was conscious of not being as enthusiastic about the planes as was expected of me, but did not know how to do better. Forty Lancasters flew off to bomb Turin, and they all returned. One of these, which I may have even climbed over, now sits outside the War Museum in Canberra, Australia.

We next heard from my father in September 1940. It was the time my mother and I were severely bombed and shot at. There were times when she was machine-gunned. Known as 'Deadly', because of her expertise in revolver training, she would be encouraged to run as fast as she could, and sometimes her companions were shot at her side. Throughout the first two years of the war, she was always accompanied by her Great Dane, which was killed by shrapnel at her side. One of her best friends was blown up on a petrol tank, and another crashed in a Spitfire in flames quite close to her. While my mother suffered from anxiety, as a child I did not recognise the daily bombing for the danger that it was. My father wrote to my mother, 'Don't worry about your reactions, darling: they are perfectly natural.' He went on to explain that the German bombs were most dangerous when they hit buildings, and she should try and get into a bunker where within a few yards they did little damage. 'As soon as you can after the bombing find a job to do.'

My mother's main job was decoding messages and teaching the WAAFs to do the same. As head of her WAAFs at Harwell, she found herself involved in increasing bureaucracy, not any longer of her own making, and indeed for the first time she had to take examinations. Later, she boasted of how she obtained 90% in examinations in nutrition, but mostly this was a period about which she remained silent for the rest of her life. She was dyslexic and probably had never sat exams before. She developed insomnia and disorderly action of the heart, symptoms of panic, and clearly could no longer cope, so was discharged as unfit for service at a time when such was regarded as failure, which is probably the reason why she never spoke about the Air Force in the later 40 years of her life.

After her being invalided out of the Air Force, my mother set up home at Galashiels in Scotland where my father's regiment was temporarily providing defence. There was occasion when a threat of invasion at nearby Dunbar resulted in my mother being temporarily re-armed with revolvers to stand under a bridge and await the arrival of the Germans. It was a false alarm.

At first remaining in Amberley and at St George's prep school, only later after my worst experience of the war with no-one's shoulder to cry on, I joined my mother for Christmas when she had recovered and became the life and soul of the party, and for the first time for two years was able to lodge with my father, now a Captain in the Sherwood Foresters, and enjoy some of the mess parties. Some of the stories of these times I, then aged eight, still did not approve, like that of catapulting blancmange with a dessert spoon onto the faces of family portraits in a well-known country house.

It was at Galashiels that I read my first book – all about animal stories – from cover to cover without stop. Some older girls put on as Christmas entertainment a five-minute excerpt from *As You Like*

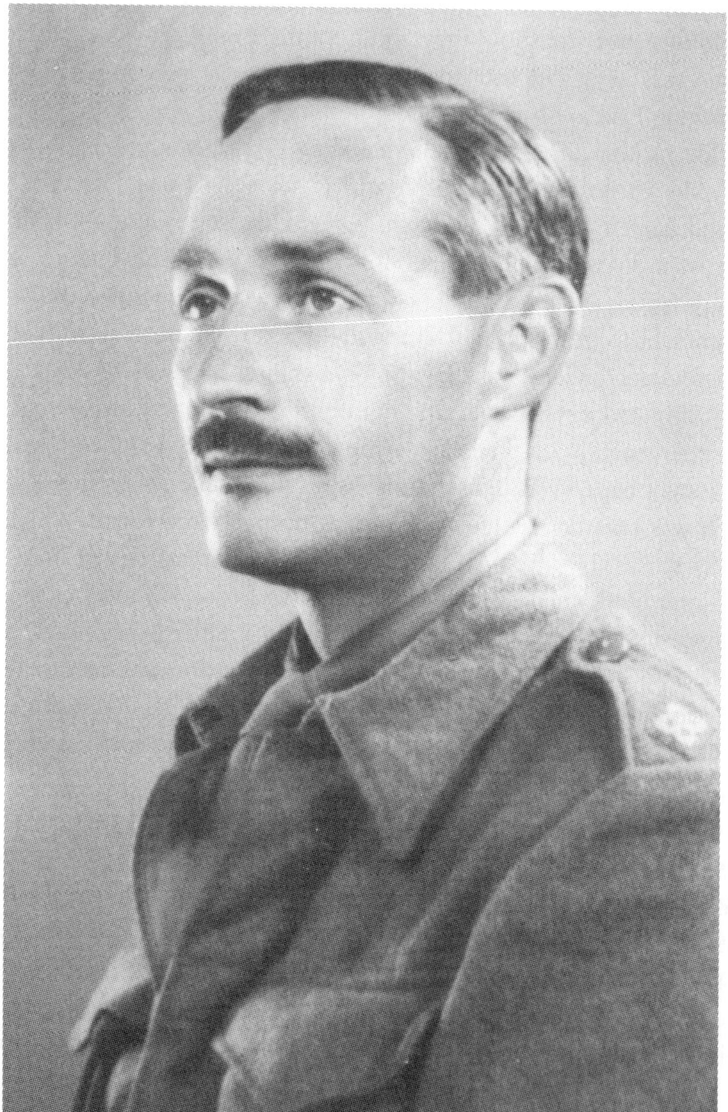

Bob Ryan dressed in his uniform prepared for Africa shortly before leaving in 1941

It, allocating to me a small part as Duke Senior, who banishes his daughter. We were asked to repeat the performance. It started a liking for amateur theatricals.

There was an obvious need, before my father went away again, to bring the family together, and while he was preparing for service in Africa over a period of six months, we stayed close by in digs at *Broome Hall Farm* on the side of Leith Hill near Dorking in Surrey. There was plenty of laughter, often shared with troops needing to be entertained.

While my father's battalion was preparing for Africa including buying tropical kit, I watched him taking church parades, and the Duke of Gloucester inspecting the troops.

There were magnificent walks through bluebell woods on Leith Hill. Riding my bicycle to an infant school run by a teacher who was Rudolf Steiner-trained, I joined about 16 other children for a very happy two terms of story-telling, painting and non-pressurised learning. The teacher, Miss Phyllis Carpenter, eventually suggested my transfer to the principal Rudolf Steiner school in the country, which had been evacuated from London to Minehead in Somerset.

It was about this time we had access to a piano and my mother's piano playing was enjoyed. Earliest memories are of stories told about music. My mother, who could never do anything without embellishment, played Rachmaninov's *C sharp Prelude*, telling me it was a man buried alive suffocating to death. She enjoyed tales of the opera on the radio, and the stories we listened to were always exciting and made more exciting by her response to them. During the war years and especially at 8.30pm at *Broome Hall Farm*, half-hours on the radio by Peter Dawson, Gracie Fields, Carrol Gibbons and Paul Robeson taught me to distinguish the music I most enjoyed as being the more serious compositions.

At Michael Hall Rudolph Steiner School, the music lessons often had an illustrated story such as that of Haydn's *Surprise Symphony* or Handel's *Water Music*. Later, listening to whole operas on the radio became a holiday occupation. Underneath the dining room table became an opera house where plasticine models would perform.

My first attendance at an opera was a Michael Hall performance of Mozart's *Bastien and Bastienne.*

While at *Broome Hall Farm*, my parents had to be an audience to some very feeble amateur theatricals prepared for my father to view in which I played a king and then, with a long wait, appeared as a queen with lots of lipstick. My father struggled to approve. My parents, steeped in war-time experiences, were given my drawings of fairies sitting on mushrooms which they interpreted as German war planes, and the mushrooms as parachutes.

In 1942, we had a short stay near Lambourn in Berkshire, close to where my father's brigade was in barracks. Our landlady, Mrs Bayliss, gave me my best friend and favourite toy, Jacko, a monkey. Already a little moth-eaten, deciding that he should be re-covered was difficult, and it was very disappointing when he did not look the same. He has survived until now in my 86th year, sitting in a display cupboard close where I am writing this account.

During the day, Jacko and I were taken round the village in a horse and trap by Miss Bayliss, and in the evening Eastbury Village Hall was the venue for seeing several Gracie Fields films.

Father's final letter of this period was from Lambourn, where he was vigorously training for service in Africa. There was little for Mother to do except worry about what might happen to him overseas. I still remember, surprisingly vividly, how I escaped into the unreal world of fairyland and the pleasure from imagining fairies amongst toadstools I discovered in the garden where we were billeted, and I continued to believe in fairies for several more years.

Then there were brief holidays, including trips to Wales, before saying farewell to my father.

There was a dash down to Minehead to fix me up with the leading Rudolph Steiner school, thinking a pacifist environment would be good for me, and to find lodgings for me now aged eight. There was the final farewell for departure to Africa. My mother drove from Lambourn back to *Broome Hall Farm* in Surrey, with me at her side, she in tears. This was more distressing than my father's departure.

The story of my father's year or so in Africa is a précis of 150 letters. He was sad at the departure by boat and he tried to provide cheer by writing every day for the next six weeks. A letter was written 14th October 1941, describing ship life with tummy upsets and being very hot in a blacked-out ship. There were bed bugs and mosquitoes but the food was very good. They arrived at Freetown on 15th October. He was chosen with one other to accompany the Brigadier visiting the other ships. Another letter was written on 22nd October as they crossed the Equator, describing an attempt by a destroyer to depth-charge a submarine lurking off North Africa. In Durban, a Zulu shield and spear was sent off to me and silk stockings to Mother. His regiment arrived in North Africa on 30th November 1941, having missed the retreat from Libya.

With my father in North Africa during 1942, my mother, short of money, joined Rex in Devon. My father had negotiated a job for him with a business contact, K.R. Osmond, the owner of a veterinary pharmaceutical firm *Osmond & Sons*. Rex with a heart murmur was unfit for the Armed Forces. On one winter's day he had blue lips and faintness after picking Brussels sprouts on a cold morning. After packing up the house, Rex had gone down to Devon in early 1940 to sell medicines to farmers there. Mother joined Rex and they lived together as brother and sister. She enjoyed the challenge of boasting her farming skills from her childhood experiences and persuading farmers to use udder creams of one kind or another. They were used on me for I know not what! Her knowledge was primitive: she spoke of but never actually used knitting needles for prodding the belly of cows that were blown.

Education at Michael Hall in Somerset, being a German Rudolf Steiner foundation, had been adapted to suit war-time England. It was vegetarian and pacifist. That meant lots of natural produce, including rose hips, but it also meant Latin without wars. There was no Caesar, there was no *miles* (soldier) or *bellum* (war), but there was *elephantus* (elephant) or *agricola* (farmer). There was much dancing and much music. There was painting with primary colours, and I got full marks for being the only one to choose to make an elephant out of purple material – whereas everyone else in the class made it out of grey or brown. The system of education tried hard not to be competitive, and there was no real way of knowing whether one was doing well or badly, since there were no examinations. But I enjoyed school time.

My landlady was Mrs Webb, a New Zealand lady who was a widow and a vegetarian, and who had elder children overseas. I was given the largest room in the house as a kind of bedsit. There was school at Michael Hall during the day, play in the streets in the evenings, and I would have breakfast and supper with Mrs Webb.

Playing as a street child, I remember stealing from *Woolworth's*, and about the same time falling through ice on a reservoir and nearly drowning, throwing stones at the windows of empty houses, and watching the fire brigade on occasions when houses were on fire – even trying to assist on one occasion in rescuing small items of furniture. I felt it was unfair of the teacher, whose class was missed, not agreeing how heroic I had been.

While in Minehead, religious tracts were sent to me from my grandmother. Building myself an altar in my bedroom, making crucifixes and attempting to be a missionary with my street friends, did not really work out as there was the intent that we should be seen kneeling and praying on the streets, but directly anyone came along, we ran away as fast as we could.

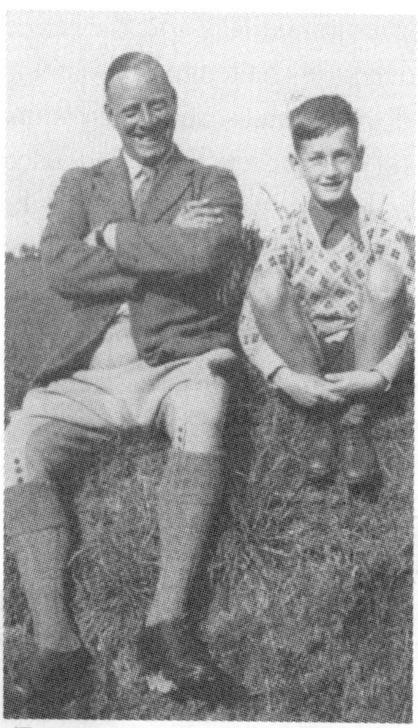

Terence on summer holiday with Rex Remington in Devon

There were street gangs which would line up to fight and I always threw stones from the back of our gang. Miss Russell, our class teacher at Michael Hall, eventually managed to steer me away from this behaviour and introduced me to the story of St Francis of Assisi.

There were three holidays in Devon with my mother in 1942, and I often arrived by coach in poor condition having been travel sick. Holiday in Devon was bliss and I enjoyed the company of

Rex, but we never stayed long at any one place.[6] There were the experiences of farm life and a few outings to the seaside and Paignton Zoo. It was a huge disappointment for my mother when a new navy blue mackintosh suffered on its first day at Paignton Zoo by having two plates of spaghetti and tomato sauce spilled on it, one after another. Rex saved my day by thinking it very funny.

It was a time when Plymouth was being badly bombed. We used to count 60 or more barrage balloons every breakfast time at Milton Abbot, from which Plymouth could be seen on the horizon.

After one year in Devon, my mother developed jaundice from hepatitis, and there was a period of two to three months' bed rest and convalescence in London with her sister with further experience of bombing.

In 1942, my father was in a difficult North African armoured retreat. Only in a letter dated 5th March did he mention any fighting.

> *I have been in two battles now and in both I have had to run away. It will be nice to do a bit of chasing for a change. The withdrawal was not all fun and on one or two occasions I missed being shot up or made prisoner – put in the bag we call it – by the skin of our teeth. Colonel Tiddles and I were alone at the time and ran smack into a Hun column which we thought was ours. They shelled and machine-gunned us, chasing us for 20 miles in armoured cars. Fortunately, we had fast cars and were able to give them the slip, but it was quite exciting while it lasted. My driver fractured his toe pressing so hard on the accelerator.*

After doing very little for three months in the desert, my father was promoted to Major and then put in charge of Massawa in Eritrea.[7] As Africa became less important in the war, Eritrea became of little significance and he felt he might as well be a civilian. He got much praise on leaving Massawa in mid-August 1943 for having done his job well. There was a tedious wait while in Cairo. He paid very frequent visits to senior staff asking for an interesting job. Eventually letters arrived in the UK via Cairo from a secret location, where my father had been assigned a special duty following his insistence for the same. He was not allowed to say where he had been sent but from the following in one letter we guessed it was in the Greek islands:

> *This is a very beautiful little place, queer little pink houses on the side of steep hills and many small picturesque bays, crystal-clear deep blue water.'*

The British newspapers were full of reports of a very foolish and unnecessary attempt to secure the Greek islands.[4]

The Battle of Leros, September to November 1943, and a special mission carrying fifteen million lira to bribe the Italians to give up their support of the Germans, is described in a full report written after the war. It covers his arrival on 18th September to his capture on 16th November. The nature of my father's mission can be read in a letter to him dated 23rd October 1945 from the HQ in Cairo, enclosing copies of letters stating that five million lira was taken ashore at Leros at night and handed personally to Major Ryan: '2nd November – Another five million lira was also carried by the commander of *HMS Dulverton* and handed over.' My father wrote on 25th October 1945 that there were three such sums. The English press reported in detail each day. Mostly they regarded the occupation of Leros as a blunder because there was no air cover and German bombing was intense. It made terrifying reading for my mother and was regarded as the last bit of good news for the German public. The headlines were 'a minor tragedy' and described uninterrupted air attack.

> *How could it be ever thought that Leros could be held? Only complete misjudgement of the Italian assistance to be anticipated, and of the forces of which the enemy disposed, could have made this scattering of troops into the blue appear hopeful at the outset.*[8]

It was not thought the Germans would get involved. In reply, my father writes after the war of three large chests sealed and locked and hidden in a cave at the top of Monte Meriviglia, and not well hidden because there was no thought in anyone's mind that the island would fall as quickly as it did. About four million lira was spent on back-paying the Italians for work done, unloading from ships and the loan of trucks, etc. On 3rd November, five million lira had been handed over to Admiral Mascupra for the Italians. My father describes very heavy bombing. He was accompanied by a junior subaltern who had a gramophone and at the height of the bombing played the Warsaw Concerto over and over again. My father buried the rest of the lira 'as best I could under a heap of stones in an alcove'. He was captured a few hours later on 17th November 1943.

On 20th May 1946, he wrote a full report to the Aegean Consolidated Reconstruction Account Dept. 10:

> *From your sketch I see that a considerable amount of excavation in the tunnel has taken place since 1943. Four alcoves are shown which were not in existence at that time. As I mentioned in my report, the money was really inadequately hidden, and as all this excavation has since taken place, the chances of recovering the money seemed regrettably rather remote.'*

As a prisoner-of-war (POW), my father was taken to Athens where an old-fashioned German battalion in charge allowed him parole and for a few days he wandered round Athens. Thereafter the discomforts of being a POW began with 24 officers lodged in a cattle truck for twelve days, let out only for twelve minutes per day. The journey was to a transit camp at Marrish Trubau in Czechoslovakia. The illustrated diary that he kept for one-and-a-half years covers his POW experience in full. He was a senior officer with some involvement in organising escapes. He did have a bayonet in his buttock on one occasion and swore revenge. Finally, in Offlag VIII in Brunswick in early 1945, he spoke on the phone to Himmler and prevented an evacuation and move.

He accepted on the 13th April 1945 the camp's Nazi flag and the sword of the German Commandant before returning to England. He wrote to us every week and we also wrote to him weekly, but only about 50 of his letters arrived, usually months late. They were heavily censored and very domestic about camp shows, sports, Red Cross parcels and learning to sketch. The first parcel he received from the UK was in November 1944.

For six months, from November 1943, he was missing, and for missing persons there was no family allowance. My mother depended on what she could earn or borrow, while for comfort and companionship depended very much on me, her nine-year-old son. She decided that her only skill was cooking, and she earned money by preparing lunches in various children's hostels in Minehead. Money was short as no income arrived while there was uncertainty as to whether a missing husband was alive or dead.

During this period, she had a number of psychosomatic illnesses, including severe mastitis and palpitations for which the homeopathic doctor of the Rudolph Steiner School provided Mistletoe. I was relied on to cope with all this and broke free only once to play with friends. It was a lonely time for my mother. Rex and her sister, Aunt Lil, visited us each for a few days only. Eventually, it was decided that she should recover with good friends back at *Broome Hall Farm* in Dorking.

Rex Remington, having made a policewoman pregnant, married her in 1943 and was not seen again.

Then, in the spring of 1944, a rag-and-bone man from North London was listening to propoganda on the radio from Germany for news of his missing son as propaganda (as the Germans broadcast names of those in prisoner-of-war camps and encouraged them to broadcast how well they were being looked after) – when he heard the name of my father! This rag-and-bone man then walked eight miles to deliver the message that my father's name had been read out during the night.

Three weeks later, while we were back at *Broome Hall Farm*, it was officially confirmed that Father was a POW, and there was once again an income. My mother and I returned to Minehead for schooling and lived in digs, with the elderly niece of the then Archbishop of Canterbury, who needed a companion. Now blessed with an income, my mother lived for the occasional letter from my

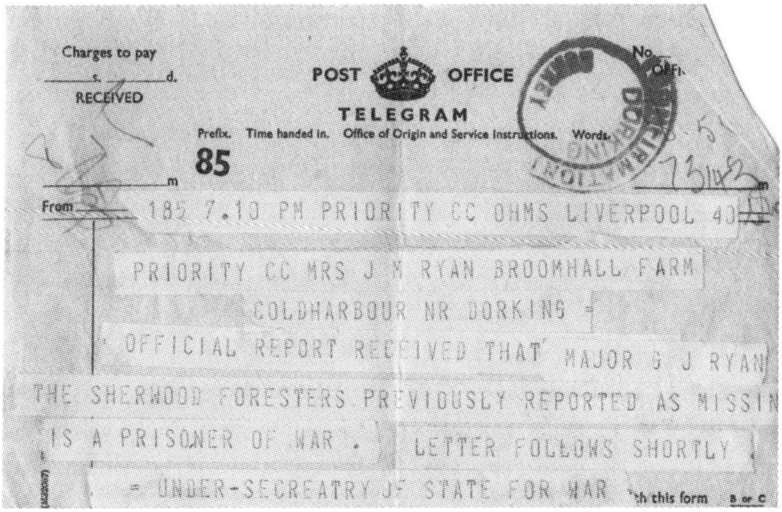

Charges to pay
s. d.
RECEIVED
POST OFFICE
TELEGRAM
Prefix. Time handed in. Office of Origin and Service Instructions. Words.
85
From 185 7.10 PM PRIORITY CC OHMS LIVERPOOL 40
PRIORITY CC MRS J M RYAN BROOMHALL FARM
COLDHARBOUR NR DORKING
OFFICIAL REPORT RECEIVED THAT MAJOR G J RYAN
THE SHERWOOD FORESTERS PREVIOUSLY REPORTED AS MISSIN
IS A PRISONER OF WAR . LETTER FOLLOWS SHORTLY
= UNDER-SECREATRY OF STATE FOR WAR

Telegram reporting for the first time after many months that Bob Ryan was a POW in Germany

father, the occasional food parcel from Australia, the packing of Red Cross parcels for sending to Germany – very few of which ever arrived – and cooking for two. It was a time of rationing, and she spent much of the day seeking ways of bypassing the system. When the war looked as though it was coming to an end, we returned to London and experienced V1 and V2 ('Doodle Bugs' and rockets), and I did not go to school for a few months.

The last letter we received from Germany was dated 13th April 1945: 'We are free – the Americans rolled up yesterday to our great joy.'

My father flew back to Northolt, and after several years of being the centre of my mother's attention, I had to manage the presence of a father. At the grand welcome home it was decided I should be the first to meet him. Although I was extremely shy, I was sent out to greet him at the roadside and to escort him into the house where there was a fireside family debrief.

He was very thin and my mother stated the next morning that 'it was like going to bed with a skeleton'. Almost immediately the rich foods laid him low. It was a while before he recovered enough to go up to London to debrief the War Office and eventually be demobilised. A letter from the senior officer of his POW camp dated 14th April 1945 states:

> *I wish to thank you for the grand work you put in on behalf of the whole of the so-called Cloak and Dagger Coy Ltd. It may at times seemed to have been farcical but it was due to your and others' efforts that so many escapes were almost successful and two of course were, even if only for a space of days and minutes.*

He had been awarded three oak leaves (that is, mentioned in dispatches) for Dunkirk, Leros and the POW camp.

My mother's early war-time achievements were unrecorded. She never spoke of them, and after 1945 my father never spoke about his army experiences either.

Notes on Chapter 2

1) On returning to Germany, Jenny Vogel married, but her husband finally died of meningitis on the Russian Front. She could not bring herself to believe that the cause for which he had fought had been in vain, and that Hitler's creed was wholly wrong, but her memories of England were so good that she brought her family back to visit us as soon as possible. I visited her in Germany once when she hosted a minibus full of St John Ambulance colleagues in an exchange with the *Johanitter umfal Hilfer.*

2) Belvoir Castle is well described by Catherine Bailey (2012), *The Secret Rooms: A True Gothic Mystery*. Penguin Viking.

3) Anxiety due to my mother's ribald behaviour. I was an anxious child well into my teenage years. I do not have vivid memories of frightening events such as bombings, but I do vividly remember times when my mother's behaviour caused me great anxiety. I did not approve of her Rabelaisian humour and frequent tales, such as the following: Bill had a habit of eating flowerpots, which would pass right through him with a clatter on the pavement: this was an occasional source of embarrassment. Much worse was his large size and male stature when urinating. He would sniff at the back of

deck-chairs and raise his leg, and a stream of water would land in the lap of the occupant. On one occasion, Pat and Bill could be seen being chased by an elderly lady in a wet black satin dress, shaking a black umbrella.

4) It was the following references written in 1918 that accounted for mother's recruitment into a senior post in the Armed Forces two years before World War II:

> *I have been driven by Miss Knight for three-and-a-half months in France, and have always found her very capable in charge of many different makes of car. She is also thoroughly versed in running repairs. When on the road, she is a very careful driver. I can thoroughly recommend her for a responsible position.*

And another:

> *I can quite appreciate your desire to find some useful scope for your undoubted ability after your strenuous work, both at home and overseas. I should think with your military training you would be invaluable to a professional man, as you can be relied on, and are capable of doing running repairs better than most men. You may refer anyone to me for a personal reference if necessary, and I wish you the best of luck.*

A 'To Whom It May Concern' letter, written by the Captain of the Royal Army Ordnance Corps, states that:

> *Miss Knight was an exceptionally efficient and reliable driver while serving under me on strength of the Director of the Ordnance Services, GHQ, France. She proved equally capable of driving several types of cars, thoroughly understood overhauling and invariably did her own running repairs. I confidently recommend her for any responsible position.*

5) A letter from the Naval and Military Club, dated 25th July, states:

> *I think it would be best for Mrs Ryan to tell her people on Monday that they are to be converted, but to say nothing about the second company, and to make no change at present in her training programme. The War Office are relieved at getting rid of the RAF companies, but rather sceptical about the officer-producing idea. They say it will be labelled another 'snob show'. Altogether, not very encouraging news, I am afraid.*

6) Accommodation in Devon in 1942:
Pen Tor, Ipplepen, Newton Abbot: January
Old Lays, Liverton, Newton Abbot: February and March
Homefield Farm, Sherford, Kingsbridge: April and May
Hillside, Ermington, Ivybridge: June and July
Glebe Farm, Dunterton, Milton Abbot: August and September
Round Hill Farm, Princetown: September and October
Orchard Hill, Buckland, Yelverton; November
Moorlands Guesthouse, Shaugh Prior near Plymouth

7) Many of my father's letters described trips up to Asmara and a visit by the Duke of Gloucester. It was fairly comfortable housing but far from the war. The Italians that were being governed there were easy and helpful. Many of his letters describe shooting grouse, duck, gazelle and guinea foul.

Towards the end of the year there was promise of further promotion to a staff post and a job in Cairo. But nothing happened till June 1943 when he was promoted to Major and temporarily held the rank of Colonel. In 1946, my father composed a well written and entertaining report about his time in Eritrea.

8) The British newspapers were full of reports of a very foolish and unnecessary attempt to secure the Greek islands. Lt Gen HG Martin, *British Aegean Strategy: To What End? Vulnerable Isles* (*Daily Telegraph*, 19th November 1943).

3: Family Life, Schooling and Planning to Be a Doctor

At the age of 45, my mother settled down to being a housewife and making a happy home for family and frequent visitors. In autumn 1945, my father was appointed in charge of road services for the AA and at first returned to his office in Brighton where we furnished a few rooms with our old furniture. During the next 25 years, he developed the AA into a very large and effective organisation and organised a review in Hyde park of AA patrols from many nations in 1980, by the President of the AA, the Duke of Edinburgh.

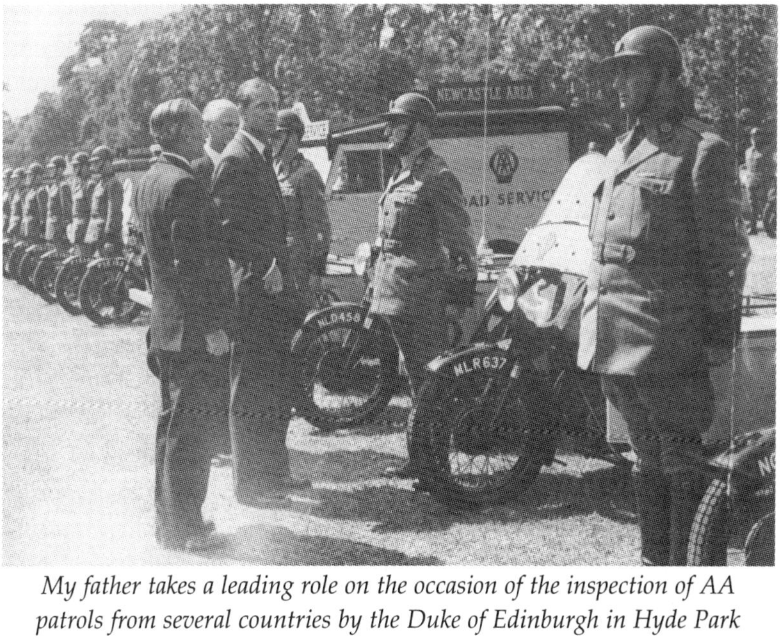

My father takes a leading role on the occasion of the inspection of AA patrols from several countries by the Duke of Edinburgh in Hyde Park on the 75th anniversary of the Automobile Association

My father thought that the Rudolph Steiner education was too airy-fairy and this resulted in an attempt to enter me into St John's School, Leatherhead. This was an abysmal failure because the Common Entrance paper was quite unlike anything I had experienced at the Rudolph Steiner School and the headmaster wrote after my interview at St John's Leatherhead, saying I was 'educationally sub-normal'.

At the age of four, I had made my mother's horses better by feeding them medicines made of nettles and whitewash. This established the view within the family that their son was to be a doctor. Now in 1945, what chance was there that this might be achieved? Was I educationally sub-normal?

Dyslexia during the next few years was to become a new and common diagnosis. It was partly a hereditary condition and my mother had signs of it. An example of her dyslexia was her difficulty remembering names. In the case of one hockey friend, Malcolm Tabernacle and his wife, who emphasised that they were not Jews, she registered them mentally as a Jewish place of worship and frequently introduced them as Mr and Mrs Synagogue. My mother, though highly intelligent, had been badly educated, and when in adult life she met examinations for the first time, she could not cope. I too had had a disordered education.

I have the same difficulties in remembering names and even now do not fully know my 'tables' nor my college or work telephone number. I have instant short-term memory which later made collating facts quite difficult. I would misname even people that I knew well, and it became a joke amongst some of my friends. However, I am visually and spatially adept. I look at a map and know instantly where to go, and can store the whole of London in my forebrain and never get lost.

Was I dyslexic? I realise that I cannot take in a sequence of names or numbers unless they are said slowly but not so slowly that I forget the first letter or number by the time I reach the last. When my wife Anne spelled out to me in front of the grandchildren 'NO CHOCOLATE', unless she spelled it very slowly and I concentrated on it, I could not tell what she was spelling. Thus, when recording a new address, I have to do it line by line, because by the time I have memorised the second line, I will have forgotten the first. Repeating it over a minute or two, however, it is recorded. I spent up to an hour each day making lists in order to sequence my daily programme.

In later years as a Trustee of *The Arts Dyslexia Trust*, once again I made contact with Brickwall School, now renamed Frewen Hall and specializing in dyslexia. I clearly had a dyslexic mother and the genetics of dyslexia are similar to those of autism and schizophrenia from which my son James suffers. The ESN diagnosis led Father to arrange schooling for four terms at Downside Preparatory School in Purley, a well-known boys' school which did not take boarders. It later was the site of Benjamin Britten's *Songs for a Friday Afternoon*. My father knew of it because it was where an old hockey friend was teaching. Because Brighton was a long way from Purley, I travelled by train every weekend, and had the unusual experience of being the only boarder at the prep school – but once again I had long periods of being alone. However, sometimes the son of the matron lived in the house and we got on fairly well together. He had a friend to visit him occasionally, and watching them together, I had my first rudimentary sex education, although did not participate in their games. As the loan boarder, I quite enjoyed the adult company of the staff at breakfast and high tea.

My musical and artistic sensibilities had been developed at the Rudolph Steiner School, Michael Hall, and at Downside I appreciated the musical interests of the Deputy Headmaster, Charles Blackburn, son of the Dean of Ely. With gramophone records of opera made available and a box of dressing-up clothes, I used to sing and dress up, and my voice was compared with that of Elizabeth Schumann, which I took to be a compliment. Charles Blackburn took me to my first professional opera at Croydon – a performance of *The Mikado*.

Then after the war, two uncles took me to hear Beethoven's *Fifth Symphony* at the Royal Albert Hall. One of these uncles had a gramophone that made Dvorak's *New World Symphony* sound very discordant, and I later made a fool of myself, saying I did not like modern music and gave the *New World Symphony* as an example.

Studies of the piano had begun at the age of nine at Michael Hall and Paderewski's *Minuet* lasted me four terms at Downside Prep School.

Charles Blackburn also took me to the cinema – *Dead of Night* with Malcolm Redgrave and Googie Withers, and following this, back at school over the staff dinner table, I heard for the first time adult critiques of the theatre and music – which were fascinating. I began to enjoy listening to concerts on the radio, and eventually began to learn the stories of opera and perform them under the dining room table, using plasticine models.

While I was at Downside, the war came to an end, and I experienced VE-Day and VJ-Day entirely alone. I remember, also, the first elections that took place after the war. We were meant to have mock elections in the school, but not one boy could be found who was a Socialist. In contrast, I happened to join the school train taking my previous classmates to the Rudolph Steiner School during the election period, and I was equally surprised that not one could be found who was a Conservative. The switch that I had made was not only educational, but cultural, and I did not feel entirely happy with it.

I passed Common Entrance after four terms and was about to go to Bradfield, a Berkshire public school, but my dislike of the plan led to a different arrangement. One of my parent's old friends from pre-war years and my godfather, Cedric Greenep, was a master at a school known as Brickwall at Northiam in Sussex. Since 1910, first located in Rottingdean, this had specialised in being a small tutorial establishment for boys that had expected to go to public school, but for a variety of reasons were unsuitable.

My parents drove me there in April 1946. I walked in with a new cricket bat given by my father. My mother heard Colin Ritchie, a partner at the school, say, "O dear, cricket bat and all." My mother quickly intervened, explaining I was not a cricketer.

I became a boarder in a Grade One Elizabethan house belonging to Admiral Frewen, the C-in-C at Portsmouth. Many of the boys at Brickwall could not read or write, one or two were from overseas, while many had experienced difficult war years. There were 46 of us, and the classes were usually no more than ten in number. Some of the school teachers were very experienced in teaching teenage boys how to read and write and had discovered, for instance, that a typewriter might ease writing difficulties. Some years later, this school became classified as dealing with dyslexia.

Brickwall was not a school that had any expectation of sending boys to university, but about half the boys were expected to take the General Certificate of Education, although not necessarily to do well. Passes, rather than credits – certainly no distinctions, and quite frequently failures – were the norm.

The arts have played a leading role in my life. I was lucky to have learned how to use watercolour at the Rudolph Steiner School I attended between the ages of nine and twelve. When I was 16, there was a trip to Holland with Uncle Cecil and Aunt Catherine and cousin Michael. A Dutch friend and artist, Grace Plokker, introduced me to the Dutch galleries. It was in the late 1940s when galleries in Vienna, Berlin and Munich were not open but their collections were on tour. I saw them all in Holland. At Brickwall, Annie Ritchie, the wife of Colin Ritchie, a senior partner of the school, was sister to Edward Burra, the leading English watercolourist. This gave me the chance to visit his studio in Rye and attend the private view of all his exhibitions. At Brickwall, I became the favourite of one of the youngest masters, who would accompany me at the piano while I sang love songs he had selected for me. He wanted me to spend some of my summer holidays with him. I was not aware that there was anything odd about this, but my parents and the school staff put a stop to this close relationship. Later I had a similar experience with another master who had taken me to several marvellous concerts including Beecham's Mozart weekends at Glyndebourne. He said that I had broken his heart. This I reported to the Headmaster and heard no more of it.

One of my dormitory mates, Pat Webb, was far more intellectual than I was, and had a great knowledge of music, and was also a Communist. He forced me to think more seriously and critically about music and about politics. He also persuaded me that fairies could not possibly exist. He told me the iron spikes on the top of the walls of Buckingham Palace were to stop the King from getting out – and I believed him. When I was given a new piece to practise for the piano, in the presence of Pat, I would play lots of wrong notes, thinking to impress him with this new modern-sounding piece. After leaving school, Pat suggested I accompany him to a Youth Festival in Warsaw. I enquired about a visa (then necessary for such a trip), but examinations were looming so I did not go. Many years later, when applying for a visa to go to the USA, I found they had copies of this application request.

The Ritchies, partners in charge of the school, were accomplished musicians, and Sunday evening and end-of-term concerts were the greatest fun with much singing of Gilbert and Sullivan. Aunt Lil bought me an upright piano when I was 13, and by this time at Brickwall School, several masters nurtured my interest. Colin Ritchie was a good narrator of his experiences in London, such as the curtain calls for Flagstad's *Isolde*, or American Shows such as *Annie Get Your Gun*. It was he who gave me the complete piano scores of Wagner's operas that eventually made me unfazed by complex key changes. One of my Brickwall friends, Rowley Holt Wilson, was another music enthusiast, and his mother took us to the Royal Opera House in 1948 for Beecham's *Meistersinger* when Elisabeth Grummer was a memorable Eva.

Radio listening brought into the home Flagstad singing the first performance of Strauss's *Four Last Songs* and the first night of *Peter Grimes*. There was also Toscanini conducting at the Royal Festival Hall all four of Brahms' symphonies and a hair-raising *Variations on a Theme of Handel*. Other teachers at the school were Malcolm Ritchie and his wife Anne, previously an actress with the Pilgrim Players. They became close lifelong friends. They organised trips to London to see Alec Guinness as the dauphin in Bernard Shaw's *St Joan*, a part I was to play in a school production. We also saw Laurence Olivier's *Richard III*, later to be filmed. Whilst there, I played many roles in school plays and on later visits.

Brickwall's headmaster, John Patterson, was more interested in character-forming. A strong Christian, he would prepare boys for confirmation and make the decisions about whether or not boys were suitable to take on responsibilities such as being a prefect. He delayed my promotion to being a prefect, telling me that I was insufficiently aware of the needs of other boys and did not know their names and would frequently give them the wrong ones, perhaps a manifestation of dyslexia.

We were prepared for the General Certificate of Education, and the exams were taken at a convent school in Hastings. There was great joy at Brickwall when about eight of us taking the General Certificate obtained credits and some distinctions. The Maths exam was an occasion when I desperately needed to urinate but was too shy to approach the nuns. I only just passed the exam.

No science was taught at the school, but I remained committed to becoming a doctor. Colin Ritchie, who had played at Wimbledon with the head of one of the Oxford colleges, J.C. Masterman at Worcester, was involved in a tennis match at Oxford and put me forward to meet this famous Provost. I had the briefest of conversations with him by the tennis courts, and was called for a college entrance examination.

It was declared that chemistry, physics and biology had to be passed before entry into Oxford to read medicine would be possible.

So, after some discussion, it was decided that I would leave Brickwall and study for one year at a 'crammers' called Bornhams next to Victoria Station in London, where the basement smelt of sewers. It specialised particularly in chemistry, physics and biology, and intensively and successfully crammed large numbers of students. Many of them had recently come out of the Army, and they were mostly older than me. They were men and women of the world, and I had little in common with them. At Brickwall, one of the boys had been expelled just for going for a walk in the school grounds with a farmer's daughter, and it was strange now to be in London with fellow-students whose main topic of conversation was about their sexual relationships.

The language of science was entirely foreign to me but we were expected to take the necessary examinations as soon as possible – and as often as possible. After three months, I failed chemistry at the first attempt but obtained biology and a second attempt secured chemistry two months later. I had to take physics four times before eventually succeeding, and I even had extra tuition from a physics master at Brighton College. At the end of my time at Bornhams, a master who had seen me on my first day there and noticed my total incompetence in lab technique, praised me in front of the whole class as an example of how to progress through working hard. However, I had now been to 15 different educational establishments and experienced many different forms of tuition. I had moved rather abruptly from the arts to science, and managed to pass its exams. However, I had little understanding of it.

From 1946 to 1951, my home was *Deaks Manor*, Cuckfield, which my parents rented in Sussex. It was a fifteenth-century house of great beauty on the forest ridge overlooking the South Downs. There were two very large oaks and wonderful woods for me and my dog to explore. My mother was never completely clear of episodes of anxiety, and was at times prescribed by Ned White both arsenic and valerian.

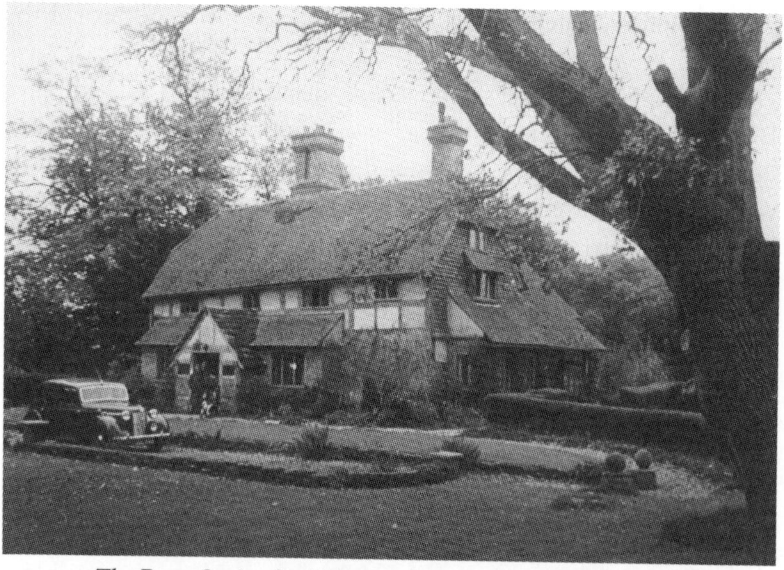

The Ryan Senior family's post-war home, fifteenth century Deakes Farm House, Cuckfield, Sussex

In 1951, coinciding with my moving to the University of Oxford, my father needed to be central in the UK, and for the first time could buy a house. It had belonged to the County of Buckinghamshire tuberculosis officer. It was convenient for Oxford, but unlike Sussex which paid for my first term at Oxford, Buckinghamshire would not pay anything towards my education. The house bordered on *Chequers* and had wonderful walks on Cymberlyn Hill. We shared the church at Christmas with parties from *Chequers*, listening on one occasion to Rab Butler, then Chancellor of the Exchequer, reading the lesson on tax collecting. It was a large house of flintstone with large barns and a tennis court. My mother was able to keep geese and turkeys, and my Aunt Lil, her sister, came as a widow to live there too. The focus of my mother's life now became entirely domestic, often as a host and partner for events organised for father or me.

4: Oxford University and Hospital Medicine at the Radcliffe Infirmary

In 1950, Worcester College admitted four medical students and I was welcomed as one of those who knew little science. Having a science tutor and a quota of medical students was a fairly recent idea for many colleges. The Provost of Worcester College, Sir John Masterman, was a polymath who, as an intelligence officer during World War II, was appointed to MI6 in charge of the *Double Cross System.*[1] Before the era of Inspector Morse, he wrote detective stories about Oxford, and was also a skilful Davis Cup player – hence my interview with him had been on a tennis court. His views on science were expressed in a novel *Teach the Senators Wisdom* – about college tutors in which the only scientist was young, inarticulate and unappreciative of Oxford's ancient beauty. At the college entrance viva, when asked, "Do you know the formula of common salt?" my answer was "No". Clearly, I was not a scientist of promise. However, the Provost told Colin Ritchie, a partner heading Brickwall School, with whom he played tennis, that my essays on *Music is the most ethereal of the arts: A comparison of Hitler with Napoleon* and on *The Romantic Revival* were approved. In a fictitious discussion of the admission system, one tutor in his book asks, 'Should we not give opportunity to those who start with handicap but may hope to improve?' Such a person, he said, would gain more from Oxford and value his gains more than most people do. Possibly I was such a person, for at a later date I was told by the college Senior Tutor, "The Provost took pity on you, didn't he, as you were at some school for the educationally weird?"

My first days in college were anxious. Post-war expansion meant that the 1950 entrants were housed in a corrugated roofed garage outside the college. There were fifteen of us with musical instruments and typewriters creating an immense amount of noise. On my first day to find the place, I had asked its whereabouts from the Australian Senior College Law Tutor. His response: "Can't you show any initiative, boy?"

Once settled in, there was a weekly tutorial[2] from one's tutor over a sherry in his panelled room, and the rest of the week was spent cycling to and from the anatomy and physiology schools on my one-pedal, lightless and brakeless bicycle, soon to bring me for the first time a fine of £3 from Oxford's well-known Inspector Quelch.

My tutorials were at 6.00pm but one had to wait before entering the room each week while the tutor, played through the same Brahms *Intermezzo*. My tutor and I were united more by music than by science, as his pupil never completely understood the concepts he was presenting to me. But it was a better experience than that of the first Director of Clinical Studies, Dr Alexander Cooke, in 1919 whose tutorial with the respiratory physiologist Claude Douglas was at 9.00am, and he read his weekly essay aloud while his tutor read *The Times* newspaper and ate a full English breakfast.

The university was famed for stories of its lack of appreciation of science. The nineteenth century Sir Henry Acland arrived by barge with 14 large packing cases on the banks of the Thames to head medicine, aiming to create a museum of medicine. The university was not so much hostile as contemptuous. Acland worked indefatigably to introduce Natural Science but there were many who spoke about the evils and dangers of science. The Professor of Anatomy would not believe what he saw under the microscope, and he did not think God would want such knowledge disseminated.

My college tutor was given little support by the college. The Worcester College Librarian, when asked by him, their first science tutor in 1946, whether he could purchase some books for his students to read in the library, was told, after a long pause, "Yes, you may, but you cannot put them in my library." In 1950, there was still no section on the sciences in the college library, and my tutor made me sign for books from his personal library. I remember reading in my room in college only three of my tutor's books. They included

Trueta on his 'Renal Shunt', Garrod on *Inborn Errors of Metabolism*, and some gastric tales pertaining to the stomach of a certain 'Tom'. Alternatively, one could borrow books from the University Science Library, having put on a gown and sworn at The Bodleian not to burn it down.

Following Masterman's belief that both student and tutor should have an idyllic life, no-one seemed too upset if one's hobby dominated one's life within the college walls. Hobbies could, for some, be the keeping of pets. A cow was kept on one occasion and Rupert Murdoch introduced Wallabies. When too many dogs appeared on site, the Dean Harry Pitt put up a notice banning them. The next day he put up another notice: 'From henceforth the Dean's *dog* is designated *cat*.'

Oxford was a rich place for the music lover and the face of my tutor was lightened when he saw me listed on the Worcester Somerville Music Society's programme as 'Speaking and Illustrating at the Piano the Psychology of Wagner's Motifs'.

Music became a preoccupation, there being recitals in the same week by Alfred Cortot and Claudio Arrau. There was Kathleen Ferrier at The Sheldonian in *Gerontius*. One could sing under Beecham in the chorus of the first performance of *Irmelin* by Delius. The college hosted the Boyd Neel Orchestra with *Brandenburg Concertos*. The Chelsea Opera Group, conducted by Colin Davis, performed *Così fan tutte*, and *The Marriage of Figaro* in Somerville College, while Alfred Deller and Julian Bream explored the counter-tenor and lute repertory in Worcester College.[3] In Oxford, The New Theatre was host to pre- and post-London shows of a high standard and rich variety.[4] Rowley Holt Wilson – also from my school, Brickwall – produced Smetana's *The Kiss* for the Oxford University Opera Club. The lead was taken by Janet Baker, her first public performance in opera. She made little impression on me, and it wasn't until I heard her sing Brahms' songs accompanied by the viola and piano at the Edinburgh Festival that she seemed outstanding. Attending her final performance as Orpheus at Glyndebourne was another occasion when she did not rise to her glorious best, but as Berlioz's Dido at the Royal Opera

House she thrilled. In 1952, a first of hundreds of visits to Glyndebourne was notable for the performance of Lisa Della Casa in *Figaro*. Later, Lisa Della Casa was to appear at Covent Garden in a Munich State Opera production of *Arabella* by Richard Strauss, fortunately now available on CD.

Rowley Holt Wilson did his military service in the Intelligence Corps learning Russian in Cornwall. He got me tickets for the visit of the Munich Opera and I hurriedly sent him a telegram which said: 'Arabella only if Lisa Della Casa.' But inadvertently tearing the telegram through the word 'only', it read: 'Arabella on ly if lisa della casa' and seemed too much like a coded message, and Rowley had difficulty explaining it to a philistine military. Rowley was not given leave for expeditions to the opera but he discovered that leave was given for playing golf. The cloakroom at the Royal Opera House became familiar with Rowley's never-to-be-used bag of golf clubs.

My opera CV was hugely enhanced when my mother decided to drive me to Bayreuth to see the now famous new 1950s productions of *The Ring* and *The Meistersingers*. The young Wagners had the musical world at their feet. My mother and I dined where they dined at *Die Eule*. We got up to leave early. It was just as Friedlinde Wagner swept in, and assuming we were giving up our seats, thanked us profusely. I have visited Bayreuth four times.

In Coronation week, Jo Penney and I began frequent visits to the Royal Opera House, watching Callas and Simionato in *Aida* conducted by Sir John Barbirolli.[5] Seeing Callas followed by Wellitsch as Musetta started a passion for divas. Returning to Oxford by the milk train and climbing into Worcester College at 2.00am were less welcome experiences as part of London opera-going, but once I moved into lodgings in 131 Walton Street with an opera-loving landlady, there would be a thermos of hot chocolate.

The interests of music and medicine clashed once or twice during midwifery. We were expected to deliver 24 babies in the homes of poorer Oxford families. Trapped in Rosehill for a long and seatless night with an Opera Club ticket for *Alceste* at Glyndebourne in my pocket, I only just made it because with it being a dress rehearsal, one did not have to change into a dinner jacket.

In 1957, I began correspondence with Harold Rosenthal, editor of *Opera Magazine*, and he published in a Christmas edition my analysis of deaths in opera. He agreed with my belief that Colin Davis was insufficiently recognised as a conductor of opera, and was amused with my analysis of 'love' in three languages in Bayreuth programmes of Wagner's *Ring*.

London opera-going saw some very poorly dressed and staged operas, particularly when small and thin last-minute stand-ins were substituting for fat giants of both sexes. For lack of money, Covent Garden replaced the set of the dying Manon by the set of the last act of *Die Walküre*. Svet Svanholm as Siegfried failed to break Wotan's spear but instead broke his own sword and dashed off-stage to get a new one.

Evelyn Waugh's *Brideshead Revisited* provided a picture of undergraduates, often 'gay' and self-indulgent, flaunting their teddy bears. At Worcester College in 1951, six of us – including one woman who married her tutor who later became head of college – enacted similar events. We called ourselves the Cabuguan Club. We had a mascot, a small wooden horse strung together with elastic, allowing one to induce a variety of postures. The elastic snapped, so one late evening we had an elaborate funeral in the college garden. On a rainy day, we set out in a punt down the Cherwell to the Thames dressed in silk dressing gowns. We had silver tableware and many soft woollen toys, including 'Mother', an ancient Teddy bear, and 'Jacko', my monkey. We were part shielded from the rain by a Hapsburg umbrella, once the property of an Archduke. Slightly tipsy and watched by a large towpath audience, we allowed the umbrella to fall into the Thames, never to be seen again.

Work in the Science Areas Laboratories was initially on Organic Chemistry. It was my first failure at Oxford and there was a second term retake. A few others accompanied me, including Dr John Ledingham, later to become the lead physician in Oxford, and Shirley Summerskill, a budding socialist politician. We had some fun and we all passed.

To get to the anatomy and physiology sessions one walked through the Natural History Museum. The Canadian Rhodes Scholar and pupil of the Nobel Prize winner Charles Sherrington, William Gibson wrote in 1938: 'Beyond the Museums, all was confusion.'[6] One was overloaded by a heavy mix of arts and sciences.

One could buy sandwiches in town for lunch but we also dashed there for snacks. It was still post-war with cheap meals available in the British Restaurant. On one occasion, the fruit salad had a human finger in the bowl. We sent it back and were told, "It's OK – it's not one of ours." Later in the hospital, in the late evening between visits of the night sister, one might cook oneself scrambled eggs in the ward kitchen. During the day, making friends with the Diet Kitchen could provide some of the snacks they made for the Private Ward. On ward rounds, there were always chocolates within touch. However, on one occasion, a patient long affected by a stroke and never speaking a word, saw me and astonished us all by shouting clearly, "Feeding yourself again!"

My parents' house in Buckinghamshire was the frequent site for my friends at Oxford to drive over for a good meal, and the scene of many parties, often for my friends and sometimes some of my parents' friends, over a period of at least twelve years. Some were the elaborate pre-war type of party with complex games such as 'murders' when all the lights were switched off, and my mother would listen for the sound of kissing behind the curtains.

I would return to Brickwall School frequently. For Wimbledon fortnight, it was useful to have me as a substitute teacher and participating in end-of-term events. I had also launched an Old Boys' Association' with a termly newsletter.

Two years later, my two years of study of anatomy and physiology was also followed by failure and there were no distinguished persons to fail with me, but there was a Pass at a post-vacation re-sit.

There were good lectures that are remembered 60 years later but there were also some extraordinarily bad ones. There were a few special courses such as one by Howard Florey on Pathology and

John Eccles on Neurophysiology. Their presence caused excitement but the content of their lectures was hard to assimilate. Fortunately, the lectures were published and could be enjoyed at leisure. Even so, Pathology and Bacteriology exams had to be taken twice.

One felt like the first Director of Clinical Studies, Dr Alec Cooke, who had been told in response to a notice of lectures in Wadham College, that he would be better not to attend because the lecturer was very old and would be much upset if anyone attended. One also recalled Bill Gibson's story of a lecture taken down by shorthand and those notes being read while the lecture was given again 30 years later. It began: "Gentleman! Since addressing you yesterday, I have changed my mind."

Alec Cooke himself gave one of the most exciting lectures of my first term, mostly because – besides his wit and capacity to hold an audience – he lectured on live problems. It was the first clinical session we were encouraged to attend. There was also in one's first term the opportunity to visit local hospitals. Particularly memorable was the Mental Hospital at Littlemore. It was still a Hogarthian Bedlam. We were shown round by a reproduction of Dr Copernicus who presented the patients like toys of his own creation. He had a very large bunch of keys and one entered crowded wards of patients with mixed conditions such as schizophrenia, mania, idiocy and imbecility, illustrating catatonia, flights of fancy and delusions of grandeur, observed in padded cells and crowded corridors – and dressed, partly dressed or nude, they were encouraged to perform for us. There was electric shock therapy, insulin convulsions, and malaria fever therapy. One of the visits most enjoyed was to an elderly white-haired psychologist who, at a children's clinic, had a dozen sand trays, each with a different set of toys, ranging from military equipment to farm animals or pink frilly dolls. The trays were in front of large mirrors. The children were observed for their choice and type of play, and especially whether they played while looking into the mirror or never looking into it. The interpretation was whether they lived a life of realism and no fantasy, or vice versa. It was clear that some children never did look in the mirror and others played while always seeing only their games reflected in the mirrors.

When women, post-war, began to enter Medicine at Oxford in the late 1940s, they were provided with more scientific stimulus and support for their studies. According to Celia Westrupp, who was appointed as Medical Tutor to all female medical students immediately post-war and was the college tutor at Lady Margaret Hall, "They were all such ladies, except at Somerville" – when it was the college that produced Dorothy Hodgkin, the Nobel Prize winner for the structure of insulin, and Janet Vaughan who advanced our understanding of haematology. There was also a chemist – one Margaret Roberts – who later became Mrs Thatcher.

The first Professor of Ophthalmology was a female, Antoinette Pirie, who wrote of how a scientific colleague described her arrival at St Hugh's as 'bringing sanity to a nunnery'.

In the 1950s, Alice Carleton was the dermatologist. She came to Oxford from Dublin in 1921 to teach a few girls, separately from the boys, about anatomy above the waist, in an attic of the Anatomy School. In the 1930s, Alice visited Paris and Vienna and acquired the skills of a dermatologist. Her practice was widespread geographically, including Swindon and Cirencester, but she was still also teaching anatomy in 1950 when I first met her. During the war she was supported by a house officer shared with paediatrics. One of these in 1945-46 was Thomas Stapleton, later Professor of Paediatrics at Sydney University. Alice was to be avoided in the Anatomy School because her wit was capable of destroying one, and I had to struggle to learn the language of anatomy and its long lists of parts. However, by 1954 it was time to learn dermatology: my father had met her brother and she knew of my existence. This made me work a little harder on knowing my spots. Later I dedicated a book to her, quoting her command: "Look, boy, look!"

The way Alice Carleton practised dermatology amused her medical students. Every patient was undressed and their skin problems demonstrated, and anyone who called a macule a papule might get hit. On one occasion, she swung round to a female assistant who was nodding a clue to a student from behind her, and punched her firmly in the chest. She had in the clinic a psychiatrist, Kenneth Dewhurst (best known for his books on Oxford's medical history), in the clinic waiting room in case a patient needed talking to. An allergist was also there in waiting. Her role was solely to diagnose and treat. All prescriptions were written by the female doctor in attendance who on other days looked after female VD. In the next room, Mary Assinder and Susanne Alexander saw the follow-ups. These clinics were held twice a week and there was a weekly ward round.

Unpredictably, my path was to cross with anatomists for many years. There were Alice and Grahame Weddell who brought electron microscopy to Oxford. Neither thought themselves as high-grade scientists. Grahame reported himself as just 'B+' and Alice as 'non-academic'. The head of anatomy was Professor Le Gros Clark who would wax eloquent on the merits of the hippocampus, reading long tracks of *The Water Babies* by Charles Kingsley where, surprisingly, it is a feature.

Corporal punishment was not confined to Alice Carleton. The bacteriologist Dr Vollum slapped you round the ears if he caught you waving in the air a bacteria-loaded steel probe or using it to scratch your head instead of firing it in the Bunsen burner. A senior technician, also known to be a rather pompous city councillor, in the respiratory laboratory, would slap you when air got on the wrong side of the mercury in some glass tubing for the third time.

I never got slapped or punched but for me mental stress was more frequent due to painfully non-productive sessions with some tutors. Hermann Blaschko, universally regarded as an Oxford 'Great', was a German refugee who worked on skin pigment. He was not intelligible when speaking in a strong accent on his favourite Furo Melanins, and it was a strain to show undiminished interest when tutorials continued for more than one hour. It did not prepare me for the Biochemical paper a year later in Honours Physiology. Unable to understand any of it, I was lucky to get a Third overall on the physiology papers when a harder working friend only obtained a fourth grade.

One contributory factor to not having a total focus on learning was not working hard enough, Another was some basic learning difficulty. As indicated above, there was also making the most of Oxford and the non-academic aspects of being there. However, interest in Medicine was enhanced by patient contact from October 1954. My journey, which later was to be into microcirculation, probably began in about 1955, with the admission to the Nuffield Department of Medicine of a middle-aged woman who had purpura of the legs and bilateral swelling of the parotid glands. As a student responsible for clerking this patient, and knowing that one might be questioned about her, a literature search found, somewhat by chance, a paper of four similar patients described by the Norwegian, Jan Waldenstrom, published in the *Norwegian Journal of Medicine* just before World War II. Later in the week, when attending a ward round led by the Nuffield Professor of Medicine, Leslie Witts – who had some visitors on this occasion – the Norwegian paper was duly mentioned by me. Leslie, after a long pause said, "Really?" and turned to a visitor and said, "What do you think?" It was Jan Waldenstrom, who was duly impressed. At the end of the ward round, it was suggested that the grand round of the week should feature this patient and that the presentation should be done by the knowledgeable medical student. Thus began an extensive reading round the topic of cutaneous blood vessel pathology, which was to remain a lifelong interest.

A period of a few weeks in Accident and Emergency was not busy, unlike anything one would see nowadays. There were very few self-poisonings and few drunks. Before crash helmets became mandatory, there were more deaths from bicycle accidents and consequently fewer cuts to be sewn up by medical students. Vivid memories include when four of us were chased down a corridor by a confused post-epileptic patient whirling a bucket of plaster of Paris.

We struggled to remember all the abbreviations used. One patient whose nose bleed had stopped by the time he had arrived at casualty was given a follow-up of one week, and in his notes was written 'WOC' meaning 'Words of Comfort'. This was misinterpreted by a discharge nurse and he came back 'Walking on Crutches'.

Although marriage as a medical student might prevent appointment to a good house job on qualification, one nevertheless had to give time to finding girlfriends and socialising at the various dances one was invited to. The Regius Professor before Sir George Pickering was Gardener who, when asked to provide a love interest in a film on Penicillin, said, "We do not encourage things like that in Oxford." I found it difficult to judge the intensity of relationships and hated sessions of tears when suspected of diminishing interest. Looking for girls as partners was never a high priority. Three of my previous headmasters could be described as misogynist, and one boy in my dormitory (as mentioned in Chapter 3) was expelled at the age of 16 for going for a walk with a local farmer's daughter, which at that time I did not consider unfair. Before going to Oxford, at a crammer in London I met more normal relationships, but lack of confidence, the need for hard work, and a mother who did not encourage girlfriends, stifled my interest in partners.

At Worcester College, my shyness and some rather bad experiences of over-confident girls telling me to join in more at parties caused me to withdraw to male company. Once entering hospital life, one or two nurses on the lookout for partners chose me, so searching for partners was not an issue. One went to the nurses' parties and we were very well behaved. Difficulties arose when one wanted to break relationships before the girlfriend had developed too great expectations. Girls in tears worried me. It was a time when the medical establishment made it quite clear that young doctors should not be married during their first jobs, and I was well into house jobs before I began to think about relationships that could lead to marriage. A good friend from Yorkshire, sharing digs with me, came from an environment where pairing off with girls had to be part of everyday life, where it was normal to sit in the back of a car 'necking'. He introduced me to the niece of a well-known comedian. We went to a New Year Ball and to the Hallé Orchestra's Annual Viennese Ball. There was the compulsory post-ball sitting in the car with one's girlfriend in one's arms – not an experience with which I was comfortable. Back in Oxford, Tessa, whose voice, looks and humour I enjoyed, was the first girl I took home and my mother said, "She is very nice, but are those her teeth?" My mother had found for me the daughter of the local GP who invited me to the Sandhurst Royal Military Academy's Annual Ball; my first night-long event, and it seemed never-ending.

I was elected as President of the medical students' social club known as Osler House, based in the Observer's house of the eighteenth century Observatory,[7] next to the Radcliffe Infirmary and now part of the Medical School. One had to keep all wheels oiled and give one's support in diverse directions, such as occasional support for the rugby team when they were short, playing like a soccer player on the right wing, and taking part in two tough games, against St George's Hospital, London, and the Welsh School of Medicine. Many of the friends one made included technicians and support staff. I have published for Medical Alumni a description of life below stairs and a description of the paint, pipes and electrics below stairs in the old Radcliffe.[8, 9]

As president of the medical students social club, one was expected to give a student opinion on the future of the Clinical School, there being a high-level debate as to whether it should be postgraduate and not take students in their first clinical year, since there were now several heads of department who preferred discussions with qualified research workers rather than teaching less knowledgeable medical students.[10]

Every Medical School puts on an annual Rag, usually as a fund-raising event. At Oxford, the event was linked with the annual Christmas festivities. Charles Fletcher (Chest Physician), Alastair Robb-Smith (Morbid Pathologist), and Ronald Macbeth (Ear, Nose and Throat Surgeon), initiated it in 1939 with a Christmas Pantomime and called the organisation 'Tynchewyke' after the first teacher of medicine in Oxford. It became an annual event which continues to the present day. Put on for a few nights either before or just after Christmas, it was initially for the entertainment of the nurses after their Christmas dinner. It was followed on the final night by a party and a Rag event.

I joined the Tynchewyke Society in my first clinical year, 1954, playing Snow White's mother in the end-of-year pantomime. In

1955 I had a part in an Asian themed pantomime, and then in 1956, on being elected as director of the next one, I began writing *Handsome and Dettol* in January. The first and fourth acts were in verse, and there was a longish ballet scene to the overture *Hansel and Gretel.* The hospital carpenter's shop was responsible for the staging of the show and the making of props, which included a gigantic steam-issuing anaesthetic machine and a large pink elephant.

With every hospital ward having increased electricity demands for Christmas tree and other Christmas lights, we had to cope with the hospital power supply fusing several times during rehearsals and during the pantomime.

After the event, all the staging had to be dismounted on the last night and was followed in the early hours of the morning by a student rag when some remarkable stunts were sometimes undertaken. Among recollections of such stunts, there was a clever exercise of putting a car on the roof of the Radcliffe Infirmary.

On my watch there was a stunt that badly messed up the hospital canteen. As a result, the police were called and I had to deal with a group of shocked hospital governors and administrators. About a dozen of us were called up before the Regius Professor and fined £20, which was paid by the surgeon elected as official advisor to the Tynchewyke Society, Ted Maloney. One student was sent down for

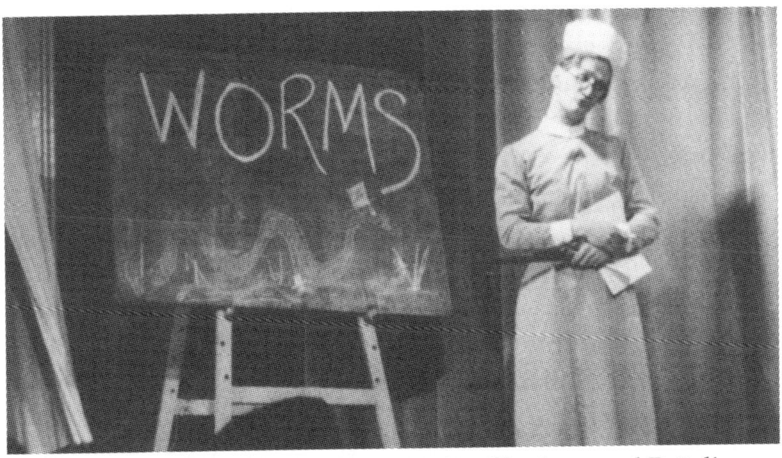

Myself as Sister Tutor in the pantomime 'Handsome and Dettol'

a week. The experience and involvement in the Rag was one of the most intense and demanding of my life. In later years, the involvement of women in the annual pantomime added more wit and converted the Rag to a less potentially damaging fund-raising exercise.

Although I expected the scene in the pantomime which was not complimentary of the new Regius Professor, George Pickering, as well as the Rag itself, to count against me, it was a surprise to be appointed House Physician to the Regius Professor nine months later.

Notes on Chapter 4

1) Masterman, J.C. (1972), *The Double Cross System in the War of 1939-1945*. Yale University Press.

Masterman, J.C., (1953), *To Teach the Senators Wisdom, or, An Oxford Guide-Book*. London, Hodder & Stoughton.

2) Palfreyman, David (2008), *The Oxford Tutorial: Thanks, You Taught Me How to Think*. Oxford, Blackwell.

Oxford, many think, is the more outstanding because of its tutorial system. I have no doubt that some who give and receive tutorials hugely benefit. My lack of benefit was because I had too little basic knowledge of science to engage in confident discussions and I was in any case shy in one-to-one relationships.

3) These college concerts required much shifting of furniture at both Worcester and Somerville Colleges. Those who helped with this were to become the UK's leading musicians in public schools, and music critics of British newspapers, and included Peter Branscombe, John Culshaw, James Dalton, Christopher Dearnley, Noel De Jong, Bob Layton, Jeremy Noble, Andrew Porter and Hans Seelig.

4) The New Theatre had the largest stage for shows touring the provinces before setting up in London. I saw *Kiss me Kate* and *Kismet* in this way. Many shows visited Oxford after their time in London, such as *Bless the Bride, Free as Air*, and shows built up round individual artists such as Joyce Grenville, Maurice Chevalier,

Beatrice Lillie, Arthur Askey and the Crazy Gang. The New Theatre was also a stopping-point for Carl Rosa Opera Company, Sadlers Wells Opera, and the Royal Opera and Glyndebourne companies.

5) We were lucky not to see the first of three performances of the Coronation *Aida* in June 1952 when Sir John Barbarolli famously conducted out of time. It was not consistently one of Callas's greater performances but Simionato was at her best. It is available on CD SBT2 1355.

6) The Natural History Museum and the Ashmolean have always been two of my favourite places. The Arts and Craft movement is much in evidence with the wonderful use of hand-made materials, until often either materials, salaries or energy ran out *viz* the outside windows of the Natural History Museum. The initial enthusiasm of some of the outer windows are wonderful. However, at various times in my life, until improvements in the last decade, I have been irritated by how the needs of the public viewer and their families must be met, in spite of the fact that, while there is praise of the concept of 'the public understanding of science', as a concept it had not been followed through. For 40 years of my viewing, there was too much naming in Latin alone, and no pushchairs were allowed so children could disappear under exhibits and be lost from their parents' control.

7) There was a belief that the Radcliffe Infirmary could be no more than a country hospital, and there being no question of it being in the first rank. Lord Nuffield thought otherwise and even bought the Radcliffe Observatory to prove it. Dr Alec Cooke took one look at it and thought it unsuitable for clinical research on patients. It eventually became the Nuffield Institute for Medical Research, focusing on the pregnancy of sheep, almost as unsuitable a place for sheep, but first class research was done there in spite of the stairs they had to ascend with difficulty. It was too cold in winter and too hot in summer. Cine radiology was also developed there under Ardran.

Ryan, T.J. and Loudon, I., 'The Observatory and the Nuffield Institute for Medical Research' in Loudon, I, and Burley, J., (Eds.), *The Tower of the Winds. A Biography of an Observatory*. Green College (2005), 134-44.

8) Ryan, T.J., *Life Below Stairs at the Radcliffe Infirmary*. Oxford Medical Alumni, Oxford Medicine.

9) The *Oxford Medical School Gazette*, during the 1950s and 60s, is a rich resource of opinion on the future of the Medical School. The Nuffield Committee on the Advancement of Science was told in 1952 by the gastroenterologist Sydney Truelove that the number of beds under the direct control of professors was inadequate. The editor in my time, David Sargeant, carried out interviews with Lord Nuffield who, by 1956, was being less consulted and we students thought him neglected. The students were also anxious to retain the rugby club supporters and thought a drift towards postgraduate medicine would be the end of it. Joseph Trueta, the Nuffield Orthopaedic Surgeon, described us students as 'half-rejected characters from other schools'. The year 1954 was indeed a low point with two intakes of only eight students.

10) One of the more complex issues was the entitlement of anyone appointed to consult in the Medical School to be attached and able to enjoy Oxford's privileged college life and high table dining.

5: Early Years as a Doctor

My first job as a doctor was as Houseman to the Regius Professor George Pickering. Much could be written about George Pickering[1] that would both illuminate and entertain. He was the Regius I knew best, perhaps the most colourful. He had recently arrived in Oxford. As his House Physician George liked to be on first-name terms, and I value his reference that was fulsome about my 'integrity and outlook'!

This Regius Professor valued William of Wykehame's motto, 'Manners makyth man', and the outlook of Sir William Osler, his early twentieth-century predecessor, in whose house he lived. At the same time, he aimed to be a great scientist, and in his younger days treasured his experience of being a co-author with the leading London physiologist, Sir Thomas Lewis, who had been one of the first clinical scientists appointed to the Medical Research Council. Finding himself as head of a great medical school at its most difficult period of development, he wished to be thought of as a great administrator. He was in many ways a model for the Medical School itself, but quite unpredictable as to which of arts, science, good administration or a heritage site worthy of display would rise to the top. He valued histrionics as a discipline contributing to success. Sir George was a master of advocacy which Burrough (1978)[2] – when writing about his attempt to make the Medical School less parochial – described it as 'a characteristic sales campaign' with 'a whiff of the theatrical'. A sentence about me in the same book spoke of the new dermatologist who had been a leading actor in student pantomimes.

As Sir George's second Houseman in Oxford, I experienced the competitiveness and quirkiness of those who conducted his rounds, and occasionally others from his temperature control laboratories. He had just published his book on high blood pressure, and there were greatly publicised debates between himself and Lord Platt about its mode of inheritance.[3] He would be pleased with today's awareness that a phenomenon such as blood pressure is dependent on a few genes interacting with the environment, and that there is not one gene for every protein, as was believed by several of my contemporaries following up on Garrod.

Pickering, a leading scientist, now the Medical School's great administrator, lived at 13 Norham Gardens (home from 1905 to 1919 of Sir William Osler, the most celebrated physician of the twentieth century), and would descend on his wards ready to play an Oslerian role as bedside teacher. He would pounce on one for using words he thought inappropriate to describe illness, and I was given a list of words not to use, for saying 'cyanosis' instead of 'blue' or being imprecise and saying 'chesty'. Other words were 'spasm' and 'shocked'. We were to give the pulse rate rather than use words such as 'tachycardia'. He shared a ward with the Consultant Physician Teddy Buzzard who used these words all the time. All George's patients with chest pains were kept in bed for a minimum of six weeks but Teddy's patients were up and about after one week. The Senior Physician at the hospital was Alec Cooke, who went round shutting windows and stopping anyone whistling. George Pickering liked fresh air and whistled Mozart's *Clarinet Quintet* on most days.

My predecessor, Geoffrey Rivett, handed me a note saying that the only way to be a successful Houseman was not to be caught out not knowing, so he recommended asking for a blood count and sedimentation rate, tests for syphilis, a urine test, a chest X-ray and blood urea on every patient. That was not approved by the Registrar Tony Mitchell, but sometimes encouraged by research assistant Dr Mike Pears. Sir George would delay surgery on a bleeding ulcer until the blood bank ran out and would repeat angiograms until a postulated stenosis was incontrovertibly demonstrated. It was not a process that made a Houseman popular with patients or laboratories. As for Ward Sisters, they dreaded it when George would himself perform procedures on the ward, such as lumbar punctures, about which he had published in earlier days. Being out of practice, he did not always impress.

Many of us would act as controls for studies such as the fever-inducing Pyrogen test. The idea was that inducing rigors would identify kidneys with pyelonephritis by flushing out white cells into the urine and lead to better therapy of all the patients admitted with high blood pressure. It was the Houseman who had to count the cells in the urine, Osler-like, using a microscope in a ward laboratory. Rigors in healthy staff controls expected shortly after inoculation of the Pyrogen seemed sometimes to be delayed and would come on when sitting with a girlfriend on the double seats at the back of Oxford's Scala cinema.

It was George Pickering who set me on the path initiated by his mentor Sir Thomas Lewis to explore the physiology of the cutaneous vasculature of the skin. George Pickering, having worked with Sir Thomas Lewis, had an extensive knowledge of blood supply. In Pickering's department there was work being carried out on the vascular responses to cold, such as during drowning at sea, and six months in his department laid a firm base for the knowledge of blood supply, thermo-regulation of the skin, and whether capillary endothelium contracts.

As a medical student, I had at one time considered an elective in Zeneca, Yugoslavia, to study forms of swaddling and hence exposure to cold in ethnic groups that were Muslim or Bosnian. It proved impossible because of poor relations between my Bosnian supervisor and the Muslims. Later, at the Royal Free, I published with Patsy Periera and Amal Kurban a study of the skin vasculature development during the first three months of life and the influence of cooling. Some sites in flexures are never cooled during this period of life, and I suggested this explained why childhood eczema is often localised to the flexures, warm sites tending to itch more.

After retirement as Regius Professor of Medicine, Sir George Pickering was asked by the Nuffield Provincial Hospitals Trust to survey medical education outside London. In *A Quest for Excellence in Medical Education – A Personal Survey* (1978), Sir George Pickering describes the problem of the proliferation of facts for a finite curriculum, and prescribed 'continuing education'. He wrote that no-one is competent over the whole field of medicine and that it was necessary to know one's competence. He decried the Heads of Departments, that 'like birds of prey snatched up the student to get their pound of flesh to instil their favourite facts'. A strong advocate of Oslerian principles, he wished for a blend of the scientific and the humanitarian, but he also advocated every student being given time for original enquiry. He is the acknowledged disseminator of the concept of postgraduate medicine. Like me, he disapproved of exams which demanded facts rather than explanation, and he had written to the Royal College of Physicians accordingly.

One's first medical job is always a steep learning curve. There were not just clinical facts still to be learned but George Pickering surrounded himself with a large team of often quite tricky colleagues. One also had to learn to be on good terms with many other hospital departments whose backs he put up.

Finishing each day at about 10.00pm with a social round, as George's patients had long stays, I got to know them well. There was only one in my age group – a namesake, Patrick Ryan – an 22-year-old Irishman with high blood pressure. He was accompanied by his priest who persuaded us to let them take a weekend away in Lourdes. While there, he drank heavily and passed into a deep sleep. Because the anatomy of his radial pulse was aberrant, the priest could not feel it. He triggered alarm throughout the British and French medical services. We organised an ambulance to Heathrow. By the time he arrived, he was fully awake though terrified by having holy oil dripped over him. The priest was given a drink in Sister's office but did not accept a diagnosis, for his Lourdes semi-consciousness ward, of 'dead drunk'.

The next job was as a House Surgeon to Ronald Macbeth and his Ear, Nose and Throat Department. Macbeth was not a surgeon, limiting himself to those sites. He operated through the nose on the pituitary gland and down to the stomach through the oesophagus. These were days when safety and anaesthesia were still primitive. Ethyl chloride sprayed onto a gauze mask was not always speedily sleep-making and there were cries of children, usually twelve in one hour from 4.00pm, having their tonsils guillotined – a session which went unheard because *Mrs Dale's Diary* was turned on fully at 4 pm. Children were bound up in green hospital sheets and sat on the floor outside the operating theatre.

In 1959, there was National Service to complete. As Oxford's Senior ENT surgeon, Ronald Macbeth was well-known to a fellow ENT surgeon, then head of the Royal Army Medical Corps, and so this led to me having two years as an Ear, Nose and Throat Surgeon in Colchester Military Hospital, the centre for all the evacuations of the British Army of the Rhine (BAOR). I performed 200 tonsillectomies and 200 sub-mucosal resections of the nasal septum, sometimes to give respite to National Servicemen who were inmates of the military prison in Colchester. One with tonsillitis had fallen asleep when on duty in Northern Ireland. His father was a General in the Army searching for an excuse for this dishonour, so removing tonsils was very welcome. At home on one weekend leave, I listened to Churchill testing new guns at neighbouring *Chequers*. A new gun was to induce deafness. I decided to test the hearing of 200 soldiers but the War Office never allowed me to publish the results showing severe deafness. Many of my patients were civilians from the local county hospital, the RAMC wishing to be seen to be helpful to the NHS.

When I signed on, I told the RAMC administrators that I was interested in dermatology and so was put in charge of that department as well. Over a period of two years, I received all the evacuations from the BAOR and discharged from the Army 50 soldiers for conditions such as psoriasis.

At Colchester Military Hospital, where all the evacuations from the BAOR tended to arrive, I was given two male and two female wards for the practice of dermatology and ear, nose and throat surgery. There was never any visit by a senior army dermatologist, and one had to cope. If there was a real difficulty, one could refer to a civilian dermatologist or ENT surgeon in Colchester, but mostly I made good by reading the *Textbook of Dermatology* by Pillsbury. When it came to prescribing – the Army having not yet purchased steroids – I prescribed pre-war remedies such as arsenic, in the form of Fowlers Solution, as well as old-fashioned tar or mercury ointments, with the help of a willing pharmacist.

Certainly, in the Army, one was plunged in at the deep end. There was the occasion when I had to do my first biopsy and had no idea how to do this, but knew that I had to excise a piece of skin. The lesion was a possible malignancy on the thigh of a young soldier, and my biopsy was three inches long and half an inch wide. Only 3mm was needed. The sample was sent to Millbank Military Hospital in London and unfortunately managed to get lost there.

While in the Army there was the wine cellar of the Officers' Mess to be run. I was also involved with a pantomime and two plays at the Garrison Theatre, and reached the semi-finals of the British Drama League Competitions. When in the Army at Colchester, Tessa, who had been my favourite ballroom dancing companion in Oxford, visited for mess dances, and my army colleagues encouraged me to take the relationship further. Tessa hoped it would end up with a proposal but I did not feel passionate nor was I ready career-wise. Ten years were to go by before it would be the right time to be married.

Conscious as a hospital employee of not experiencing the Army, I joined a Signals Regiment next-door as a Medical Officer (MO) from 6.00am to 10.00am. The CO was a very tall fast runner and in my first week took new recruits on a long run without paying attention to regulations about stopping after an hour and adjusting footwear. The MI room was filled with servicemen unable to walk because of severe blisters, and a visit to the CO followed when I put in an official rebuke. He took it well. Later, playing soldiers, there would be night visits to Norfolk forests, and it was fun to camouflage my medical inspection tent with branches of fir and pine trees. The 'soldiering' was playing bridge in the CO's van.

On completing my two years as a National Serviceman, I was given a farewell dinner by the Commanding Officer and returned home to Buckinghamshire for a period of domesticity and more music-going. When I was a House Physician, a dying patient had bequeathed me £21 for purchase of records. This started the hobby of record-collecting but only of opera. When I was 21, my mother had a bumper year selling turkeys, enabling her to purchase a much-valued gramophone plus the *Furtwangler* recording of the Flagstad *Tristan and Isolde* and the Schwarzkopf *Merry Widow*. A Belgian friend, Yves Van Schoote, who had been a visiting elective student to the Radcliffe Infirmary when I was a House Physician, invited me a couple of years later for a Vienna State Opera production of *Figaro* and *Salome* at the Brussels World Exhibition. There was also an excellent *Boris Godunov* to an empty audience because of an overcrowded schedule at that event. We were to meet almost yearly either in the USA or still later, once we were both married, in their Ramsgate Summer abode, or most often in their very attractive Ghent and Latem Belgium homes.

Rowley Holt Wilson, my friend from school, later produced an excellent Britten edition of *The Beggar's Opera* at the Oxford Playhouse at the command of Miss Penelope Sweeting, who later directed the Adelaide Festival Theatre. Meeting her years after her retirement, she was charmingly grateful for being remembered for both. László Heltay, later to be New Zealand's chief conductor, was the Musical Director.

On an early experience of Glyndebourne Opera, Josephine Whalley from the Department of Dermatology, who was known at Oxford for her knowledge of wines, had invited two of her friends – one from Avery's and the other Freddie Price, well-known in wine circles. I had been commanded to produce smoked salmon sandwiches. Not having prepared such an item before, I found new bread did not cut finely so used old bread. In a voice redolent of Edith Evans and the 'Handbag', Josephine said, "*That* was a great mistake." Wine enthusiasts have been part of the story at other times. The wine and opera lover and historian Felix Markham at Hertford College asked me to meet Josephine Veasey after her performance of Dido in Berlioz's *The Trojans*. Her husband Anderson (a producer of opera and soon to lose her to another) and I spent the meeting listening to him clearly besotted by his wife's performances. I became a friend of the President of the Wine Society, Penning Rousell, and had some alarming meals with failing to guess what I was drinking.

Some musical experiences were when the cosmetic industry's *L'Oreal* invited leading journalists from women's journals to listen to me lecturing about the skin and a production at La Scala in Milan, of a contemporary opera by Tesi – *Richard III*. It was not the appropriate audience – but then *L'Oreal* had a habit of taking over magnificent settings and ruining them. Once I lectured for them in a prefabricated Greek temple in front of Leonardo da Vinci's *Last Supper* to background music of *Also Sprach Zarathustra*. On another occasion, it was the Palace of Versailles for 'Ballet in the Gardens', which included elephants, artificial grass and hedges, but although it was midsummer, it happened to be freezing and there was a rain storm.

In London, I heard Geraint Evans and Joan Sutherland in all their minor and later major roles. I only once queued all night at Covent Garden in the rain. It was for Maria Callas and it was for a performance that she cancelled.

After the experience as a National Service officer, the struggle of examinations for 'Membership' of the Royal College of Physicians began. Most doctors were tutored by a Dr Papworth in London who, like Pickering, was a critic of the physicians in London and taught exam techniques that matched some of their eccentricities and beliefs. I went to a local student of Papworth, Leo Wollner, a consultant at Stoke Mandeville. The taking of 'Membership' followed eleven times! The problem was sequencing and giving the right name to the right condition under pressure. There was fabrication and transposing of names. In the higher medical examinations, I would know what I was looking at and everything that was necessary about it, but could not name it or would give it the wrong name.

Although a skilled confabulator, giving a made-up name to a 'short case' was not allowed, however well recognised the syndrome. In examination, lack of confidence was covered by an act of over-confidence which was often not liked by the examiner, one of whom took me aside and counselled me helpfully after the short case examination.

After my National Service, I lived at home in rural Buckinghamshire and worked nearby for 18 months on Leo

Wollner's wards at Stoke Mandeville, Amersham and High Wycombe, mostly on pressure ulcers in the elderly. I tried to travel by double-decker bus as I had not yet learned to drive. I had been put off by driving into my father's precious lawn-mower and into a house when in the Army. I was not enthusiastic about cars and would hasten to get in and out of them. This might explain why on two occasions I suffered the shock of getting into the car and finding the steering wheel had been stolen and while planning what to do about it, I found the solution by noting I was sitting in the back seat!

I aimed to apply for a dermatology job in Oxford. Oxford's dermatology inpatient department had once been the 'septic ward' of the Infirmary, where penicillin was first used in 1941, but now consisted of 40 beds at the Infectious Diseases Unit outside the city. It was in the idyllic surroundings of an isolation hospital. The occasional lumbar punctures for cerebral syphilis were done there (more whenever the ballet visited Oxford!), but students visiting this outlying unit were rare and saw only special cases such as leprosy or anthrax. Alice Carleton played a considerable part in the history of this department. During the war, she wrote papers on British Anti-Lewisite (BAL), used for mustard gas, and published a few significant case histories. She was one of the first to write about hereditary factors in venous leg disorders and was the first British dermatologist to visit Japan, about which she published a few anecdotes. Her photographer, Tugwell, was superb and pre-1940 black-and-white photos in the *Oxford Textbook of Dermatology* in the 1990s are regarded as outstanding. The originals, now lodged with the History Section of the British Association of Dermatology (BAD), include cattle ringworm which was commonplace, and drug reactions from arsenicals, mercury, gold and iodides.

When frequently asked why I took up dermatology, the explanation given was that it was through fear of her in the Anatomy School which later in her dermatology clinic made me read up about skin diseases before attending her clinics. Consequently, with greater knowledge, I found greater interest in this topic and later very often attended her clinics electively.

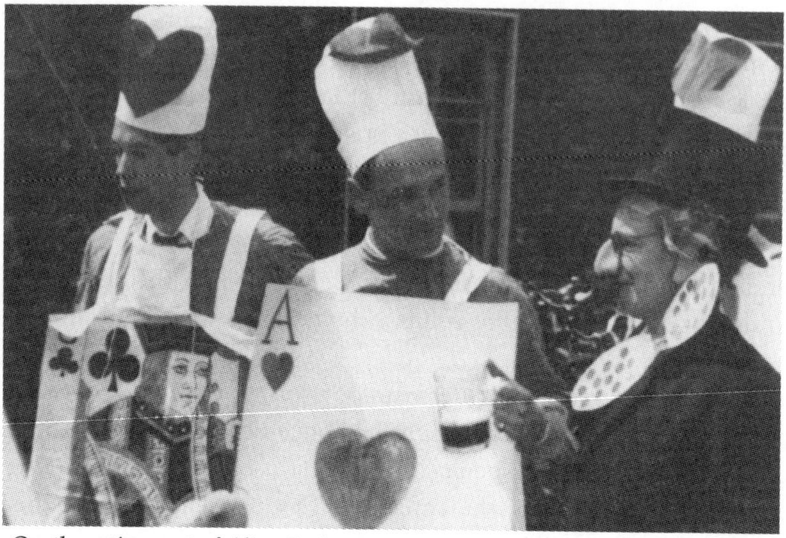

On the retirement of Alice Carleton. Medical students dragged her car from her home in Banbury Road to the Radcliffe Infirmary. I'm in the middle as the Ace of Hearts and Josephine Whalley as the Mad Hatter.

As a student, when Alice Carleton retired, and dressed as a pack of cards with four other medical students, we dragged her car to an 'Alice in Wonderland' farewell at the Infirmary on the occasion of her final clinic. Later in her retirement, there were holidays with Alice in France with introductions in the late 1950s by her to the Hôpital St Louis in Paris, the Mecca of French dermatology.

Alice was correct in saying that she had advanced dermatology very little, but because she was a brilliant raconteur, even in French, she was well-known in Europe. The Harvard dermatologist Tom Fitzpatrick, who studied pigmentation with Blaschko in Oxford for one year, was also a good friend, and Alice was appointed as the Prosser White Lecturer at the Royal College of Physicians while he was in Oxford. She was very nervous about this – feeling that she had little to offer, but knowing that she was expected to be amusing. She spoke about the history of scabies but it was not a good performance, and Tom and I had to cheer her up at a small dinner party afterwards. Tom became Professor of Dermatology at Harvard, and knowing him through Alice proved an important link when later visiting the USA for the first time. A memorable experience was lying on a bed at his beautiful home, listening to stereo vinyl records for the first time.

Renwick Vickers came from Sheffield to Oxford in 1957 when Alice retired. He had learned his dermatology as a very young man from Rupert Hallam in Sheffield. The war saw him as a dermatologist in the Royal Navy. His philosophy, partly learned from his friend Professor John Ingram, was that dermatologists should first and foremost be physicians and must therefore pass the 'Membership' exam. This view, supported by Charles Calnan, was a major influence on British dermatology and a reason I had to pass this exam in spite of Pickering's views. It was also the reason Renwick carried around his neck a golden stethoscope presented by the students as their favourite teacher.

In 1959, Renwick Vickers gave the prestigious Watson Smith Lecture at the Royal College of Physicians, focusing on clinical dermatology and general medicine, closing with a reference to myself as 'a student with an interest in dermatology', describing it as 'the least specialised of all branches of medicine'.

In a letter to the Nuffield Professor of Medicine, Leslie Witts (8th March 1965), Renwick wrote that he was concerned about the need for research into skin disease, and asked for research opportunities to be funded as part of future consultant activities to be considered during the next five years. He also stated that 'the amount of pure clinical work is not enough to keep a second consultant actively employed'. The Senior Registrar was also encouraged to work for a DPhil.[4]

Eventually, in 1962, a registrar post became available in the Department of Dermatology at Oxford, and there, under Renwick Vickers, I learned the trade according to his practice. My parents provided the money for me to rent a semi-detached house in Eynsham. While there, I bought a grand piano at £12 per month for two years, and I still play it on most days half a century later. At that time, two doctors shared my Eynsham house: Alasdair Smith, a family practitioner, was a fine tenor and we practised Schumann *Liede*. Arnold Freedman, an ophthalmologist, was also a violinist, rather more accomplished than I was, but we had many enjoyable sessions. Arnold once asked me to accompany him and the actress Eleanor Bron to her first Janacek opera. Left alone with her having drinks, I had to reassure her that holes in her long black gloves really did not matter. Later, R.S. (Charles) Wells shared my house while he worked on families with ichthyosis – at first in the Oxford Region, and later nationally. He was later to become the Dean of Dermatology in London, guiding many young people through their training. An easy lodger, he possessed a small table, which I have kept, and a packet of *Kellogg's Cornflakes*, which I have not.

While living in Buckinghamshire, my father commuted to London most days and enjoyed his role as Road Manager of an enlarging road service. He organised a major celebration of the Automobile Association's 75th anniversary. He disliked its marketing activities with the *Readers' Digest* but enjoyed helping many nations develop road services. It led to holidays in Europe, with the *Wegen Wacht* in Holland, *Touring Secours* in Belgium and *ADAC* in Germany. I joined them in Holland on several occasions. Patrols and their motorbikes from many nations were on display in the celebrations in Hyde Park for the 75th anniversary.

My mother developed breast cancer, and after surgery in London recovered well and was driving again within three weeks. She remained cancer-free for 20 years but later developed and survived spinal metastases, dying eventually of heart failure in her mid-eighties.

My parents moved to a seventeenth century cottage, *South Heath Farm* near Great Missenden. This was where my father in retirement could cope with a garden and successfully enter flower shows. They always had two or three dogs taking up much of their attention. It was not far from a prep school where Anne Merry, an Australian, was teaching. My mother's brother had lived and married in Australia and Anne, his wife's niece, came to England in 1963 as a school teacher. It was natural for her and any visiting friends to lodge frequently. We met often, sometimes going to plays and operas together.

During two or three years, there were struggles with the membership exams, taken in London, but sometimes in Glasgow or Edinburgh.[5] In spite of these struggles, I was nevertheless given several good opportunities to develop dermatology skills. It was the days of patronage – one would only get invited to the British Association of Dermatology (BAD) annual meeting if one had a paper to read on behalf of one's patron, in my case, Renwick Vickers, and he was expected to pay for the three-day occasion.

While the World Congress took place in Washington, there was a link by *Telstar* to the UK. The link was based at Land's End, and Renwick Vickers went down to represent the UK, with Geoffrey Dowling, the doyen of British dermatology and the senior dermatologist in London, with the most influence on training.

The discussion was about folic acid antagonists as an alternative to steroids, and patients were seen for the first time by satellite. Rees, the initiator of this therapy for psoriasis, spoke from Washington. On return to Oxford, folic acid antagonists were deemed worth studying, and as a junior doctor in the dermatology department, the study came my way – with a small team of senior consultants: Sheila Callendar (haematologist), and John Badenoch (gastro-enterologists), as well as dermatologists. The outcome was my giving the first paper on folic acid antagonists in the UK at the BAD meeting in Leeds 1964. On one evening, I found myself hosting my first international guest list: Leonard Juhlin from Uppsala, El-Hafnawi from Cairo, Elenor Feuerman from Tel Aviv, and one or two distinguished consultants of other nationalities.

During my time as Registrar and Senior Registrar, it was realised that electron microscopy in the Anatomy School, focusing on leprosy, needed fresh material, skilfully taken and frozen – and not material sent from Nigeria in formalin. Renwick offered the leprology team two beds for the programme, and soon the department became a centre for leprosy research. First, Dr Frank Allenby, Senior Registrar, and then I, organised quarterly meetings for experts on leprosy. Attending these were the leading world leprologists: Robert Cochrane, Paul Brand, Stanley Browne,

Michael Waters, John Pearson, Dick Rees, Roy Vollum and Jamison, as well as Graham Weddell.

It was at this time that I hit international dermatology headlines. The hypothesis was that everything the epithelium required was on the inside, like its blood supply, and it was really very unlikely that it would regularly migrate towards the outside away from everything that it needed – which was the classical view of epithelial cells being lost from the skin surface. At the next BAD meeting in Bristol, I gave a paper on 'The Direction of Epithelial Growth'. This was published and led to a published blitz from the leading American dermato-pathologist Herman Pinkus, and thereafter we had a regular correspondence about what we meant by the direction of growth. At the Dowling Oration shortly after that, Ian Magnus spoke of the 'Two Lateral Thinkers' in dermatology: Ian Whimster, a zoology based dermato-pathologist, and myself. This, for a junior, was very flattering. Seeing the epidermis as inwardly-looking was a somewhat dyslexic view of things, with its known facility for spatial orientation, as is my easy memorisation of maps, and perhaps a facility to recognise the patterns of skin disease – though less so to name them.

In the Department of Dermatology there was the physician in charge of Venereology, Josephine Whalley, the aforementioned renowned expert on wines and a close friend of several of Oxford's experts on wines.[6] One of these was Gordon Sanders, a close colleague of Lord Florey and assistant to the Nobel Prize winning team for the development of penicillin, but also a leader in the field of studies of blood supply.

Once my interest in blood supply and lymphatics began to advance, Gordon Sanders invited me to be a member of the British Microcirculation Committee with members Howard Florey, Henry Barcroft (of St Thomas's Medical School), Joseph Trueta (the orthopaedic surgeon whose vascular shunting systems described in the kidney following crush injury had made him an acknowledged expert on blood supply), and other colleagues. We initiated the British Microcirculation Society; with me very aware of being their junior.

During the following two years, I kept a notebook in which any idea and relevant fact about the blood vessel was written down. It

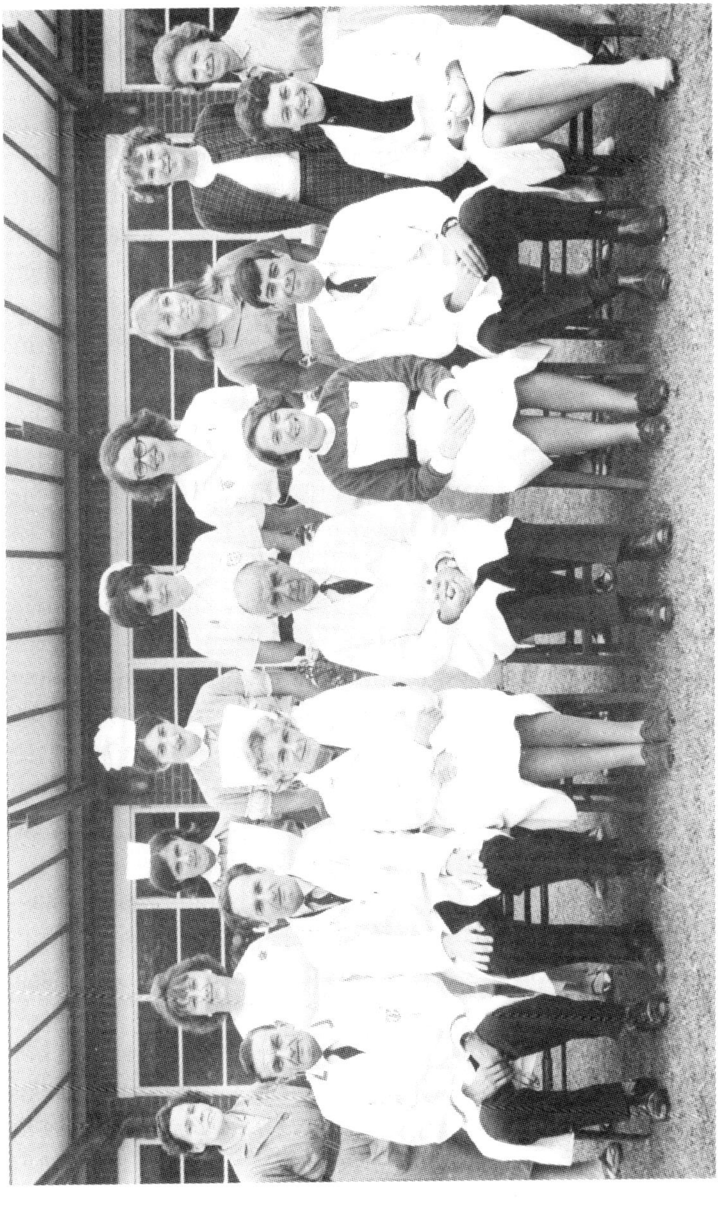

The Department of Dermatology on a cold winter morning in 1967. Front row left to right: Nurse Eric Haines, Terence Ryan, Josephine Whalley, Renwick Vickers, Sister Cox, Keith Durrant, The Almoner

culminated in a number of large notebooks eventually shown to Gordon Sanders. It was suggested that they should also be shown to Margaret Jennings, later the second wife of Howard Florey, about how exactly to organise them into a *Doctor of Medicine* thesis

The British Microcirculation Society met twice yearly, and it was thought appropriate to have a meeting in Oxford. I was the co-organiser, with Joseph Trueta, Nuffield Professor of Orthopaedics, of a two-day meeting on skin and bone blood supply, held at the Nuffield Orthopaedic Centre. Very gradually, the idea was evolving that the best way to explain the various patterns I was observing in blood supply in the skin was that they were correlated with demands and other influences relating to the epidermal/dermal junction.

Gradually, the theory was put together that the epidermis influenced the blood vasculature, and the vasculature determined some of the behaviour of the epidermis, but other influences such as nerve endings, the connective tissue and the mononuclear phagocytic system, had to be taken into account in order to explain all the variations. Particularly important was the concept of a spectrum of atrophy to hypertrophy, in which both the epidermis and the blood vessels jointly atrophied or hypertrophied.

All this began to come together into a good story, and the British Association of Dermatology meeting under Renwick Vickers was being planned for Oxford in 1966. Renwick Vickers was to be the President and Ken Crow of Swindon was to be the local secretary. Ken suffered from an anxiety syndrome, and there needed to be a back-up, which was me. It was agreed that I should prepare for the clinical case discussion a number of patients showing problems with blood supply of the skin, with a demonstration of capillary microscopy so that everybody could see what it was that I was observing in the skin. It was also agreed that there would be a symposium on the factors controlling the blood supply to the skin.

The time of the meeting arrived. The Oxford Playhouse was the theatre in which the symposium was presented – it was fashionable to call it a 'teach-in'. I put on a two-hour symposium with speakers, including Gordon Sanders and Grahame Weddell.

The organisation of several patients with vascular disease to be seen under the microscope on the Saturday of the conference was an unusual event, and it launched my reputation for being an authority on blood supply of the skin.

As a registrar, and then as a senior registrar, after Renwick had become well-established, I had the job of helping to set up regular monthly meetings, which were attended by regional dermatologists, by American dermatologists from the Upper Heyford Air Base, and by occasional visitors to the Department of Biochemistry (such as the American Lowell Goldsmith who lived with his family in a wing of my country house).

In the Region we had considerable expertise and initiatives. About twice a year we would have a Saturday morning visit to one of the outlying consultants. Under Renwick Vickers, the study of skin blood vessel disorders was encouraged and I quickly made an international name.

Ken Crow at Swindon made a name for himself as an advisor on dioxin and the *Sevesco* disaster. Dowlings' London graduates were spread throughout the Oxford Region. Bob Bowers at Cheltenham had an interest in haemangiomas. Dickie Coles in Northampton was starting his Group Therapy for psoriasis and used hypnotism for warts. Hugh Calvert in Reading was the most widely read, and he had an interest in French texts. Darrell Wilkinson, Aylesbury, High Wycombe and Amersham, who had been a guerrilla in the Greek underground during the war and whose clinics I used to attend while I was a registrar at Stoke Mandeville before joining Renwick, had multiple interests and was the region's most prolific writer. He started me on the topic of leg ulcers. Renwick was single-handedly attempting to give Oxford dermatology its general medical flavour; he was conscious that Cambridge had the academic lead through the courses on 'Biology of the Skin' that Arthur Rook was organising. My efforts were regarded as a contribution to science from the Department of Dermatology in Oxford. I was quite unaware of this at the time.

At last I passed the membership exam and the Professor of Dermatology at the Institute of Dermatology, and St John's

Hospital for Diseases of the Skin, Charles Calnan, discussed with Renwick Vickers and with Professor Ingram of Leeds how best to further my training. I was encouraged to apply for a registrar's job at St John's Hospital for Diseases of the Skin, the British Mecca of dermatology. At the interview, while waiting with three others on a bench in a waiting room, I was approached by Adrian Ives – who was already a registrar there – who said, in a very loud voice, exactly which clinics I would be doing. I had, at that point, not been interviewed, nor had my other companions, but it was an omen that the job had already been decided.

Within three months of my presentation to the annual conference of the BAD, I had a post of Lecturer at the Institute of Dermatology, London University, where money was obtained from the Dunhill Trust to finance a vascular laboratory in Homerton Grove. This was a period of consolidation of the learning of dermatology, but presentations at the British Microcirculation Society followed at six-monthly intervals. I was given my own vascular laboratory for five years.

At St John's I learned all the finer points of dermatology. It was a place for wonderful discussions, with good colleagues such as Edward Wilson-Jones, Harvey Baker, John Turk and many others from the UK and overseas.

It was while in London that I seriously began to think about marriage. Anne Merry, with whom I had spent many hours as a guest of my parents, had arrived from Australia in 1965. I enjoyed her enthusiasm for seeing places and visiting the theatre and opera. Anne's favourite evening was the 1967 Visconti black-and-white *La Traviata* at the Royal Opera House. We went to the first night attended by Maria Callas sweeping in through the front entrance to applause, and watched and listened while Miraella Freni played nervously her first *La Traviata.* She burst into tears after great applause at the first interval.

Anne and her friends, Judy and Margie, were made very welcome and, unusually for girls whom I took out, evoked no criticism from my parents. The three of them toured Europe including May Day in Moscow. After about two years of frequent meetings, I began to

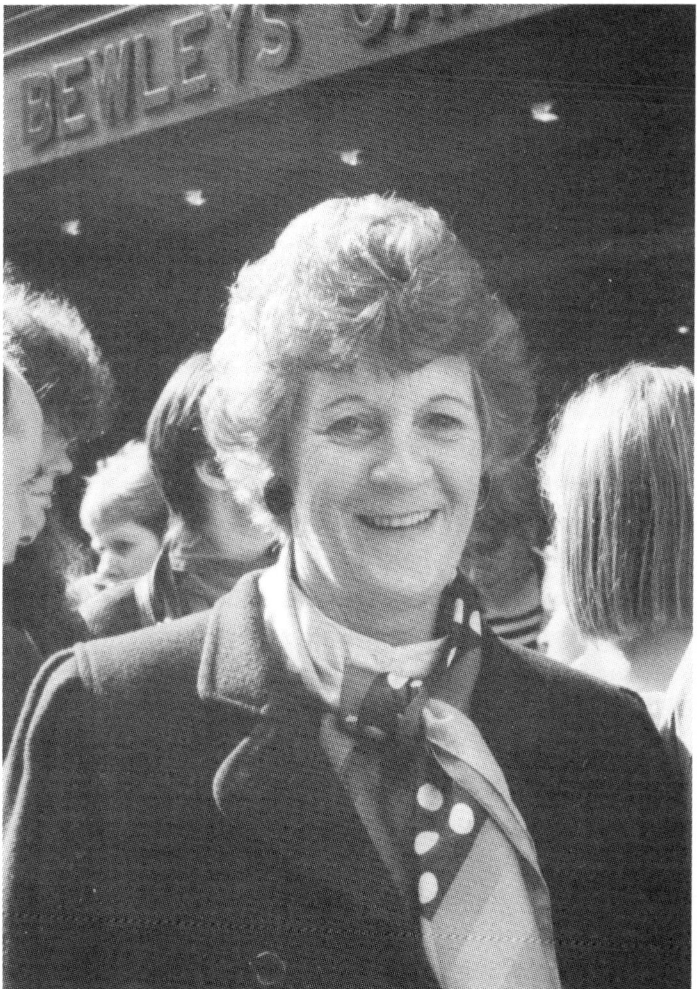

Anne Merry in 1965 to whom I was to propose marriage

wonder about Anne as a wife but had no idea how to take it further without risking not being able to break the relationship. We were visited at home by a Czech dermatology colleague, Paul Bartak, who fielded a number of questions about me from Anne and which he interpreted as interest. It was actually Anne's usual technique of finding a topic of common interest for the purpose of putting people at ease. Paul spoke to me about his conversation, and as a result I wrote a letter to Anne asking her to marry me. It actually came as a complete surprise to her, and she was within a week of leaving for home to take up a career as a teacher in Adelaide. We met at a pub for an anxious session: she told my mother, who was enthusiastic, and Anne agreed to consider it. We then parted for a year! The announcement of the engagement was in *The Times*.

The year 1967 became a period of preparation for marriage in Australia, and I planned to take advantage of the trip to meet as many experts as possible who might further my career. To get there, I would go through America and spend a few weeks meeting with the leaders in the field of microcirculation studies. These included Herman Berman in Boston to look at hamster cheek pouches, which could be adapted to study the blood supply of skin grafts; there was Roe Wells to examine the viscosity of blood, also in Boston; and then there was a few days with Edward Bloch in Cleveland, whose spectacular laboratory for looking at the blood supply of every organ had become very well-known. There followed a period at the Mayo Clinic with Peter Copeman, from Westminster Hospital, London, who was having an elective year there to discuss our mutual interest and publications in preparation on vasculitis, and some potential publications on the effect of cold on the skin as well as vascular patterns. Other visits were to Curt Wiederhelm in Seattle to examine the bat's wing. This is an animal of which the wing is transparent under the microscope, and when hibernating, it will spread the wing under the microscope for several hours.

Interspersed with all this was a meeting of the American Microcirculatory Society at Atlanta. 23,000 people were at the biology meeting, my first experience of the large size of American meetings. While there, I remember waking up with a robber in my room about to escape through the window onto a balcony with my suitcase, which he fortunately dropped. He was probably a member of hotel staff dressed in white, but because of outside lights being yellow, I described him to the police as dressed in a yellow suit.

On arriving in Sydney, Australia, I visited Dintenfass, an expert on blood viscosity, and Arnold Palmer, well-known for his simple techniques of examining blood flow which I thought could be applied to the skin.

The Vicar at St Jude's, Brighton, Adelaide, Australia, the Reverend Peter Hopton, said it was a pleasure to marry a 'mature couple'. I was aged 36, and Anne was nine years younger.

Our marriage took place in Adelaide on 16th May 1968. My parents were on their retirement world tour. The Stage Manager of my 1956 pantomime in Oxford, Bob Porter, then Vice-Chancellor of Monash University, was my Best Man. We drove Anne's *Holden* to a holiday house on the sea coast 400 miles to the west to begin our honeymoon, which continued as a three-month lecture tour beginning in Singapore where I gave a course on the blood supply of the skin. We lived in the university's guest accommodation. After eating off a stall in China Town, I managed to lecture with a severe stomach upset and a high fever. We then went on to India where I lectured on psoriasis at the Calcutta Medical School. Anne was taken off by a British Council wife to see Mother Teresa who, taking her into her office, took her by surprise saying, "What are you going to do about the Australian Aborigines?" Mother Teresa did build a care home in Queensland. We went on to Delhi where Anne was expected to speak to a group of women sociologists.

Our flight from Delhi to Warsaw landed in Tashkent and then in Moscow where, without a visa, we were guarded securely by a uniformed and rather hefty female – even watching me using the toilet. On arrival in Warsaw, we were looked after by a previous student of Graham Weddell, Andrew Pavlowski, who had been an acquaintance of mine and his famous boss, Professor Stefanie Jablonska. We flew on to Prague to stay with the Bartaks and experienced the beginning of Russian manoeuvres which were to take over Czechoslovakia. Finally we arrived in Gothenburg for a

Microcirculation Conference where we sold our very expensive banquet tickets to help us get home.

Once back in England, Anne and I lived in several houses, such as my parents' home at Great Missenden while they were still in Australia and New Zealand, returning via North America. Anne was to teach at Brickwall School where we were given accommodation for a while. Professor Charles Calnan had both a central London house and a house in the suburbs which he lent us. In 1969, we found a flat in Morden Road, Blackheath. It was ideal for entertaining as the main room was large and acoustically suitable for my piano. There were bangings from below on the first night as we had as a guest a strong mezzo-soprano, wife of a dermatologist from Adelaide. At one of our parties, Dr Francisco Costa Martins from Brazil telephoned Sao Paulo. It was very expensive and we were a little annoyed. However, on his return to Brazil, he sent Charles Calnan and me plane tickets for a superb clinical meeting rich in tropical dermatology.

We were met off the plane and did not go through customs. In the middle of the week, we found ourselves to be illegal immigrants! It was the time of the Great Train Robbery and it was believed the robbers were in Brazil. A girlfriend of the Chief of Police was found, and in one of the grandest offices in which I have ever been, we watched her while she used her allure to get our passports signed.

Back at work for the first time, I was responsible for the lives and work of employees in my new Vascular Laboratory in the Eastern Fever Hospital in Homerton. The development of a Vascular Unit was based on the technique of fibrinolysis autography. There were studies on platelets, studies on cold-induced disorders, and the setting up of a Hamster Cheek Pouch Laboratory to explore, *in vivo* and under the microscope, the relationship between epithelial grafts and their blood supply. Helpers at this time included Robert Turner, from Portland, Oregon, Amal Kurban, an established Professor of Dermatology from the American University of Beirut, and Kiyoshi Nishioka – only the second Japanese dermatologist to visit the Institute of Dermatology in London. The first Japanese-trained dermatologist to get a postgraduate degree in the UK (1968-72) was, in fact, later to become Professor of Dermatology in Taipei, Taiwan. C.K. Wong studied in Sapporo, northern Japan, and later, in the Department of Dermatology at Oxford, did his DPhil on field defects of the melanocyte. Both C.K. Wong and Kiyoshi Nishioka had British-born babies. Kiyoshi's child was born in the same hospital as my daughter and where Geoffrey Dowling was doing a locum after his retirement. C.K. Wong named his son after Roger Vickers, the son of the Oxford dermatologist, Renwick Vickers

In Japan in 1967, Charles Calnan met the young Kiyoshi Nishioka who indicated his hope of working in England. It is probably relevant that this was a period of unrest in the universities around the world, and at the time of the Expo '70 in Tokyo, Japanese students were particularly restive. Kiyoshi was one of these. They wished to achieve the independence to determine the course of their careers, and dermatology in London under the influence of Geoffrey Dowling was perceived as unusually democratic.

Kiyoshi Nishioka arrived in London in 1971. Collaboration with these two Japanese dermatologists, Aoki and Nishioka, confirmed the nineteenth century impressions of their politeness, good humour and industriousness. They became good friends of many in the UK. Before Kiyoshi Nishioka arrived in England, to work initially with me on inhibitors of plasminogen activators, I visited Tom Fitzpatrick in Boston on the way to get married in Australia, and noted the same qualities of the Japanese in his department. Kiyoshi learned how to study angiogenesis and set up the Hamster Cheek Pouch Laboratory at the Institute of Dermatology, London. The cheek pouch vasculature could be converted to a blood supply to serve tissues placed on the cheek pouch. In order to do this, he first had to learn the technique from Gordon Sanders, who worked with the Nobel Prize winner Howard Florey in Oxford. It was an unforgettable ordeal for someone whose English was not yet proficient; as a guest at the High Table of Lincoln College, Oxford, at which conversation is valued, he had a hard time. Later, with the pathologist John Turk, Kiyoshi Nishioka developed his career as an immunologist, for which he has become so celebrated.

These were productive years, with another combined meeting of the British Microcirculation Society – this time with the Dowling Club – at which, once again, I showed many patients with vascular diseases using a new microscope, that unlike older microscopes, used a lens within a few millimetres of the skin and could examine the skin from a distance of several centimetres. With my colleagues, we published in 1970 a supplement of the *British Journal of Dermatology* entirely devoted to blood supply. It was as a result of this that I was invited to provide several chapters for the series *Physiology and Pathophysiology of the Skin*, edited by Jarrett. I was also a co-editor of the *Handbook of Microcirculation Studies* for the British Microcirculation Society.

While in London, one attended monthly the pub-based Journal Club, known originally as the George Club but in my time renamed The Dowling Club after its founder Geoffrey Dowling who by this time I knew well.[7]

There were still very few dermatologists interested in microcirculation, but blood supply had to be included in any major symposium, so it was gratifying to be asked in September 1975 to help with the celebration of the 25th annual Montagna Biology Symposiums in Portland, USA. Al Kligman wrote that I should prepare a review of blood supply: 'A tone poem of moderate length. Anyway, glad to have a true artist on the program.' I was later invited to write the vascular sections of *Physiology and Biochemistry of the Skin*, edited by Lowell Goldsmith and a major USA textbook. During this time, I continued to develop ideas about vasculitis, which culminated in the book *Microvascular Injury* (1976).

One of the more prestigious dermatology jobs in London was that at the Royal Postgraduate Medical School. Stephen Gold, the Secretary of the British Association of Dermatology, was due for retirement, and I was appointed to take his clinic two days a week. For two years, I was the dermatologist there and experienced all the stimulus of the Postgraduate School at one of its most active periods. However, my first clinic was marred by a minor accident.

While treating *molluscum contagiosum*, the dish of carbolic acid I was holding received a jolt as my coat caught the edge of the examination couch, and some of it spilt down the female patient's neck. She brought a claim against me, and she received £300 for distress, although after a few weeks there was nothing to see. The Royal Postgraduate Medical School was sympathetic, and it proved no blot on my career.

While at the Institute of Dermatology, I looked after several clinics at St John's Hospital for Diseases of the Skin, including the Leg Ulcer Clinic. I took over from Mitchell Heggs, one-time secretary of the World Congress in London. He was a well-known Mason and every letter about every patient was written in Masonic language. The best experience was the Saturday morning clinic at St John's, attended by Geoffrey Dowling, Charles Calnan, Imry Sarkany and Louis Forman, amongst others, when unusual and undiagnosable cases were presented and discussed in exquisite detail.

Another experience resulting from being at St Johns Hospital was the contact made with an eccentric American, Bill Reed, I had first heard of him when on holiday in Holland. He was to be a generous funder of several trips to the USA and a fellow opera enthusiast.[8]

Eventually, the time came to consider returning to Oxford, as a registrar in dermatology job became available. At the interview, questions were posed about many subjects unrelated to dermatology. I was even asked about the relative merits of William Byrd versus Monteverdi! For at least six months after being appointed, I continued at the Royal Postgraduate Medical School two days a week, spending the rest of the week in Oxford.

Our daughter Josephine was born in London. One vacation shortly after her birth, Malcolm Ritchie produced, in aid of The Sussex Churches, *Ring round the Moon* by Jean Anouilh. I took part in this and Anne was in charge of costumes. We also visited the school for musical events, one of which was for the harpist Melissa Robles. She had recently had a car accident and asked me to examine her arm which had a thrombosed vein from an injection of

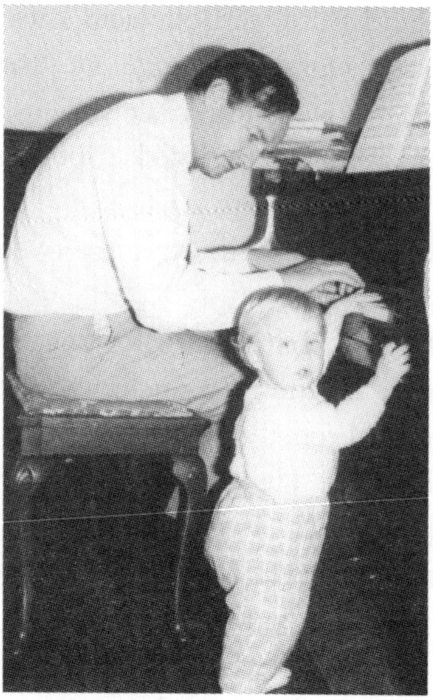

At the piano with Josephine in 1971

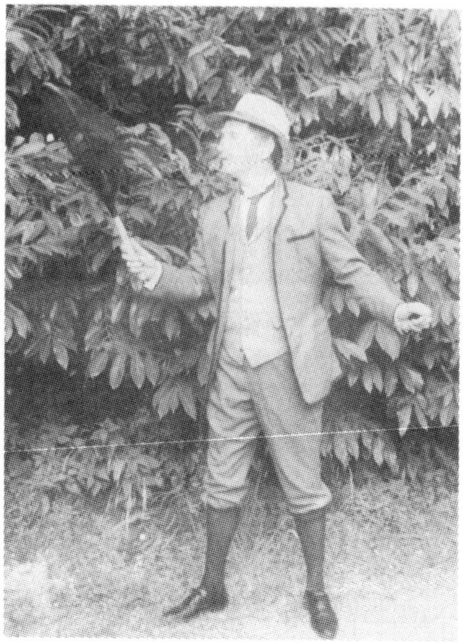

Playing the role of a butterfly catcher in 'Ring round the Moon'

pentothal. I knew nothing could be done and told her it would resolve which fortunately was the case.

After a happy four years at the Institute of Dermatology developing microcirculatory skills, on returning to Oxford as a consultant dermatologist and aged 39, I maintained my links with the British Microcirculation Society – which, in turn, led to my appointment as Treasurer of the European Microcirculation Society.

Renwick retired in 1976. He had been joined by me as a second Consultant in 1971 and was now replaced by Rodney Dawber. In Oxford, Renwick published little, and after he had retired, he took a tour to Australia, gave time to the Royal College of Physicians, and became the Chairman of Oxford's Medicine Board. He followed me and Rodney at the Royal Postgraduate Medical School when he wanted a retirement job. Chris Booth was delighted to have such a distinguished 'physician' taking part in the well-known grand rounds.

Notes on Chapter 5

1) Fitzherbert-Jones, Rosemary (2014), *Sir George Pickering (1904-1980)* in *Oxford's Medical Heritage: The People behind the Names*. Oxford University Press.

Pickering, G.W. (1959), 'A Study of Medical Education in Great Britain', in *Journal of Medical Education* 34: 11.39.

Pickering, George (1978), *Quest for Excellence in Medical Education:A Personal Survey*. London, George Allen & Unwin.

2) Burrough, E.L.R. (1978), *Unity and Diversity: The Short Life of the United Oxford Hospitals*. Privately printed by the author.

3) Parnell, R.W., Pickering, G.W., Davis, E. (1963), 'Hereditary in Hypertension' (the state in which any animal finds itself at any time is determined by two prime factors: its inherited constitution and the effects of the environment), in *The Lancet* 281: 1213-14.

4) Renwick Vicker's first Senior Registrar in Oxford was Tony Cowan, who studied silver staining of the cutaneous nerves in psoriasis, working with the anatomist Graham Weddell. Duncan Macmillan studied platelet aggregation, The first DPhil had been C.K. Wong from Taiwan in 1960.

5) After one trip in 1967 to take the exam in Edinburgh, I treated myself to lunch on the train – the Flying Scotsman – and chose turkey. As it was chicken that was served, I wrote and complained. A General Services Manager eventually wrote to me and told me I had uncovered a long-lasting scam. Years later, inexplicably, Frank Dickens, a cartoonist of 'Bristow' in the *Evening Standard*, featured 'Let us raise our cup and toast Terence Ryan'. 'Who the devil is he?' 'He exposed the Great Luncheon Voucher Swindle of 1975.' Not the right year, nor really a voucher scandal. Was the Terence Ryan mentioned really me?

6) Typically for Oxford, I was appointed as an equal as a wines member of the wine committee chaired by Gordon Sanders at Halifax House, the social centre of the Science Area, even though very junior in all other respects. Dr Gordon Sanders was a bachelor, particularly anxious when it came to entertaining women at the High Table, but with the middle-aged Josephine Whalley he felt secure. Gordon Sanders had at one time been part

of the penicillin team, and had been responsible for taking news of how to develop penicillin to Russia and China. His special interest was the microscope and examination of blood vessels *in vivo*. Josephine told him of the young dermatologist in Oxford who was looking at the blood supply of the skin. Gordon Sanders was about to become a President of the newly-formed society called the British Microcirculation Society. It was to have its first meeting, and I agreed to give a paper on my findings in the skin, using the Jobson Horne probe to shift tissue fluid. I had not yet mastered any technique for taking photographs, so drew some slightly inadequate drawings and managed to take one black-and-white photograph of the vessels in the skin, using the new technique. The presentation went sufficiently well to result in a request from Geoffrey Bourne, an established editor of technical books to include the work in a book on *In vivo histopathologic techniques* that he was editing, and shortly after that I was invited onto the newly-formed committee of the British Microcirculation Society – Gordon Sanders being the President and P.A.G. Munro, the anatomist from Cambridge, being the Secretary. Other members included Henry Barcroft, the physiologist, and Sir Howard Florey. My contribution was lightweight in comparison with these giants.

7) When Geoffrey Dowling visited Oxford, we had not spoken about dermatology but had discussed the biography of Benvenuto Cellini. Later, in the year of his death, I was to be President of The Dowling Club, and my wife and I entertained him at home before he fell ill. I was a frequent visitor to his house in west London. Anne and I worked hard for The Dowling Club and took a coach-load to our friends, the Agaches in Besançon. Unfortunately, Geoffrey Dowling was unwell for that trip. In April 1976, after hosting the Dowling Club at home, Geoffrey Dowling wrote, 'It was the most elaborate and most happy of the events up to now.' 'Your home is beyond belief.' 'Perhaps I ought to say that I have never heard more austere Brahms being read by a non-professional straight out of the book.' When I played it to him, I was trying to make it romantic and anything but 'austere'. Geoffrey Dowling admitted in a Prosser White

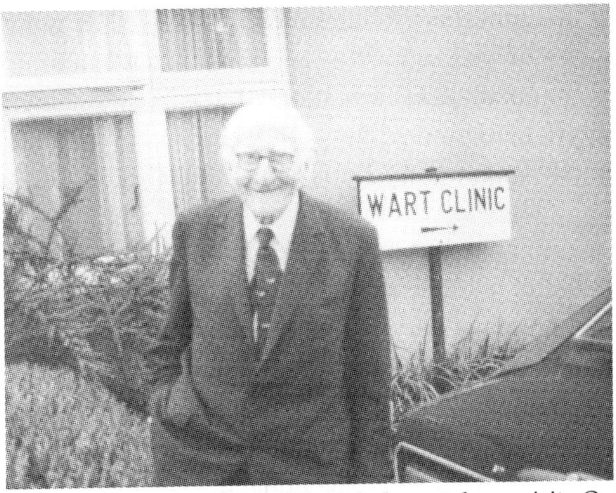

Geoffrey Dowling, the doyen of British dermatology, visits Oxford

Lecture at St John's (1958) that he was fond of expressing opinions freely and frequently, but was not always right.

8) It was in the summer of 1948 that I was staying with my parents and some good friends who lived in Haarlem, Holland. During the previous two years, their son and daughter had received a scholarship at Columbia University, New York, supported by Dean Macintosh – a famous name in paediatrics. On the day of our arrival, our hosts were bursting to tell us about the visit of an American medical student. It was Bill Reed, whose visit to the household was like a whirlwind, and somehow he managed to put out of action their upstairs toilet and kept them awake for two nights trying to remedy it. That was my first encounter with the spirit of Bill Reed.

As a young registrar, it was extraordinary to be with this American dermatologist, for whom the world was his stage and the players there in were dermatologists of many countries. Their names would be introduced into almost every conversation. He was very proud of his friends, which in the UK included Edward Wilson-Jones and later Martin Black, the Oxford biochemist, Martin Francis, being the only non-dermatologist. Bill's dermatology seemed, like himself, to be over-the-top and slightly flawed. At that time, his products mostly consisted of rather poorly edited movies of yellow rarities, and while I understood that cine films were an advance in technology, I was busy cataloguing pre-World War II black-and-white photographs of very much better quality which 30 years later I was actually able to use in the *Oxford Textbook of Medicine.* Notwithstanding his weirdness and his enthusiasms, Bill will be remembered in the UK for his generosity and the range of experiences, from the sublime to the ridiculous, which in his presence one found oneself committed to.

Bill discovered that I had a passion for opera and had probably been to more operas than he had with a passion similar to mine. Almost every week, I would receive a gramophone record that he had purchased from the local secondhand record store, and I would receive telephone calls – not about dermatology, but about opera – at four o'clock in the morning. At the opera, he was not always a comfortable companion: at a performance of *Parsifal* in Bayreuth, a place where every performance is a religious experience with no applause, Bill was the sole applauder. I was happy that we had single tickets and I was separated by about twenty rows, but that didn't stop him – immediately the interval had started – wishing to carry out a conversation across 20 rows, giving his opinion on what had been happening.

He was the first to show me *Disneyland*, and I was impressed – most of all by his enthusiasm for everything there. I remember watching the Gettysburg Speech by a robotic Abraham Lincoln, and being much nudged and expected to respond to a very loud stage whisper, saying, "Isn't he wonderful? Don't you think he's wonderful? Isn't it a great speech?"

Bill was generous in his support of my visits to the States, and always managed to organise a lecture or two for me. Sometimes earning what in those days was the useful sum of $100-200 was a bit of an embarrassment. In particular, I remember a very hot day at the Naval Hospital in San Diego when I was given a two-hour slot to talk to two sleeping sailors – but the $200 was greatly needed. There were no secrets in his clinic, however famous his Hollywood visitors, such as Marlon Brando, may have been.

I remember, too, a burglary in Bill's department where I was staying: although he reacted and talked about it in his manic way, it did not interrupt his preoccupation with wanting to play his latest records, to which I was required to listen before finding out whether the burglar was still in the house. On another occasion in London, we attended a lecture at the Royal College of Physicians and he left his cine camera and dollars on the front seat of the car. Inevitably, the car was broken into and these disappeared, but it did not seem to worry him too much and we drove back to my house for him to meet my wife for the first time. One hour before that event, there was a death in the next-door flat on the same level as our apartment. We managed to cook Bill a meal and cater to all his needs while dashing in and out to support the widow. He was on top form, and Martin and Anne Black, who lived above us, remember to this day the loudness of his voice while he enjoyed the meal and told us about his latest ventures.

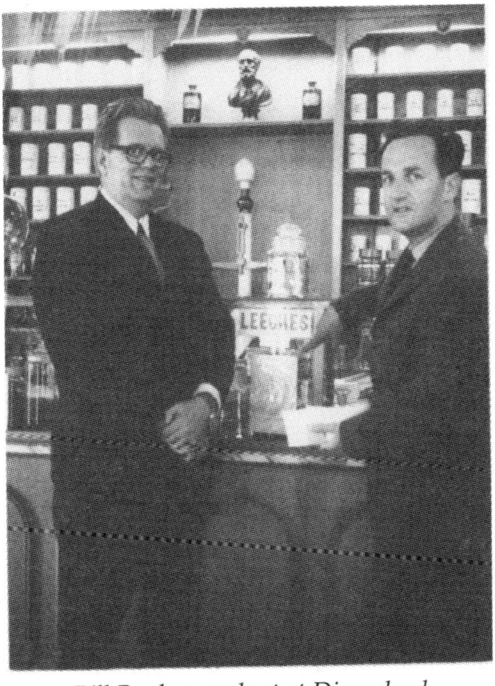

Bill Reed as my host at Disneyland

I have always applauded Bill Epstein of the University of California, San Francisco, for recognising that this was a man worth commemorating by a *Friends of Bill Reed Club.* Years later, at St John's Hospital for Diseases of the Skin and the Institute of Dermatology, he appeared with a cine camera, wanting to photograph a patient in Oxford with Gunther's Disease – a description of which I had just published. At the same time, I showed him a patient in Oxford with a very large skin cancer associated with *epidermolysis bullosa*, and this cemented our relationship. I introduced him to my colleague, the biochemist Martin Francis, who was actually the first to show that there was a collagen defect in that disorder. Bill Reed whisked him off to America to introduce him to Victor McKusick, the leading geneticist, and papers were published jointly in 1975, but never got much into the news until anchoring fibrils were recognised and shown to be collagen.

6: Consultant Dermatologist at Oxford: Laying the Foundation for a Great International Department

The Oxford Medical School can claim that dermatology was there right from the start. In Saxon times, St Frideswide cured a student from York of his leprosy by kissing him. In addition, John of Gaddesden, Chaucer's *Doctor of Physic* in *The Canterbury Tales,* had a stall in St Giles marketplace where he sold his perfumes, hair dyes, greases and powders for the skin. His textbook makes good reading for dermatologists (Rosa Angelica). He was a founder of photobiology, treating the smallpox of the King's son with red light.

However, no-one could claim that there was much interest in the skin before the nineteenth century. The Medical School owned little teaching material apart from a piece of skin from a criminal. Bearing in mind that the Clinical School did not begin until 1939, and that previously the hospital in Oxford was an infirmary overseen by general practitioners, one could not expect much expansion in the nineteenth century. There was no great regional community, and the nineteenth-century Oxford Medical Society attracted its members from no further away than the Cotswolds. Dermatology developed during the nineteenth century and in Oxford at the turn of the century, Ernest Mallam Senior practised it a little.

When William Osler arrived in Oxford, he gave his name to several skin conditions, having discovered most of them while he was still in North America. His paper in the *British Medical Journal,* which described patients from Oxfordshire attending his clinic with vasculitis, has been widely quoted).[1]

My first introduction to dermatology in Oxford was through Alice Carleton, a well-known teacher of anatomy who was only part-time and who also practised in Swindon and Cheltenham.

Two years after his arrival in Oxford in 1957, Renwick Vickers worked hard to expand his team by getting a second consultant. This was originally proposed in 1967 as a combined dermatology VD appointment but the VD component was removed in 1969. I was appointed in 1971.

Top departments of dermatology have great histopathology provision. In Oxford, histopathology of the skin was initially provided by Alastair Robb-Smith. He was replaced by Peter Millard, sharing the role for a while with Ken Fleming, who had worked with Herman Pinkus, the American pathologist who had argued with me over the direction of growth of epidermis (see Chapter 5). There was always debate (as yet unresolved) about how to ensure the expertise of both dermatologists and of general pathologists in the interpretation of skin biopsies.

In describing my role as a consultant dermatologist based at the Radcliffe Infirmary and the Slade Isolation Hospital, it has to be said that working in buildings that everyone likes makes a big difference, even though the 40-bedded unit was finally reduced to only twelve beds. They were overlooking lawns and trees, and there is evidence that such an environment makes people feel better.[2]

How Oxford Became an International Centre in the Field of Leprosy.[3]

During 1970-71, Renwick had extended the facilities for leprosy research at the Cochrane Annex. In 1982, increased workspace at the Slade was made possible by a grant from the Oxford District Hospital Development Fund of £22,000, with a new laboratory for histopathology and extension of the seminar/library room. A further £6,000 allowed extension of secretarial space. Much later we had a *Portakabin* to give more space for the nurses to have coffee.

Dr Colin McDougall had joined us in 1971 after 14 years in the tropics, and was given the task of admitting, investigating and treating patients affected by leprosy, in the Cochrane Annex. Such patients were always immigrants, and were referred from consultant dermatologists around the country. One 20-year-old was the first

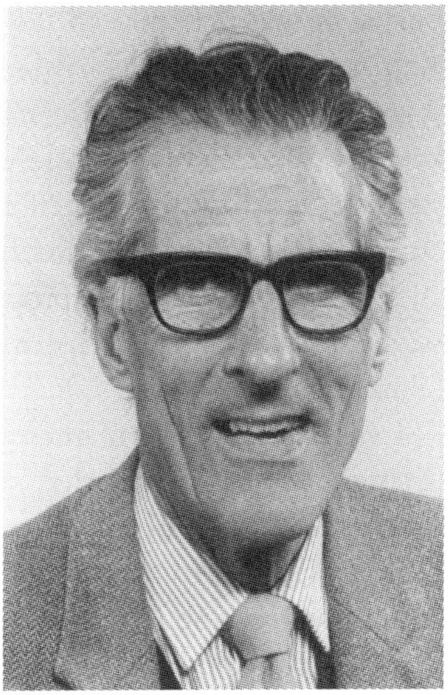

Dr Colin McDougall, distinguished leprologist attached to the Department of Dermatology, Oxford

patient in whom we proved resistance to dapsone. She was the last resident of the Home of St Giles for Leprosy in Chelmsford when we sent her there for one year. One Chinese woman from Banbury, rejected by her Chinese restaurant community, was housed with us throughout her pregnancy while we prescribed trials of dapsone, chlorfazamine and rifampicin.

A major event was the retirement of the Professor of Anatomy, Graham Weddell, and his relocation to the Department of Dermatology with all his equipment that included a *Siemens* Electron Microscope. The laboratory was processing histopathological specimens from Bamako, Mali, Chingleput in India, and Malawi. The International Leprosy Elimination Programme (ILEP) and Leprosy Relief Association (LEPRA) funded histopathology technicians, first Richard Jones and then Chris Gummer. Richard did his thesis on elastin stains and the lymphatic in leprosy; Gurmohan Singh in Varanasi, India, hosted a study there with Peter Mortimer and I looking at the lymphatics in leprosy. It was the first such study. To do this, we had to inoculate radioactive isotopes and measure their movement with Geiger counters. It required the importing of a molybdenum generator which our host risked carrying and guarding on a train journey from Delhi to Varanasi.[4]

Chris Gummer did his thesis on the ultrastructure of hair with Rodney Dawber, also describing some changes in leprosy. After the successful 'Blue Peter' TV appeal for Leprosy, Chris Gummer was sent to Hyderabad in India to set up the Blue Peter Lab for Leprosy. Colin's work and his editorship of *Leprosy Review*, the leading British journal in that field, placed the Department to the fore of the new campaign to eliminate leprosy, as it was clear from the histopathology of drug trials that rifampicin, chlorfazamine and dapsone were lethal for the mycobacterium. There was a collaboration with the National Institute for Medical Research including the production of a leprosy vaccine. Kate Schomberg later became the histopathology technician for the bulk of the leprosy programme, and funds were found for an excellent academic secretary, Margot Cook, in support of me and Colin McDougall.

Even for leprosy, my interests remained for a while in the field of microcirculation. In the late 1970s, I had the help of Wajdi Kanan from Kuwait, interested in the localisation of a number of tropical diseases to the blood vessels of the nose. Wajdi Kanan's DPhil involved the localisation of carbon in the nose of rats after injection into the blood vessels of the tail under the influence of cooling or ovarectomy, and the measurement of oxygenation of the nasal mucosa. These studies were of substantial interest, and kept alive a potential for studying the big tropical diseases of the world, such as leprosy and leishmaniasis.

With Colin McDougall's interest in leprosy, some studies could be focused on blood supply. About this time, the Department of Physics at the Churchill gave us Aga Thermography equipment with which the predilection of mycobacterium leprae for the cooler areas of the face was confirmed, and we learned much about environmental temperature and its effect of breathing cold air on the blood supply of the nose and teeth.

Microcirculation Studies

For a junior, some of the early meetings of the British Microcirculation Society were difficult. The secretary, P.A.G. Munro, a Cambridge anatomist, was extremely pedantic, and managed to annoy everybody. On one occasion, Henry Barcroft, Professor of Physiology at St Thomas's Hospital, London, stormed out, never to be seen again at microcirculation meetings. Howard Florey simply preferred not to turn up. As the years passed, my role as the European Microcirculation Society Treasurer was something of a success since exchange rates, when banking in Switzerland, had proved a good investment. On my appointment as the second dermatology consultant in Oxford, there was an unwritten belief that I would lead the academic development of the department. as an international authority on the blood supply of the skin, and maintain that role mostly by reading the non-dermatology literature in that field and taking up senior roles in microcirculation societies. Two books were examined by the anatomist Graham Weddell and the dermatologist Sam Shuster, for which the Oxford Doctor of Medicine was awarded. These were written in 1973 and 1976, the first being *Physiology and Pathophysiology of the Skin, Volume 2* – half of which was concerned with the blood supply – while the second, *Microvascular Injury*, was concerned with localisation of disease processes.

When elected President of the Third World Microcirculation Congress, the European Society having the opportunity to host the event, the American scientists were at first not too happy about this; they, having hosted the previous two World Congresses at five-yearly intervals, had expected a proper scientist to be in charge of it in Europe. The only such scientist who might have done this was also an Oxford figure, Charles Michel, a distinguished physiologist, but he had not been a member of the host European Microcirculation Society. Preparations for the World Congress in Oxford began by employing a conference organiser, who after one year was bankrupt and had disappeared, embezzling some of the funds. George and Chris Cherry, of the Department of Dermatology's Wound Healing Foundation, took over. Running Congresses was to become their forte and a source of income for them in the Department.

Eventually, in 1984, the World Microcirculation Congress was successfully held in Oxford, with a very full meeting and by far the largest number of microcirculation experts ever to have met in one place. It was the first use of the full facilities of the new academic centre of the John Radcliffe Infirmary for a congress. My wife Anne spent several weeks making sure all the rooms were properly blacked out for lectures.

Ultimately, about 900 people came to the Congress, and we entertained them all at home on one evening, with several marquees

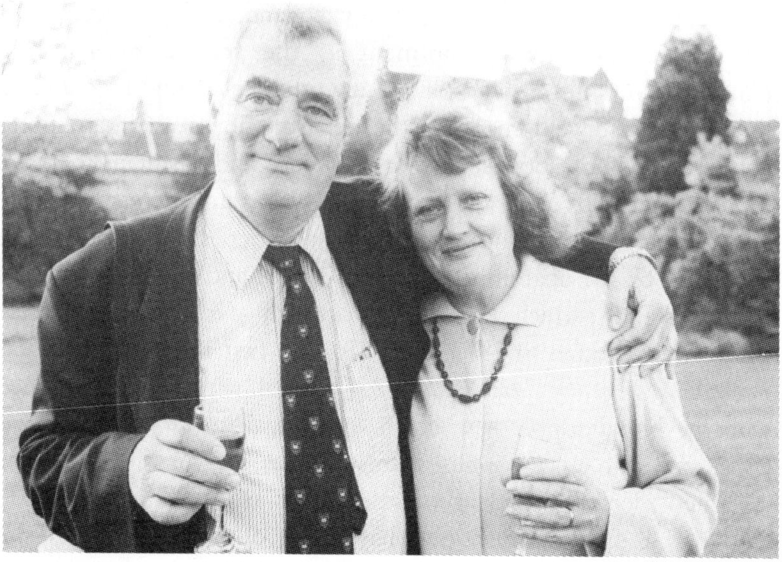

George and Christine Cherry who established programmes on wound healing and succesfully ran many conferences

and a lot of folk events. The St John Ambulance Brigade produced all the salads, the Upper Heyford American Air Base produced the hamburgers, and Anne cooked 2,000 tarts during the course of the year, which were stored in a local farmer's deep freeze. The Duke of Edinburgh was the Patron. He didn't come to the event, but he did write his own preface to the programme book after rejecting the one we had prepared for him. Margaret Jennings, now Lady Florey, opened the event explaining that the lymphatic system had been her husband's first love. We had an award-giving ceremony in the Long Library of Blenheim. David Lewis, the treasurer of the European Microcirculation Society, gave a speech of thanks, stating that if he had known he was coming there, he would have brought his library ticket. There were many evening events, and much wine was drunk. All the wine was bought four years ahead of time, because wine is a good investment and could be sold if all else fails. A Swiss nutritionist, who claimed rye bread was good for the circulation, provided 900 loaves, but they arrived only after the conference creating a dilemma solved by using them as gifts for the very many helpers!

BUCKINGHAM PALACE.

All the participants in the Third World Congress for Microcirculation are most heartily welcome and I use the word "heartily" quite deliberately. Even before William Harvey's discoveries, the heart was known to have a particular importance in human life. A great deal more has been learnt about the circulatory system in the last 200 years and today with all the benefits of rapidly developing technology, the potential for research and treatment is changing all the time.

I am certain that the Congress will prove to be highly valuable to all participants but I hope it will also be the occasion for making many firm and lasting friendships.

Philip

1984

A letter from the Duke of Edinburgh with which to open the 1984 World Microcirculation Congress

Following this event, I was elected chairman of an International Liaison Committee, to meet regularly with all microcirculation societies, and to decide such issues as where the next World Congress should be, and the way forward for the field of microcirculation. It gave me, at a young age of 52, considerable international authority. Ten years later, this role was handed over to John Tooke, later Sir John Tooke of the Peninsular University, Exeter.

My microcirculation studies continued mainly with human material as the basis of study, except when in London we had used the hamster cheek pouch, the blood supply of which would support skin grafts. At the Slade Hospital, we needed for a brief period a study of the chorio-allantoic membrane of the egg, a preparation of no concern to animal rights activists and which could be housed on the inpatient unit of the Dermatology Department. Only once did we accidently hatch chicks, allowing their escape on to the ward.

Following the studies on fibrinolysis in London, having moved into the field of wound healing, it seemed that an area to develop

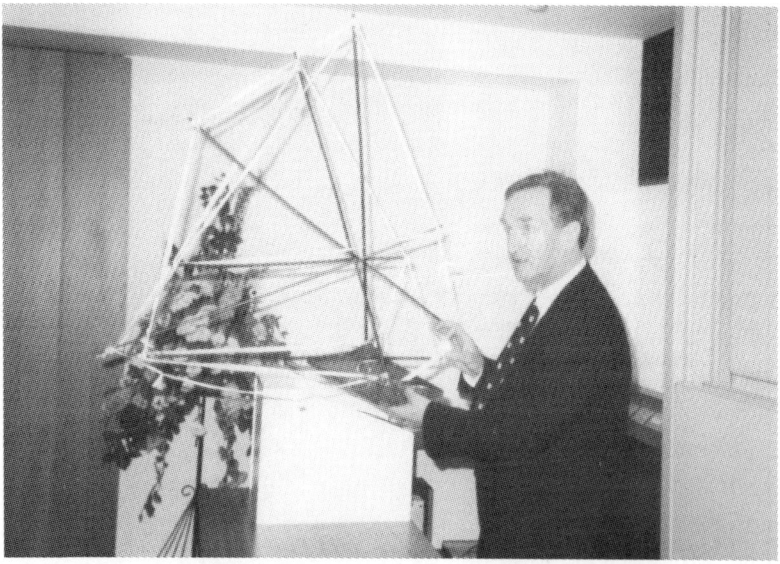

Preparing for the Dowling Oration in Edinburgh in which the affect of mechanical forces on cell function was discussed and a tensegrity model was demonstrated

an interest in was the role of mechanical forces in the transduction of biochemical signals, a field of cellular 'grip and stick' sensitive to proteases. I gave the Dowling Oration in 1985 entitled *Morphosis, occult forces and ectoplasm – the role of glues and proteolysis in skin disease.*[4] With the help of a number of Japanese colleagues – in particular, Mikio Masuzawa, Yasu Horiuchi and Hiroshi Kakinuma – we began the cell culture studies which were later to blossom into a useful cell culture laboratory for a number of wound healing studies. Based on these studies, I gave the Annual Dowling Oration.

Lymphatic Studies

The field of microcirculation studies cannot ignore the lymphatic field, and after the success in 1973 of writing Volume 2 of *Physiology and Pathophysiology of the Blood Vascular System* for Jarrett's series of eight textbooks, published by the Academic Press, he requested in 1975 the inclusion of the lymphatic system. This provided an opportunity for a full overview, the first of its kind and well received in the USA. It opened up a new field for dermatology and another society to belong to – namely, the International Lymphology Society. When, in 1987, this society met in Adelaide, Australia, where I had got married many years earlier, it was obviously a suitable event to attend, and I found myself as not only Editor of a consensus document on the lymphatic system, but appointed also as Assistant Editor to the *International Journal of Lymphology*.

Throughout a career of interest in microcirculation and lymphatics, my main role has been to tell people about the skin – when attending microcirculation or lymphatic societies – and when visiting dermatology societies, to tell them about blood supply and lymphatic drainage. The value of the society meetings has been as a place for discussion and learning, and it has not been difficult to keep abreast of the field – and, for some reason at that time, almost no-one else in the field of dermatology wanted to play a similar role. Molecular biology was to change this, as the endothelial cell became recognised as a factory of important cytokines, underlying inflammation and influencing the behaviour of the surrounding tissues. These discoveries led many people to become much more interested in blood vessels. Peter Mortimer, while a registrar in Oxford, developed an interest in the lymphatics and later became a distinguished authority in this field at St George's Hospital, Tooting, London.

As my interests moved from the study of blood supply to the study of lymphatic drainage and of wound healing, the Department became the centre for a number of new initiatives. Thus, with Peter Mortimer as Senior Registrar, we worked with Bob Twycross in palliative care at Michael Sobell House, Oxford, to meet the cry of help from the *Post-mastectomy Society* for the better management of lymphoedema. We therefore set up the *British Lymphology Interest Group* and gradually took on leadership in this field – locally, nationally and internationally.

The first Nishimara Award for lymphatic studies was presented to me by the Japanese Microcirculation Society, and a gold medal was presented by the German Society of Microcirculation.

Leg Ulcers and Wound Healing

There has always been a high prevalence of leg ulcers in Oxfordshire, and the Department of Dermatology has shared them with several other departments such as geriatrics, rheumatology, vascular surgery and physiotherapy. Alice Carleton was interested in their inheritance. Until the 1970s, bandaging by application of traditional cotton bandages, often soaked in zinc or tar paste, was the classic intervention but difficult to apply properly. Eric Haines, the Department's male nurse, learned the skills of bandaging and eventually developed a reputation for healing difficult ulcers. Renwick Vickers arranged for Eric Haines to receive an MBE. During the 1970s and 1980s, it was made clear internationally that wounds do best if left moist. Major bandaging industries were developed, based on new materials encouraging moist wounds such as colloids and seaweed.

George Cherry came from Louisiana where he had worked with leg ulcers as a zoologist. He did a DPhil on ischaemia and reperfusion in the Nuffield Department of Surgery, and some of his studies were done with me. In Cape Town, he worked with Christian Barnard on the hearts of baboons. He pioneered skin expansion with a group in Michigan where I was invited for an inaugural session.

In 1984, the Edward Abrahams Research Fund grant of £50,000 seeded academic development, employing George Cherry, with Richard Jones as his technician. Richard, a country boy and son of a primary school teacher, had found the Cirencester Royal Agricultural College too much like a public school in flavour, and joined us as a carer of George's pigs, on which research on healing supported the leg ulcer service. Richard took advantage of the leprosy research and obtained a first class in the Institute of Medical and Laboratory Science's master's on Leprosy and the Lymphatics. For several years from 1979, he was funded by LEPRA and later, in 1992, achieved a First Class BA in Business Administration and Management/Computer studies. By finally obtaining George's salary from the District Health Authority, we were able to build up a wound healing specialty with a research programme, mostly funded from industry, and with trials of new dressings.

Huge developments in the wound healing field were led by George Cherry, spreading the influence of the Department worldwide.[5] Later, George brought in many colleagues such as Frank Arnold and Margaret Hughes and, from military burns units in China and Vietnam, more than a dozen trainees to learn wound healing skills, and to further develop the cell culture laboratory.

He established an annual weekly course on wound healing for up to 150 young European investigators, and then we joined in and led the establishment of the *European Tissue Repair Society*, which collaborated with the *American Wound Healing Society*. Dermatologists played a leading role in both. I became President of the *European Tissue Repair Society*. George Cherry continued to develop the nursing profile in wound healing up to an international level.

One person who provided fuel for all my activities was the High Wycome orthopaedic surgeon John Church. One had only to spend ten minutes with him to be re-invigorated. He initiated and part funded the studies of the use of maggots to debride wounds in the department of dermatology and at the Regional

Dermatology Training Centre (RDTC) in Tanzania. He had several projects of his own, such as sniffer dogs to detect cancer and hypoglycaemia, and he designed scooters for the disabled.

Traditional Medicine

While President of the World Congress of Microcirculation, familiarity with studies of the effects of traditional medicine on the blood supply of the skin due to presentations from China, opened up another field – an interest in complementary and alternative medicine, as well as traditional medicine. Both the Chinese and the Japanese were particularly supportive, and honorary appointments to the Institute of Microcirculation in Beijing – as well as one or two international medals – fell into place. The Development of this field is described in Chapter 7.

The Psoriasis Association and Patient-Centred Approaches

Renwick Vickers and I supported the Northampton dermatologist Dickie Coles' interest in founding a National Psoriasis Association, and we became the first department in the UK to set up a local branch. Renwick wrote to all British consultants. Not all supported the idea. Some thought intermarriage would strengthen the gene, and others that it might become an anti-dermatologists' club. We were also much involved with the founders of the Eczema Society. When the Disabled Living Foundation moved from general classes of disablement through visual and then mental handicap, they turned to Renwick Vickers in 1979 for their first meeting on skin conditions. I entered into discussions with Margaret Agerholm, working with WHO on polio, on her term 'aversive handicap', and introduced the concept of being unwelcome because of skin disease which eventually led to the 'look-good feel-good', 'confident when nude' and the 'quality-of-life' fields. Oxford did much to explore this and its role, leading to employment with funding from patient associations. The Psoriasis Association funded a sociologist, Sandra Jowett, for a two-year study, and Andrew Findlay, in Cardiff, took up the theme and made it a major field of medicine.

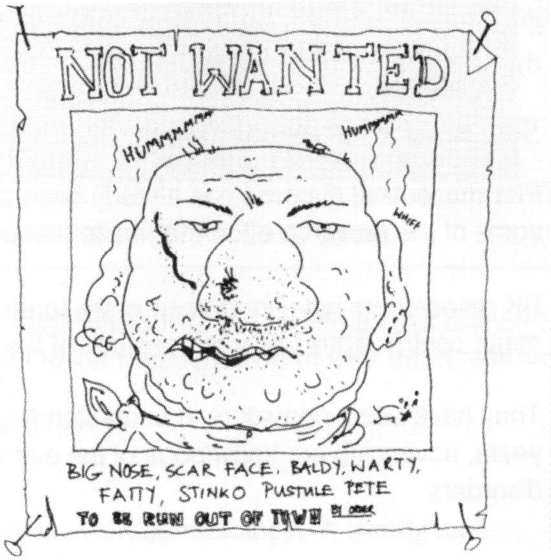
NOT WANTED
BIG NOSE, SCAR FACE, BALDY, WARTY,
FATTY, STINKO PUSTULE PETE

Drawing by David De Berker to illustrate the developing themes of 'Quality of Life' and the 'Look Good, Feel Good Factor'

Funding of research equipment was always difficult because we were essentially a department with a full-time service commitment rather than a research one. One of the first grants I received was the first grant ever from the National Psoriasis Association. It was £120 for a centrifuge.

Renwick had a fatherly regard for his patients, and after a formal ward round, would do his own round alone, socialising with them. When the term 'Lady Almoner' was in vogue, Renwick insisted that one was appointed to dermatology and she was always on his Friday morning ward round. The terminology changed to 'Social Worker', and eventually their help evaporated, partly as a result of NHS reorganisation, but also because the welfare role of doctors and nurses with patient participation and associations increasingly managed social problems.

Another change that was taking place was the evolution of litigation. It was departmental policy to steer complaints into improvement of the service. When, in 1978, the Psoriasis Association was asked to provide evidence on steroid side-effects, it declined to do so because of the effect it might have on their relationships with the medical profession. From its beginning, our policy was to guide the Association into being a lobby for the medical profession rather than, as at one time in the USA, a collector of evidence against the profession.

Apart from the development of patient associations requiring our support, a few patients became long-term colleagues and a few delighted us with their eccentricity. Thus Mr Potts arrived in dermatology outpatients, suffering from pemphigoid, a disorder presenting as blisters. His skin disorder was easily controlled but, being elderly, he was a frequent visitor for having his therapy monitored. Approaching the age of 80, he had spent his life in a Liverpool 'lunatic asylum', having been placed there at the age of about 14 for pinching some family money, but he was otherwise mentally normal. Mentally he had been released after 40 years when a mental health act made it possible. Big asylums in the North of England had prestigious patrons who would be visitors to whom the mentally normal and well-mannered Mr Potts could, as a young man, be safely introduced. There came a time when he was given weekend passes and he consequently, as a guest, visited a few country houses and got to know their owners.

Mr Potts was a showman who liked being the centre of attention in outpatients, and on one occasion when I walked out of the hospital, the Oxford traffic could be observed coming to a standstill while Mr Potts walked slowly and diagonally across the road, smiling and thanking all those in cars or on the pavement, assisting him in a slow progression across the road.

One day, several doctors and nurses received invitations to sherry at his St John's Street apartment. We all took pity on him and decided that, out of duty, we should attend. On arrival, we were ushered into a red velvet-lined establishment like a stage set from a Verdi opera. We need not have worried about neglecting him. The apartment was filled by Dukes and Duchesses, Lord Lieutenants, Chief Constables and leaders of the people of Great Britain, some from far afield and owners of some of the country's finest castles, dutifully in attendance.

Threatened Closure

In 1974, the local branch of the Psoriasis Association was steered into being a strong lobby to oppose the Department of Dermatology at the Slade being turned into a site for a laundry. From time to time, the Health Authority, wishing to reduce its multiple site occupancy, threatened to close this site without appropriate planning for re-siting, suggesting first at the Radcliffe Infirmary, where there was no outlook for inpatients, some of whom were long-stay, and then at the Churchill, linked with infectious diseases, but without space for special clinics and research. Closure of the Slade was fought with the help of MPs, patient associations and the press. The Health Authority was displeased and Renwick was told by one chairman that any proposal for a 'national honour' for him would be blocked. After his retirement, a second attempt to close the Department was fought with the help of the Community Health Council and the media as well as by patient associations.

Later, beds for skin conditions world-wide were lost as hospital costs increased and day care became more feasible and effective. The use of the inpatient department for long-term care was much discussed. In an earlier publication on Methotrexate (Ryan and Baker,

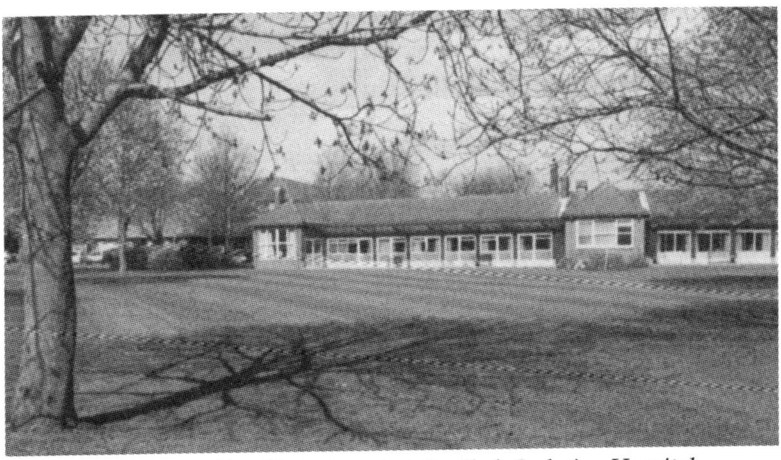

The Dermatology Department at the Slade Isolation Hospital, showing its wards and much-loved lawns and trees

1969), I wrote that three months of skin care for psoriasis in dermatology beds by good nursing in hospital was preferable. It is a view that is unthinkable today. We had long-term patients; one young man with generalised Morphea and an older man with Buerger's Disease, each for at least two years, as well as the above-mentioned pregnant Chinese woman affected by leprosy. Beds were used for psychological respite and for teaching all grades of staff. In 1976, under Renwick's guidance, the Department of Health produced a 'Design Guide for Dermatology Departments' based on the inpatient unit at the Slade Hospital. It proved a useful document when the Health Authority imagined it could move this department to lesser facilities. Its location at the Slade on the Oxford Ring Road, with its extensive lawns and mature trees as well as adequate parking, was popular with patients and staff alike. As special outpatient clinics developed – viz. leg ulcer, ultra violet light, biopsy and minor surgery, patch testing, leprosy, camouflage – they were based at the Slade.

An NHS technician for regular electrolysis of the beard for sex-change patients from the Warneford was also needed, and this too was done at the Slade. Regular monthly plastic surgery and radiotherapy clinics had been held at the Churchill since the earliest days of radiotherapy.

It was natural for Oxford to become the home of the first Camouflage Clinic for birthmarks and vitilgo run by Mrs Savage, all the way from Glasgow, and we were later to formally set up a consultancy with the British Red Cross.

The Wart Clinic

Before Renwick Vickers the most active department for the treatment of warts, highly prevalent in children was the physiotherapy department. Here there was a wicker seat with a copper base on which, after moisterisation of trousers, one was sat so that an electrical circuit allowed electrocution of warts. 'Find a witch to charm them' was alternative advice. At the Royal Postgraduate Medical School, a previous dermatologist had managed to assign the wart clinic to a reluctant senior neurology registrar. Dickie Coles in Northampton employed hypnotism.

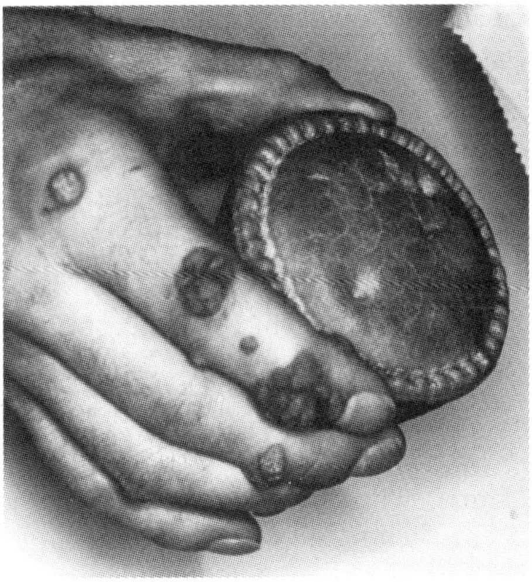

Warts are not trivial to those who have them, as in the case of loss of customers when the hands of this butcher are observed handling food

This Wart Clinic was set up by Renwick Vickers to focus treatment round once-weekly provision of freezing, using liquid nitrogen. When Renwick started the Wart Clinic, it was the Registrar's job to drive in the early morning to pick up liquid nitrogen from Harwell. Occasionally, it tipped over, causing ice clouds and some interest by passers-by. There were times when the Wart Clinic was trivialised by administrators, and thought to be an unnecessary cost and one that could be lost in retrenchment exercises. We emphasised that warts were not trivial to those who have them, and that they could affect work and social interaction. Eventually, as liquid nitrogen became available throughout the week, the special clinic was stopped. However, in 1989, the Family Practitioners Medical Committee complained about its closure. In 1989 they were also having to accept other policy changes, such as referral to the Department rather than to an individual consultant, and managing long waiting lists due to staff shortages, and to the increasing rate of referral. For a while, warts were a focal point on which to persuade 'the authorities' that the need for skin care was based, not on severe morbidity but on quality of life. At the

Churchill Hospital, the management of warts was eventually covered by a procedure-trained senior nurse.

Adipose Tissue and Cellulite

Towards the end of the twentieth century, it became clear that there was a story to tell about, not only the neglected field of lymphatics, but also about another tissue neglected by the Health Service. It was adipose tissue which seemed to grow when there was lymphatic failure, causing difficulty with the management of lymphoedema, and which seemed to be a tissue poorly endowed with lymphatics. In the field of microcirculation, there was an Italian, Sergio Curri, who had unusual theories about adipose tissue, and had written about unusual valves and shunts in the blood supply of adipose tissue. He was large and ebullient, and greeted all males with a hug and a kiss on both cheeks, and all females with a bow and a kiss to the hand. Both his writing and lectures were complex, overlong and wordy. His research, backed by the cosmetic industry, seemed of questionable reliability, but some of what he claimed was very interesting and he had data which, if separated from his style of writing, seemed worth advocating to a wider audience.

I decided to spend time getting to know the science underlying adipose tissue, and then to write a book with Sergio Curri as a co-author. It was well liked by a small audience of interested readers – viz. by Michael Foldi, the German doyen of lymphology, who wrote: 'Thank you for sending me your phantastic (sic) book; it is a pleasure to read it.' But Lippincott, the publisher, made a mess of it – with even the title page taken from another publication. It was also poorly distributed but Sergio and the cosmetic industry were very pleased. In particular, *L'Oreal* seized on my view on impaired lymphatic drainage as an excuse for a new massage device. They involved me with their system of advertising which was, in all respects, over-the-top. As mentioned earlier, there was a lecture in the chapel housing Leonardo da Vinci's *The Last Supper* in a edifice built to mimic the Acropolis and to the background music of Strauss's *Also Sprach Zarathustra.* After listening to me, all the fashion journalists were taken to Tesi's ultra-modern opera *Richard III* at La Scala in Milan. Most walked out in the first interval.

On another occasion, my wife and I joined journalists for a night at the London *Savoy Hotel* and were taken a few hundred yards in Bentleys to The Royal Opera House to see *Giselle*.

Being a writer on adipose tissue on several occasions gave one some cause to be consulted on cellulite. Few conditions take up so much space in women's journals. The cosmetic industry markets all kinds of manoeuvres to manage this lumpy bumpy appearance of the contour of women's thighs and buttocks. I have signed many confidential agreements not to divulge knowledge of new cures.

One day in 1995, I was visited by a certain Peter Cooper, also known as Peter Foster – dressed in a long black coat with a fur collar – with Samantha Fox, a fashion celebrity, on his arm, to arrange the trial of a new thigh cream for his company *Foremost Bodycare Co. Ltd.* Its formula included a vasoactive agent called carnitine that I was interested in. He handed out a report of its previous use in Australia which made wildly exaggerated claims. As head of St John Ambulance for Oxford (see Chapter 8), I was not only in touch with female volunteers who had big thighs but I was in need of money to support their cadet force's summer camp. My Indian colleague, Vineet Kaur, who needed funds to attend a congress, agreed to measure their thighs, one of which would have the active cream massaged into the skin each day for a month, while the other thigh would be treated only with the base. At the end of each week, I was slipped an envelope full of 200 or so £20 notes.

Towards the end of the study, which showed a slight reduction in circumference of both thighs but more on the side of the active principle, there was a call from the *Daily Express*, telling me that Peter Foster had been in gaol in Australia for marketing fraudulent agents for cellulite. For a week, the Department of Dermatology was bombarded by the national and international press. There were eleven radio and TV interviews, and it was difficult to maintain a reputation of an honest scientist and to emphasise our findings that the cream worked a little, but probably because of massage rather than the active principle. Apart from a police interview, the Department of Dermatology was not troubled after one week. My Medical Defence Union and the university were not worried on my behalf. Nor was George Cherry, our Department's acting Chairman at that time. Peter Foster went to prison for obtaining the packets of pound notes under false pretences, Vineet went to her congress and the St John Ambulance cadets had a successful summer camp.

Several years later, in 2002, Cherie Blair, wife of the then Prime Minister, was alleged, as a high court judge, to have intervened in Peter Foster's fight against deportation. He was the boyfriend of her exercise guru, Carole Caplin, who had introduced him to advise the Prime Minister, Tony Blair, on buying two London apartments.

Thigh creams are still one of the commonest problems for the advertising agency but, most years, they provide a little of my income from advice to *Which?* magazine, and it is about the only topic that gets me quoted in the press. In 2007, Peter Foster went to prison for borrowing money to develop a tourist resort off Fiji, where he is known as 'the big tongue man'.

New Consultants

Rodney Dawber worked on fibrinolysis with me in 1970 at the Institute of Dermatology in London, and then was Senior Registrar at the Royal Postgraduate Medical School where he later took over from me as consultant. In my letter of December 1971, recommending him for the consultant post at Stoke, I wrote:

> *His honesty and integrity I greatly admire, and in conversation I have been surprised by his vigorous championship of causes such as the monarchy and the countryside. The quality which makes him most appealing is his energy which he directs at many different interests.*

When Renwick Vickers retired in 1976, Rodney Dawber was persuaded to join us from his successful post in Stoke, Staffordshire. Over the next 20 years, he established leadership in three fields: cryosurgery, hair and nails. Not only was he a national consultant in

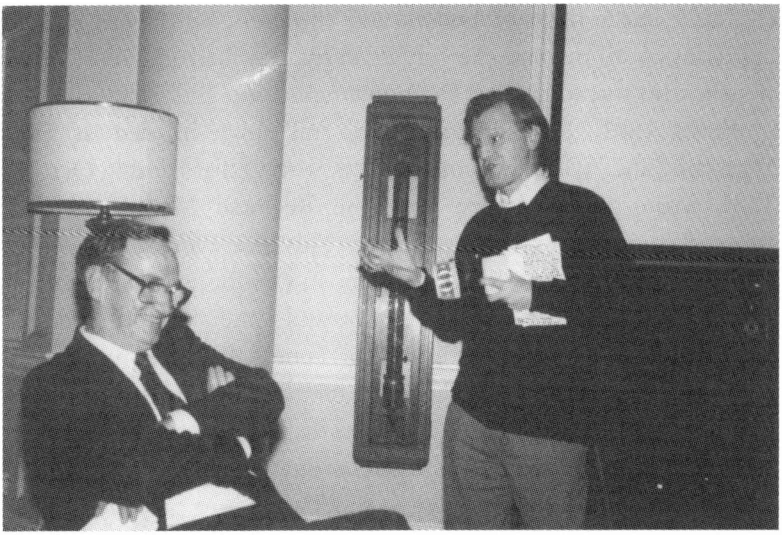

Rodney Dawber Consultant Dermatologist at the annual Christmas show, on this occasion singing Gershwin's 'Embracable You'

these fields, but his many publications and lectures spread his influence world-wide. Locally, he promoted developments in his interests and organised a restructuring of the administration of the Department leading to a rotating chairmanship. He abolished the Wart Clinic, amalgamating it into cryosurgery. Two hours per week were sufficient for all skin 'surgery' at that time. Later, this was to change with increasing demands for skin surgery and pigmented lesion clinics, and Rodney did much to set up the new systems. He was responsible for bringing Dr Neil Walker from London into the Department to improve the surgical skills. Rodney was especially successful at exciting the younger members to take up research and bringing overseas trainees into the Department. Between us, we added more than 1,000 publications to the literature. Rodney was also a well-qualified rugby referee and popular with the medical students. We were fortunate in having a good relationship and never a cross word.

When we were able to add a third consultant, Fenella Wojnarowska, further national and international kudos followed, especially in the fields of bullous and vulval diseases. Sheila Powell's appointment to manage the contact dermatitis field added one more person who was to achieve a national reputation and leadership.

From 1981, Darrell Wilkinson, still single-handed at High Wycombe and Aylesbury, sought a link with Oxford and in October 1981 wrote to Rosemary Rue, the Regional Medical Officer, proposing such a Consultant's post. This was eventually filled by Fenella Wojnarowska. Fenella's link post, with only four sessions in Oxford and seven in High Wycombe and Amersham, fulfilled the hopes of Darrell Wilkinson, but for Fenella home commitments following the birth of Freddy, and giving more than a part-time commitment to two departments, was difficult. Her major interests were research, for which she made additional time. In 1991, hers was the first A+B appointment – a mechanism to provide funding to give time to NHS consultants for research. She obtained travel fellowships from the British Association of Dermatology (BAD) and from Oxford to provide time to develop her research interests overseas. She supervised many honorary and full-time junior staff at High Wycombe and in Oxford.

Getting Sheila Powell fixed up with a consultant post was one of the most complex activities undertaken. A consultant post for Contact and Industrial Dermatology, specifically with Sheila Powell in mind, was funded for three sessions in 1987; it was essentially the same work as she had performed under the Part-Time Married Woman (PTMW) scheme as a senior registrar – the first such post for contact dermatitis outside London. Renwick Vickers regarded himself as expert in this field, and there were regular visits for junior staff to the motor and other industries as part of our training. Sheila's interests in industry were welcomed and encouraged. Her career was unusual, and contribute to the archives of part-time married women. She had been a Registrar from 1971. Her husband was employed at Shrivenham, a suburb of Swindon, and so in 1974 she was appointed to a Consultant post in Swindon to take this into account. However, at the appointment it was realised she had not received accreditation for sufficient training, and she was required to continue to work in Oxford for one further year. A case was made that she could learn enough under the guidance of Ken Crow at Swindon, but she became pregnant and resigned the post. Rosemary Rue recommended she went part-time as a senior Registrar from 1974 till 1984, becoming accredited for a Consultant post only in 1981, and we skilfully extended her on the PTMW scheme at six-monthly intervals for three years. She was then part-funded on research money, obtained while I was on the Area Research Committee because of a public demand for allergy clinics funded by health authorities.

Another major issue in the 1990s was the suggestion in the 1970s that she could be usefully employed as a liaison dermatologist for community hospitals at Witney, Thame, Wallingford and Wantage. Over many years, we played on the fact that Sheila needed more training but at the same time, for other purposes, we had to keep telling everyone how expert she was. On the PTMW scheme, she became the only five-session Senior Registrar. Sheila found even this too much for her family commitments, and resigned from attending the Dermatology Section of the Royal Society of Medicine (RSM). This caused alarm at the RSM, no Senior Registrar having resigned before. As one of her part-time jobs, we gave her the job of teaching our nurses as an investment for the future as we developed the dermatology nurse.

In 1995, Dr Chris Sharp was appointed honorary Senior Clinical Lecturer to the Department. For two years, he was Head of the Medical Division of the National Radiological Protection Board at Harwell (the link with Harwell included informing us on the disappearance of the ozone layer), and he was a clinician in the Pigmented Lesion Clinic.

A survey by Muir Grey of the staffing levels in this Region in the late 1980s proposed that dermatology needed five extra consultants. My appointment as a dermatologist at Banbury was initially a single session but GP assistants, and later, a two-session expansion allowed for contact dermatitis clinics and reading of patch tests 48 hours later, as well as a wart clinic. It was much helped by GPs who supported the Department, often for many years: McKissock Leach, Peter Middleton and Sarah Wookey were especially loyal and reliable.

As the Department developed, we explored ways of contributing to the education of part-time married women, general practitioners and visiting researchers and trainees from overseas.

Nursing Development

When Eric Haines retired, we asked Benedict Wilders, who ran the dermatology outpatients at the Radcliffe Infirmary, to take over the inpatients, She was a mature Danish nurse who had trained under the famous dermatologist Haxthausen. She brought stability to the Department, first in outpatients and then in charge of inpatients. Stalwarts of the early days were Audrey Couldrey, Joyce Eriksen and Eleanor Kuht. Benedict had a motherly way of looking after both patients and junior nurses. After her retirement, there was a succession of young nurses in charge. In 1979, the General Nursing Council (GNC) suddenly decided to withdraw us from training young nurses, as we were geographically too far from their training school.

I was asked by nurses working in several fields, including diabetes, to help to set up a Nursing Research Group, and to facilitate their development through the university. I got myself onto the Regional Authority's Nursing Committee, and was also appointed to the Board of the new Institute of Nursing, and from this was able to appoint more senior nurses to the Department of Dermatology. Steve Ersser was the first to develop nursing beyond its traditional roles. He managed to persuade the authorities to allow him to recruit a team of nurses with higher qualifications. He brought in academically inclined nurses such as Julie van Onselen and Rebecca Penzer. George Cherry had recruited and paid for a wound healing nursing team of equal status.

Over a period of seven years, attempts were made to get the University of Oxford to approve the nurses' intellectual development – partly to keep them in Oxford and in the nursing profession – there being at that time a huge loss both during training and once qualified. I worked with the radiologist Basil Shepstone, whose wife was a district nurse, and several senior nurses but, partly because their language was educational and sociological rather than science-based, the University of Oxford's Medicine Board refused to allow them entry. So they went to Oxford Brookes University, where they flourished. By this time, I had become a committee member of the International Foundation of Dermatology, under the aegis of the International League of Dermatology Societies and its International Committee. The aim of the International Foundation was to take skin care into the developing world. While negotiating a contract with UNESCO to generate a global programme for dermatology, UNESCO had difficulty in understanding why, as head of a department with an Oxford address, with whom they wanted a relationship, I had no professorial title. The contract would carry the title of Professor. When this was raised with the Health Authority, they thought it advantageous, provided any locums needed were paid for. I had attempted to get myself an *ad hominem* chair when the University of Oxford began to open up this possibility to NHS consultants. The very strong Department of Medicine took the first of these. Oxford Brookes gave me the *ad hominem* title of Professor, but the Regius Professor, Henry Harris, called me into his office and told me not to use it! After a couple of years, based on a review of my research, the University of Oxford appointed me as Professor, and this was an important step forward for the academic reputation of the Department.

With a senior and academic nursing team, the Department once again began to develop its teaching skills, both within and beyond Oxford. The nurses took on some higher technology skills, such as sorting out allergies to medicaments and enhancing ulcer repair, using grafts. Once we moved to the Churchill, it was decided to combine ulcer healing, lymphoedema management, skin care for eczema and psoriasis in a curriculum beyond the walls of the Department. The British Skincare Nursing Group was formed and led to a National Organisation.[6] The International Skin care Nursing Group was founded, once we had managed to get funding from *Smith Kline Beecham* by awarding (at an international congress in Cairo) senior management with a certificate of appreciation for their gift of albendazole for the elimination of lymphatic filariasis. We arranged nursing help in the morbidity management of lymphatic filariasis in islands off the coast of Tanzania. Funding was also obtained from the Department of International Development. Later, the ISNG became affiliated with the International Council of Nurses and a Member of the International League of Dermatology Societies (ILDS). There were several major initiatives: Dr Vineet Kaur took on a study of British dermatology nursing, and then began setting up a dermatology nursing programme in India. There were visits of Steve Ersser's team and George Cherry's nursing team to the Regional Dermatology Training Centre in Tanzania. There were successful initiatives to set up regular workshops with the European Academy of Dermatology and Venereology (EADV) and with World Congresses.

New Hospital Building

The Dermatology Outpatient Department moved from the old Radcliffe in 1986 to the new John Radcliffe Infirmary and continued to function separately from its inpatient, administrative and research bases at the Slade Hospital. Space was adequate after a fight to get it for teaching the increasing number of medical students and the need for nursing space for leg ulcers. Later, Fenella Wojnarowska initiated a combined Oral Clinic at the John Radcliffe with the odontologists and a combined Dermatology Genetics Clinic. Combined clinics had been initiated in Alice's time for cancer therapy and the need for teamwork. Much later, Fenella also had a clinic for transplantation disorders, and a vulva clinic with gynaecologists. Her technician, Jill, built up immunology studies, contributing much to Fenella's portfolio. George Cherry's Leg Ulcer Clinic link with the vascular surgeons was another collaboration.

Apart from the above-mentioned extensions and, for a few years from 1980, the addition of a *Portakabin* for wound healing and nursing administration, and a staff tea room, all these activities provided the background to persuading a number of donors to fund a new building.

We began the process of fundraising by emphasising the need to improve our services, which by 1987 were already overstretched, and by 1989 a letter from the Oxfordshire Local Medical Committee found plenty to complain about, waiting times for appointments having become unacceptably long.

The political background of the 'Thatcher era' allowed us to plan to have private practice on site and to initiate unrestricted fund raising. We soon found that donations to improve the service would be difficult to get but support of research was a better bet. The Oxfordshire Health Authority set up a Radcliffe Medical Foundation to raise five million pounds sterling. This would enlarge the Transplant Centre, develop bioimaging (magnetic resonance), build a Dermatology Department at the Churchill and support facilities for AIDs and tropical diseases.

Half the money for the Oxford building came from the Dunhill Medical Trust, which had funded my time at the Institute of Dermatology in London from 1967-71. Although originally a tobacco related industry, there had been no such relationship for half-a-century. A substantial grant of $1,000,000 also came from the wound healing industry (*Squibb/Convatec*) partly to fund our collaboration for new wound healing devices, and another £600,000 from selling the Slade. The local hospital development fund (ODHIDF) provided £30,000 and £200,000 came from local land-owning friends such as Robin Fleming, our neighbour in North Oxfordshire.

Steifel were to provide £50,000 but withdrew for tax reasons, and then later helped staffing with £10,000 per annum for two years.

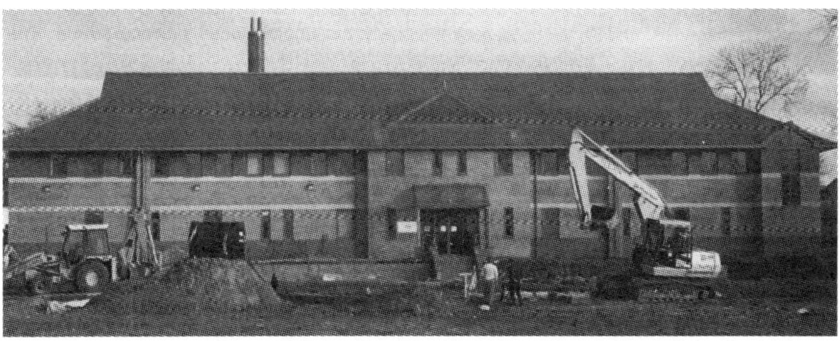

The new Dermatology Building at the Churchill Hospital

Seton Health Care added £50,000 to help with running costs. As a result of the success of the building appeal and receiving from the university some new 'White Paper' money, in 1988 Richard Jones was promoted to be the Department's Business Manager and was paid as such, after almost losing him, due to the fact his technician's salary could not be raised. He did a magnificent job in supervising our upgrading to the new building at the Churchill, and moved on to senior administrative posts at the John Radcliffe, eventually being in charge of a hospital in Kimberley, South Africa.

A very fine new building was constructed at the Churchill Hospital – for the first time linking outpatients with inpatients – in time for a 'Celebration of Dermatology' at the 1992 British Association of Dermatology meeting in Oxford. Enough money had been raised to provide a departmental car park, a corridor to the main hospital and a lift. In the 1990s, an interest in using art in hospitals was on the increase, and long corridors in the Oxford hospitals were decorated with many pieces of artwork, including many pieces of artwork given to the Dermatology Department, framed by my son James, as well as Indian cushion covers, Thai silk scarves and many Japanese wrapping papers. I communicated with other hospitals such as Charing Cross and Southampton which were well-known for art investment. For the Department stairways, I collected artwork by dermatologists and their wives. It included the doodles of well-known members of the International Committee.

The garden had been a feature of the Slade Hospital, much loved by staff and patients alike. A case was made that inpatients especially required such a facility. Land and fencing was provided by the hospital, while Katherine Shock, the garden designer, and Paul van Onselen, the landscape designer, built the basic features, including a pergola. Money was raised from the proceeds of the BAD Annual Meeting and the League of Friends. Anne organised a team of volunteers to dig and plant a substantial donation of plants from *Nicholson Nurseries.*

Wound healing studies now developed and played a role in enhancing our national and international reputation. It was strongly funded by the devices industry.[7] The Dunhill Medical Trust continued to support the Department with grants for 'research' into maggot therapy with the salary of Molly Courtenay, while from the support of nursing we bought some equipment, and computerised the Department. There was support for some of Fenella's research as well as for Eric Lamont Gregory (see Chapter 9).

The increased space of a new building allowed desks to be provided for visitors attached to the Department. Several of these had an interest in Traditional Complementary and Alternative Medicine. George Cherry had several Vietnamese and Chinese researchers with such an interest. Dr Gerard Bodeker (who had worked for the World Bank in Vietnam), Professor Jeff Burley (Chairman of several international plant science organisations), and Dr Merlin Willcox (who was interested in herbal remedies for malaria), and I supported the recently launched Global Initiatives for Traditional Systems (GIFTS) of Health, and studies of utilisation and preferences were initiated in the outpatients. Herbals were studied in the laboratory under the supervision of Margaret Hughes.

The new building had space for private practice: Renwick Vickers had practised at home and Dr Rodney Dawber had sessions at the Acland, and for a while, the Churchill Hospital provided a Day Surgery Unit elsewhere in the main building, used mainly by Neil Walker. I rarely saw private patients.

Concurrent Domestic Life

Even more important is it to have a home and family one enjoys sharing one's life with. When Anne and our one year old daughter Josephine and I moved to Oxford and bought *Abbey Willows*, a house of faded elegance, which had a fine rural view with a small river at the bottom of the garden. It was situated halfway between my two places of work, Banbury and Oxford. It was a house that had many pots in the attic collecting rainwater. Over the years we had it re-roofed, rewired, the asbestos removed, fitted new windows and had much else done. We hosted three large conference barbecues. Eventually we sold it, at 18 times what we bought it for, to the Head of *BBC1*. The only thing we lost during our time there were two toes on my left foot to a rotary mower.

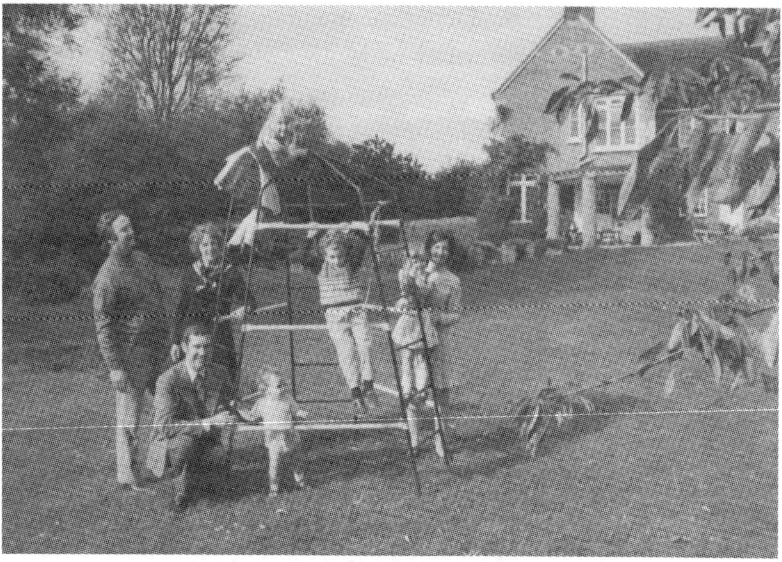

Abbey Willows, our first Oxford home.
Terence, Anne, Josephine and James entertaining Anne's twin brother David with his wife Judy and children Philippa and Peter

Abbey Willows had a wing, let at first to the American Air Force, and then to dermatologists such as the Polish dermatology refugee, Pavlowski, and from the USA, Lionel Goldsmith and Mark Kaiser, Rodney Dawber and family, the Australian Rodney Sinclair, relatives from Australia, and finally, my father with two caretakers sharing a rota. For two years, we had the stepson and daughter-in-law of James Stewart, the film star.

James Stewart must be one of the best-loved film stars, and certainly his visit to our home made news. During the war, he gave up his Hollywood salary and joined the American Air Force as a pilot at £5 per week. He ended the war as a Colonel with a DFC, and being proud of that career, continued in the reserve as a Brigadier. His salary for Hitchcock's *Rear Window* was £450,000. He married Gloria McLean when she was divorced at the age of 31 and he was 41. Gloria had two sons by her first husband and twin girls by James. During the Vietnam War, one of the sons was killed and the other, Mike, took up an anti-war stance, much to James' disappointment. In the late 1970s, Mike decided to study Law at Oxford, and he and his wife Barbara, lodging in the wing, became good friends but did not tell us about their family connections. After about one year, Barbara was pregnant and towards term announced apologetically that she feared media interest when the child was born, and why!

Indeed, this was very much the case because James and Gloria came for the Catholic christening. Barbara told us not to bother too much about entertaining them as James Stewart 'only eats soup and ice cream'. Memories fade but they include the picture of the tall and lanky film star choosing to sit on our very low poof which had little firm stuffing. Gloria joined me in our green garden overlooking fields, while I explained that it had been a meadow with cows for probably more than a thousand years. The eminent writer about the history of the countryside, Hoskins, had lived in a neighbouring vicarage and had said just that. Gloria said, "If the cows have been there that long, how come it is still so green?"

The christening was in Woodstock in a rather small and undistinguished new church. The priest, Father Walsh, was similar. He happened to share the name of Walsh with Barbara's maiden name, and the boy was to be christened Benjamin Walsh. Father Walsh was hugely pleased. James Stewart was asked to read the responses which were written as 'He/She' and 'His/Hers'. The famous reader of film scripts managed to stumble his way through the responses making several stuttering mistakes, and there was a certain nervousness overriding the christening of his first grandchild. The moment came for the naming of the child, and Father Walsh named him Benjamin Franklin!

We had a small post-christening party in an upstairs room at the *Bear Hotel* in Woodstock, and with Anne's brother, Paul, we were three of a very few guests. Downstairs, my secretaries had booked dinner in order to see the Stewarts and there was much media attention.

Benjamin grew up at *Abbey Willows*, and on a later visit as a three-year-old experienced his first stinging nettles. We said, "Get dock leaves." He then disappeared for a while, and after a search, we found him in the house in his bedroom waiting for Dr Leaves to arrive.

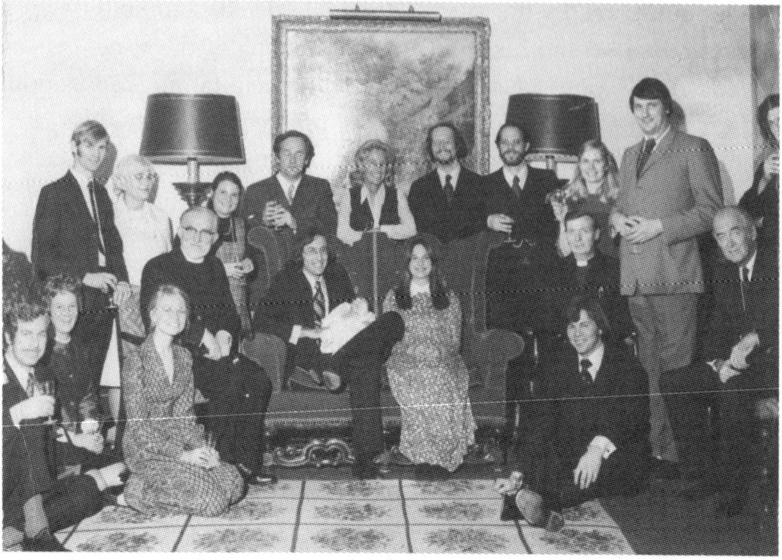

The Christening of James Stewart's (seated far right) first grandson and its party at the Bear at Woodstock. Anne and her brother Paul far left, Terence stands with Gloria Stewart behind the baby and his proud parents.

Some years later, we made a few visits to Mike and the family in Phoenix, Arizona. James Stewart, still living into old age, continued to be admired and was the recipient of many gifts which he rarely unpacked. On one occasion, we were there as baby-sitters as Barbara had to go to Alabama. We helped unpack a magnificent telescope and spent a long late evening lying on our backs searching for planets. We were surprised to find some IRA literature at our bed side.

Anne's own career as a school teacher was interrupted by bringing up two children, and eventually by giving me support at frequent travels overseas. Her career was briefly enhanced by studies and courses on dyslexia. Her longest job was as a primary school teacher in our village of Middle Barton. This, being a role central to village awareness, helped the family to be part of the local community while I worked long hours in Oxford. The children later went to school in Oxford and Abingdon. Anne learns people's names and does not forget them as I do. It is a wonderful asset in a wife.

In 1994, Martin Norton, the Headmaster of Middle Barton School, wrote:

> *I am very sorry that you feel it is time to cease being a school governor, I can't describe to you how much I have valued your support over the years, when there has been so much change in education. I think without your support you and the other governors have given me, I would have fallen by the wayside years ago. I'm grateful to you for your encouragement and support, for your enthusiasm and dedication, and for the way in which you quietly took on so many unseen tasks about the school.*

Anne, always a match-maker, brought Martin and another teacher, Lucy, together. Martin wrote:

> *As well as being a good member of the 'team' you have been a really good friend to Lucy and me. We both have so much to thank you for. You may not realise how much your friendship has helped us both before we were married and when Jack and Peter were born. Many thanks, Anne, for all your loyal support and friendship both to the school as a governor and to our family.*

Anne's interest in the Dermatology Department led to much entertaining and helping with its décor. A high point was always a massive production of home-made sweets at Christmas for many collaborators, and entertaining at home for up to 900 participants at international meetings.

Anne's role in the three villages where we have lived – Middle Barton, Iffley and Great Bedwyn – has led to many very important initiatives such as the village shop, and a community centre in a village that meets regularly over food and wine, and which maintains a well cared for profile.

Josephine was born in Lewisham Hospital in 1969, and James in the Radcliffe Infirmary Maternity Home in 1971. I was present at the births – and those were the days of staying in hospital for up to two weeks. I disappeared for dermatology events for a few days.

With James, it was to South Africa. Josephine was a beautiful, much-admired baby. Both James and Josephine were normal children in good health. Schooling began at the village school but we felt their education needed to be upgraded. Josephine went to Grey Coats, and James to New College School. Josephine passed into Headington and James to Abingdon.

Josephine's interests lay between the arts and farming, and she did jobs at *Cobbes Farm* in Witney. She did the Australian impressionists as a special subject at school. She played the flute well, had ballet lessons and danced well. James was a good trumpet player.

We took the children on overseas visits, and holidays in Australia and Japan were special successes. Josephine eventually opted to take up farming and joined my farming cousin John Knight in New South Wales for one year. His letter describing her year after she had returned home was full of praise. She then went to Seale Hayne Agricultural College in Devon but decided the economics of farming was unattractive. By taking an extra certification in English, and with an Australian mother, she was able to get a place at Monash University in Melbourne to study arts, and followed this by studying museum management at Deakin University Melbourne. While in Australia, she developed a close relationship with a pleasant young farmer. After several years – to our relief – she returned home without this relationship. She took further training to be a teacher and taught at New Hall in Essex. She married James Del Mar who became a *Knight Frank* advisor on estate management to Arabs and pop stars, and they settled in Pewsey, Wiltshire, with two children, Cosmo and Adelaide. We moved near them after retirement.

Our son James at Abingdon School took drugs and gradually after leaving school developed schizophrenia. He lost motivation for studies and job-seeking became psychotic and unhappy. It was all slow to develop and to be diagnosed. Unable to make best use of higher education, he did many helpful creativities at home, such as framing pictures for the Churchill Hospital. He did some excellent wood-carving and helped with manufacturing some new medical thermometers and with projects on waste to energy. At times, he showed behaviour which was unacceptable to his community and for a while he was admitted to the Warneford Hospital. Eventually, under control with fortnightly injections, he lived independently in an ideal detached cottage and was able to produce three really delightful books of poetry. He was unable to sustain a job but medicaments rid him of hallucinations. He was always subject to disturbing and realistic dreams.

By marrying an Australian, as I said in my bridegroom speech, there was a commitment to visiting there often. The first trip to Australia was for our marriage. We tried to go back to Australia about every three to four years. Our first trip included our farming cousin in Deniliquin. Always, there were dermatology sessions planned. A weekend course for the Department of Medicine at St Vincent's, Sydney, was one of the first. There was a course at Lidcombe Hospital, also in Sydney, headed by Kate Georgouras, whose husband had a huge collection of the oldest 78 records of opera which we later taped and exchanged. Later, there were visits to Hugh Molloy's practice in Sydney; he also spent many months at the Slade Hospital in Oxford, working on overheating and sleeplessness due to duvets. Hosts in Melbourne included Peter Cowen and Rod Sinclair, both of whom worked with us in Oxford. In 1989, there was a month in Perth,

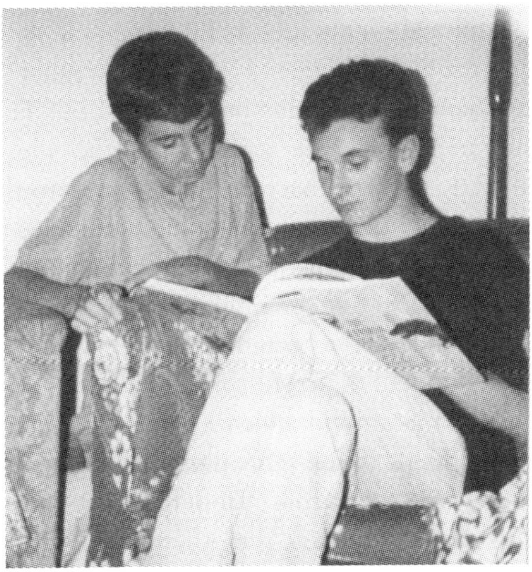

James Ryan and Peter Merry in Australia planning where to find fossils

appointed to community medicine at the Sir Charles Gairdner Hospital, with a weekend further north in Galveston teaching nurses about leg ulcer management. This was linked with staying at Guildford Grammar School in Perth where Paul, Anne's brother, and his wife Lyn taught. There were National and World Congresses of Dermatology. John Caseley Smith of Adelaide, who had worked with Howard Florey in Oxford, organised an International Lymphology Congress which took us to Alice Springs and Ayers Rock. He had the misfortune of his house being burnt down due to inadequate fire control by the local County Council. I was back in the UK, lecturing in Cambridge, when his Australian lawyer flew in just for breakfast, to ask me whether he was important enough to claim that the loss of his papers in the fire substantially reduced his marketing value. There was a second much larger lymphology congress organised by Neil Piller in Sydney. Invitations to wound healing congresses took us to Fremantle and Bendigo. The last trip in 2017 revolved round a lymphology congress in Darwin. We had thus become familiar with all the states of Australia. Anne's younger brother moved to Toowoomba, inland from Brisbane, where we also had two enjoyable holidays.

Over the years, familiarity with the art galleries of Sydney, Adelaide, Melbourne and Perth gave much pleasure. There were some notable musical events such as Prokofiev's *War and Peace* at the first season of the Sydney Opera House, and Wagner's *Ring* cycle in Adelaide, in which the Valkyries had cricket bats! The director of The Playhouse in Oxford had moved to run the Adelaide Festival.

Back in the UK in earlier bachelor days, the Oxford Professor of Music, Fred Sternfeld and his wife Sophie befriended me and, with them, I met Michael Tippett on several occasions. I first sat with him as a schoolboy on a train to Brighton. He always sent his scores to Fred and I once spoke with him at length about his support of music in the schools of Leicestershire. Finally, in 1990, I acted as chauffeur to Fred Sternfeld to the first night of *New Town* at Glyndebourne, and sat in the same row, next to the producer Peter Hall, as well as Fred and Michael Tippett.

I watched Benjamin Britten, the other great British musician, as a conductor of Mozart but not of his operas. I finally went to

Aldeburgh after the death of Peter Pears. The caretaker of The Red House was a patient of John Chalmers, a surgeon friend from National Service days. I played Debussy on the famous piano, and Pears' little terrier – straight from the well-known *HMV* gramophone label – howled and howled. Apparently, he had got used to pop music played by Britten's nurse and later caretaker, but Debussy recalled too many memories.

Another lover of music from the field of dermatology was Professor George Findley from Pretoria. He knew Vaughan Williams, and I was chauffeur to a memorial concert for him organised by Ursula Vaughan Williams and Christchurch School in their small local church.

We lived happily in North Oxfordshire gradually improving our home and garden. We made good friends. One of these was Helen Ryan, the actress who became a neighbour. Family names discussed with her father were alike in both our families and we assumed a very distant cousin relationship. We enjoyed seeing her many stage successes such as *Lettice and Loveage* and her appearances in films such as *The Elephant Man* and in television such as Queen Alexandra in the *Edward VII* series. Her son borrowed material from me for his thesis on Neitzche and Wagner and became a successful opera director for Opera North, Glyndebourne, Santa Fez and Geneva.

Notes on Chapter 6

1) In *Microvascular Injury* (1976), published by Lloyd Luke, I tried to show the importance of localisation factors in blood vessels as underlying many skin conditions. I found in the *British Medical Journal* a report by William Osler of cases of vasculitis which he had seen in Oxfordshire, and found that we shared an opinion of mechanisms: Osler, W. (1914), 'The visceral lesions of purpura and allied conditions', in *British Medical Journal* 1: 517-25.

Microvascular Injury was a very comprehensive history and analysis of the literature on vasculitis. It was about inflammation, and included chapters on the influence of cold, venous hypertension

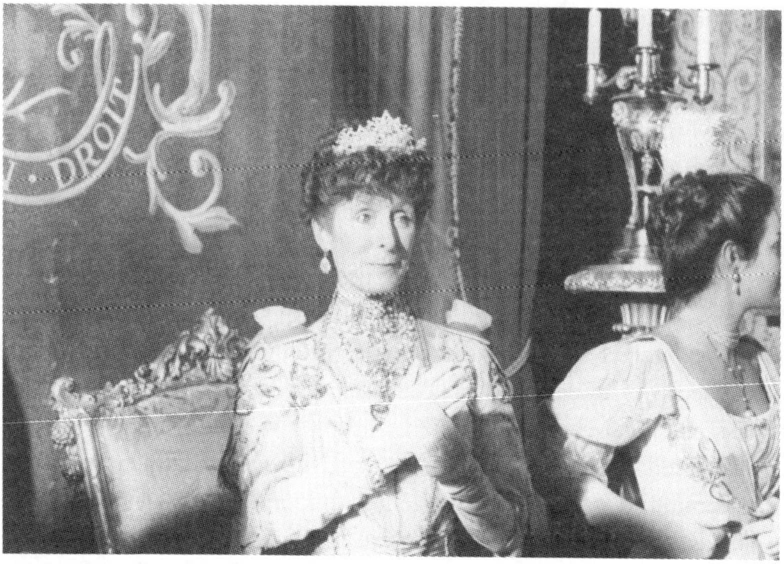

Helen Ryan when acting as Queen Alexandra in the TV series Edward VII

and the psyche on the behaviour of vessels injured by immune complexes or infectious agents. It also examined localising factors and ischaemia-reperfusion, fibrinolysis and coagulation. Later, it was in part continuously updated as a chapter in successive editions of the principal *British Textbook of Dermatology* by Rook, Wilkinson and Ebling.

2) Ryan, T.J., Matts, P.J., Snyder. B., Orr, V. (2014), 'A Seminar on Gardens for Health', in *International Journal of Dermatology* 53: 593-600. It included a review of how trees benefit the health of people admitted to hospital.

3) *Further Notes on Leprosy in Oxford.* The subsequent history is lodged with the *Global Project for the History of Leprosy*, in the Wellcome Unit for the History of Medicine: www.leprosyhistory.org – and in documents held at 13 Norham Gardens in Oxford. There is correspondence in 1960 with Cochrane, the top man of the field, that marks the difference in research focus between him and Dr Rees, at the Mill Hill Medical Research Council research centre, making clear Cochrane's desire to establish a unit at Oxford. In this correspondence, Cochrane expresses his interest in leprosy and

dermatology in general health services (23rd Feb 1965). There is also correspondence on his retirement from the Directorship of the Leprosy Study Centre, and as a Consultant Advisor in Leprosy to the Ministry of Health (letter dated 22nd Jan 1966).

There are the clinical records of me as Registrar in the Department of Dermatology in Oxford, with extensive notes and very detailed descriptions of discussions about the patients affected by leprosy admitted during 1963-65, including records relating to a case that was the first to establish dapsone resistance in Europe (Notes: 11th Jan 1965). There are notes on debates between Cochrane and Dr John Warin, the Medical Officer for Health for Oxford, on the question of contagiousness of a Chinese patient on our ward with a foot ulcer who was seen by many experts, including Paul Brand, Professor Trueta, Robert Cochrane, Graham Weddell, Dick Rees and Michael Walters.

There are extensive teaching records, including those related to teaching clinics and six-monthly seminars attended by Robert Cochrane, Stanley Browne, Dick Rees, Graham Weddell, and occasionally by Michael Walters and Paul Brand. There are records of the teaching activities of the Oxford unit – for example, clinical demonstrations given at the Institute of Dermatology in London, and the School of Hygiene and Tropical Medicine.

There is correspondence with Paul Brand when he was advising a rehabilitation centre in Croydon; correspondence with Dr D.J. Harman from the Leprosy Studies Centre, and with the Ministry of Health (including Dr Albertine Winner) from Renwick Vickers, concerning the establishment of a research unit at Oxford. On this matter, there is an extensive record of proposals and negotiations, including correspondence from Dr Robert Cochrane to members of the Department of Health; from Renwick Vickers to the Vice-Chancellor, the Regius Professor of Medicine and the Medical Officer of Health, Nuffield Foundation, for funding support, to dermatologists canvassing support for a leprosy centre (1963-67).

There is correspondence with Dr Dick Rees on the use of patients by the National Institute of Medical Research, and with

Stanley Browne on the possibility of a six-bed unit at the Slade Hospital. There are records of the opening of the Cochrane Annex at the Slade Hospital, and a letter from Cochrane sent from Shinyanga in Tanzania on its opening (8th April 1971). There is also correspondence from Renwick Vickers on the staffing and management of the annexe (1970-72).

Other correspondence relates to the role and status of the Cochrane Annex, including a proposal for an honorary consultant in tropical medicine, with a special interest in leprosy; Graham Weddell and Renwick Vickers' 'Intended Programme of Research' proposal; correspondence with Dick Rees to me about transferring the Leprosy Unit to the Department of Dermatology, and the importance of continuing the leprosy group at Oxford; the transfer of funding for the Unit to LEPRA, and an exchange between Francis Harris (Director of LEPRA), Dick Rees and me on my reports on experimental work on wound healing and the issue of generalising leprosy research. This marks the separation between increasingly focused leprosy research and dermatology's broader interests.

There is a record of changing British legislation for the management of leprosy, including the 1965 Public Health (Leprosy) Regulations which were more sensitive about protecting the privacy of patients, and which established a panel of practitioners designated to assist Medical Officers of Health.

There is also a record of the troubled relationship between leprosy and dermatology, including correspondence with dermatologists in Britain on the competence of Cochrane; extensive records of my efforts in bringing about an integration between leprosy and dermatology; records of my work in London (1967-72) at the Institute of Dermatology, and my collaboration with John Turk who was working on lymph nodes from leprosy; and correspondence from Dr Noordeen on the role of dermatology in leprosy (8th October 1998).

There are records of leprosy work such as that of Dr Dick Rees, and Dr Colin McDougall's work on dapsone resistance, using the mouse foot-pad model, and on the use of rifampicin as an effective eliminator of the leprosy bacillus from the nose; of a symposium on the role of B663 (September 1968), following Stanley Browne's claims of the effectiveness of B663 on untreated lepromatous leprosy; on Colin McDougall's research on light and electron microscopy with skin and nerve biopsies; and records of the work of Richard Jones, our histology technician, who was winning prizes on his work with leprosy in India. There is also a record of my work as Honorary Medical Adviser to the St Francis Leprosy Guild, my membership of LEPRA's Medical Board, and the initiation of the IFD (International Foundation for Dermatology), with Regional Dermatology Training Centres (the first of these being the Dermatology, Sexually Transmitted Diseases and Leprosy Collaborating Centre of WHO in Tanzania).

There are also records of my study trips to Uganda and Pretoria in 1971, meetings with Dr Convit in Venezuela and Clovis Lombardi, the Pan-American Health Organisation Advisor on Leprosy, and with Turkan Saylan at the Leprosy Unit, Istanbul. *The Lancet* of 4th July 2009 wrote an obituary on Turkan Saylan, which explains why Turkan was such a good friend. She led the fight against leprosy after spending time in the Cochrane Annex in Oxford. She was a leading women's rights activist and a generous host to 21 St John Ambulance cadets that I led from Oxford. See Chapter 8.

In the field of leprosy, there were numerous visits to leprosy centres supported by the St Francis Leprosy Guild, on some of which I was accompanied by medical students. There were visits to leprosy activities in China, In connection with the IFD training centre in Tanzania, there was Upendo, a small leprosy home created in Arusha in Tanzania.

Interest in leprosy took me also to Sineccio Talhari in Manaus in the heart of the Amazon, and to a leprosy congress in Iguasso.

4) Ryan. T.J. (1985), 'The Dowling Oration: Morphosis, occult forces and ectoplasm – the role of glues and proteolysis in skin disease', in *Clinical and Experimental Dermatology* 10: 507-22.

5) George Cherry benefited me and the Department by setting up The European Tissue Repair Society, The Oxford International Wound Foundation, The European Pressure Ulcer Advisory Panel, The Oxford Annual Young European Wound Healing Course, and

recruiting a young military burns surgeon from Vietnam and China. A few remarks about his achievements at a world congress in Florence, a few months after his death, received a prolonged standing ovation.

6) Nurses had begun to develop a National Dermatology Training Programme in the late 1980s from St Thomas' Hospital, London, and were given a slot in Saturday morning sessions of 'What's New?' at the Annual British Association of Dermatology Meeting. With the nurses in the Department, we set up a committee to take their role forward. When I was President of the British Association of Dermatology, 1992-93, we had a combined meeting with the Canadian Association of Dermatology, and I seized the chance to have a plenary session on 'Dermatology in the Community' (*British Journal of Dermatology* 1993, 129: Supplement 42: 68-70) that included a major contribution from nursing. In the meantime, our programme in Africa was fast developing, focused on the training of allied health professionals, and in the Department of Dermatology we set up the means of bringing nurses from Tanzania for a few weeks' exposure to dermatology nursing. We set up the British Skin Care Nursing Group and the International Skin Care Nursing Group. The former soon became affiliated to the British Association of Dermatology and is now its largest branch. The latter is still small but affiliated to the International Council of Nursing. (See Ersser, S.J. and Penzer, R. [2000] 'Meeting patients' skin care needs: harnessing nursing expertise at an International Level' in *International Nursing Review* 47:167-173.) Its members have lectured world-wide and have aided the development of several of international dermatology's and tissue viability programmes, most significantly in India by Vineet Kaur and in South Africa by Pat Kelly. Stephen Ersser has moved through several national promotions but remains the ISNG's leading force. Rebecca Penzer has played a supportive role in many of the IFD programmes. It is an organisation that seeks to work collaboratively to improve skin health world-wide by developing nursing education, practice research and policy. Its first meeting was in Cairo and it has met in Paris, Malta, South Africa and Argentina.

7) In 1979, the research income from the MRC, Wellcome Health Authority Psoriasis Association and industry was £100,000 per annum. By 1981, LEPRA was providing £65,000 for three technicians and Colin McDougall. The Edward Abraham Cephalosporin Fund provided £50,000 in 1984 and £150,000 in 1989. From the mid-1970s, an increasing number of research posts and visitors from residency programmes in the USA resulted in more publications and long-term studies being supervised by Colin McDougall, Rodney Dawber and me.

Opportunities for travel were opened up so that, in 1971, an Oxford dermatology registrar, Gerry Guerrier, worked in Paris on electron microscopy on the melanocyte with Professor Prunieras. We began to arrange visits overseas for most of our junior staff. Alan Marsden visited Tom Janssen and Bert Myers in the USA, Peter Mortimer studied lymphatic function in leprosy in India, and Julia Ellis went to Harvey Blank in Miami for one year. Susan Burge went to Duke University in North Carolina, and Caroline Wilson spent 1991 at the University of Pennsylvania, studying the hair follicle cycle with Bob Lavker, and later pemphigus with JC Pasricha in Delhi.

We began to increase the number of those doing pure research. Raymond Barnhill from the USA worked on angiogenesis, David Salter on skin impedence, Jonathan Shepherd on cold injury – and from Japan, beginning in 1983 with two-year appointments for Mikio Masuzawa, Yasu Horouchi and Hiroshi Kakinuma, who helped to establish a cell culture laboratory. The first Commonwealth Fellow was Dr H.S. Girgla from Delhi working on electron microscopy. Pauline Marren's DPhil was on lichensclerosis of the vulva. Several of Fenella Wojnarowska's protégés were funded by the District Research Committee and NHS locally-organised research schemes on which I served for many years. Opportunities for Fenella to take up more funded time for research with a grant of £125,000 in Oxford in 1993 was resisted by her employers in Buckinghamshire. She took the role of Chairman of Department first at the Wycombe General, 1986-89, and later in Oxford. Fenella, as an advocate for Women's dermatology diseases, set up a significant Vulva Clinic in 1987, and trained several leaders in the field for the UK and 23 overseas Fellows. Through contacts I have in Oxford, we gained entry to the Chairman of a major charity that funded this project in the late 1990s for a few years. She had supervised 23 overseas Fellows up to the year 2000. She obtained her Oxford DM through publications. In 1991. she was awarded the *ad hominem* title of Reader and, later, Professor.

Opportunity was also given to Senior Registrars to develop the Department in Oxford. Thus, Alan Marsden arranged that Oxford was the first to try out a prototype longwave ultra violet light apparatus used with the ingestion of a psoralen to make the user more sensitive to its effects in the management of skin diseases, such as psoriasis. As Registrar, Graham Colver introduced Infra Red Coagulation. Tim Sonnex had a brief trial with *Thorn Electric* on the effects of lighting on accuracy of diagnosis. Surprisingly, it proved that lighting was less important than room size. Small rooms reduced accuracy of diagnosis. Sue Burge founded the 'Pigmented Lesion Clinic', and was also the recipient of our first Arthritis and Rheumatism Grant, allowing her to take a year off for the study of lupus erythematosus, 1986-87, and to employ Kate Schomberg. As a British Association of Dermatology research fellow, she entered the field of cell adhesion molecules studies of Darriers' Disease, 1989-90. She was later funded by a cyclosporine trial. She also supervised a study of lupus erythematosus by Elisabeth Mbuagbaw from Cameroon. Susan played a significant role in the Medical School, preparing for a review by the GMC. She was awarded an OBE.

In 1998, John Wilkinson developed the Contact Dermatitis Clinic. Ian Ralfs took up injecting tritiated thymidine into the eccentric elderly nutritionist (Hugh Sinclair), who ate only seal meat as we thought there might be a change in the rate of epidermal turnover.

In 1986, the Royal College of Physicians nominally allocated a second Senior Registrar but funds could not be found to support this post.

One of Oxford's unique pioneering schemes was the 'Part-time Married Women's Scheme' of Rosemary Rue, the Regional Medical

Officer. Renwick worked with Rosemary and took full advantage of the popularity of dermatology for the woman with a family. Consequently, this was one of the first ways in which an increase in staffing was obtained. There were to be some 20 staff members introduced by this scheme, including Anne MacPherson, Margaret Rice-Oxley, Sheila Powell, Hilary Fawcett, Elspeth Young, Susan Burge, Vanessa Venning, Jenny Powell and Pauline Marren.

The GP Trainee Scheme evolved from the early 1970s with prospective GPs organising their own schemes and finance. Some, like Anne MacPherson, entered through the part-time women's scheme and joined the Department for a year, while others like Peter Middleton and Norman Watson visited one or two sessions per week for many months. Initially, the formal scheme was for three-month appointments but it settled down to two months with two appointments at all times. Thirty GPs received training through the scheme.

Training GPs was not confined to this scheme. There was a drive in the late 1980s to take teaching into the Family Practice. Rodney Dawber demonstrated cryosurgery and Susan Burge talked about pigmented lesions.

Increased secretarial support was needed for the new Consultant, and for Renwick who was now Consultant Advisor in Dermatology to the Department of Health, Chairman of the Dermatological Committees of the Regional Board, a member of the Government Committee on Borderline Substances as well as Chairman of the Section of Medicine of the United Oxford Hospitals. At the same time, there was the gradually increasing demand for dermatology services and the enlargement of the Medical School. The NHS Secretaries were Cynthia Weedon and Katie Baker, and later Jean Boyd and Sheila Carroll. A significant milestone was the introduction of *Macintosh* computers in 1988. In 1995, Olga Gold was appointed as Secretary to myself following the retirement of Margaret Cook.

7: Contributions in Five Continents Generating Global Policy

Darrell Wilkinson, practising 20 miles from Oxford at High Wycombe and Amersham, was the leading international figure of the Oxford Region's dermatology team. While writing, with Arthur Rook and John Ebling, the first major British textbook of Dermatology in 1968, he frequently asked regional dermatologists for help. I had attended his clinic as early as 1960, and was invited to contribute to the second edition of the textbook, on vascular disorders and a chapter on radiation, It was realised that more international data was needed. In 1970, before returning to Oxford as a Consultant from my post as Senior Lecturer in London, I had written a comparison of London, the USA and Indian Dermatology. It addressed the differences in the approach to taking skin biopsies, how to manage large numbers of patients (as in Calcutta), procedure training (as in the Armed Forces), and the fact that the UK was well behind the dentists in our contribution to hygiene. It discussed teaching a patient-centred approach to medical students and pointed out, quoting the Danish dermatologist Gunnar Lomholt's appeal at the World Congress of Dermatology in Munich, based on his experience in Malawi and Uganda, that dermatologists should not congregate only where there is money, and that this was not the case in the UK, with its National Health Service. I wrote: 'The need for dermatologists to be involved in the contemporary changing face of medicine is urgent. More dermatologists are needed for a public health role and teaching.'

Darrell Wilkinson had previously circulated a call for more dermatologists in the UK so that all patients could be given at least 15 minutes for their first appointment. Arthur Rook of Cambridge, as President of the British Association of Dermatology, took my paper

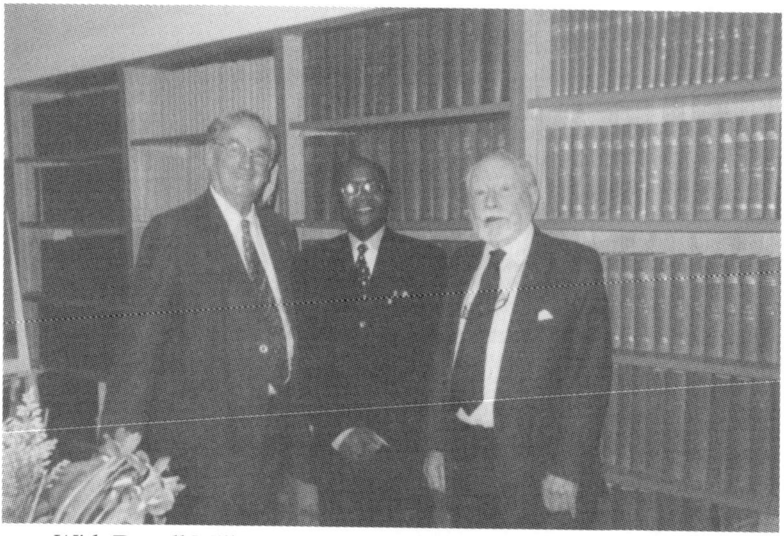

With Darrell Wilkinson at Amersham Department of Dermatology entertaining an African currently appointed to the Court of St James

to a working party on the future of dermatology. By this time, Darrell Wilkinson had begun to think of the need for a separate organisation to address international public health issues. He appreciated the need for epidemiology, and I approached the Oxford Record Linkage Group to examine disease associations of the skin, suggesting a tool such as the well established Cornell Medical Index.

While at the Institute of Dermatology, when put in charge of the British exhibition at the World Congress in Munich, I was invited to several of the organising committees of that event. At this time, Hugh Wallace at St Thomas's Hospital in London was a member of the International Committee of Dermatology (ICD) which organised the programme of quinquennial World Congresses, and he had begun to sow the seeds, provided by Darrell Wilkinson, for an international organisation to be initiated to manage the global need for developing world studies. He began also to groom me to take over his role on the International Committee. In 1976, the British Association of Dermatology proposed me for election to the ICD. Members of that committee, Rudy Baer (USA), Felix Sagher and Eleanor Feuerman

(Israel) and Rudi Commane (the Netherlands) wrote welcoming me, but on the day of the election at the World Congress in Mexico, the International Committee felt I was too young and unknown and would not get the number of votes needed to be elected, and they requested Darrell Wilkinson to put his name forward.

During the next five years, Darrell Wilkinson and I had many discussions. There was a meeting in Oxford of the International Committee, hosted by Darrell Wilkinson, at which several sessions were attended by me, while the St John Ambulance band from Banbury, of which I was its senior officer (see Chapter 8) was provided as entertainment. The concept of an International Foundation of Dermatology began to evolve, and many who were not on the International Committee, such as Francisco Kerdel Vegas, a Venezuelan dermatologist, who was also an Ambassador in London, and Orlando Canizares, the leading American specialist in tropical skin diseases, wrote in with suggestions. In 1981, there were again letters from around the world welcoming me as a candidate for the International Committee. There was a debate in my Oxford department, where research was funded largely by LEPRA, as to whether leprosy world-wide should in the future be managed by the dermatology profession, a view Francisco Kerdel Vegas was to promote strongly many years later, as a *Sine Lepra* campaign (a world without leprosy campaign generated by by the Venezuelan Professor Francisco Kerdal Vegas proposing that dermatology as a profession should take over leadership). In the previous year, a meeting of the African Association of Dermatology (AFRAD), at a workshop on training and research policy in Dermatological Sciences in Africa, had come to the same conclusion. Renwick Vickers, as President of the British Association of Dermatology in 1966, had also written to the International Committee of Dermatology, appealing for more involvement in leprosy.

In order to activate the ICD, Darrell Wilkinson proposed that there should be 'extra-congressional activities', A Glossary of Dermatological Terminology, chaired by the senior Mayo Clinic dermatologist Winkelmann, was one of these. Greater involvement of national organisations would be sought through re-designation of delegates from dermatology societies of every country with the title of International Secretary. A letter I received in 1983 requested me to take on this job, and I was so nominated by the British Association of Dermatology (BAD) in 1983. A supporting letter from Jose Mascaro of Spain, recently elected to the International Committee, approving such a concept, hoped that an International Foundation would be launched at the next World Congress. In the meantime, John Petit, one of the few dermatologists regularly lecturing on tropical dermatology, who was based in Malaysia, wrote to the BAD and to me, hoping that the next World Congress in Berlin would pay more attention to the developing world.

From 1968, my main travels had been the tour via the USA to Australia to get married and the three-month honeymoon via Singapore, India, Poland, Czechoslovakia and Sweden. There was a later return trip to Australia with lectures on blood supply of the skin which took me back to the USA and Australia. Several meetings on blood and lymphatic vasculature were to take me to Japan.

Visits to Japan[1]

In 1967, Charles Calnan, who was Professor of Dermatology at the Institute of Dermatology in London, helped *Glaxo* with the introduction of Betnovate to Japan; others of us later assisted *Stiefel* and *Squibb* with introducing their wares, while at the same time assisting with links in the UK for some Japanese pharmaceutical companies.

It was Toshiyuki Aoki from Osaka who deserved the credit for initiating the welcome habit of the post-war visits of young Japanese to the UK to gain experience in British dermatology and research. He had read a chapter on contact dermatitis by Charles Calnan in the *Textbook of Immunology* by Philip Gell and Robin Coombs. This was at a time when cell-mediated and transplant immunity was bringing immunology to the fore. Toshiyuki Aoki had started his own research in that field, and wrote to Charles Calnan, who arranged for him to work in the Institute of

Dermatology in London. Very soon the UK became as favoured as the USA for overseas experience!

Both the British and the American friends of Japan were concerned that the young should learn the English language. It was first believed that the Japanese dermatologists were merely copying and, like the early travellers, were becoming the teachers of dogma without developing free thought. However, all that was rapidly changing, and an apparent lack of free thought may in fact have been a limitation of language rather than of ability or interest. Learning English was always one main objective of visiting the UK: this was not just in dermatology, but social. One of my Japanese visitors to Oxford thought that 'something smells good' was an appropriate remark when visiting any English house, even when no food had been cooked!

From the mid-1970s, it was clear that the rapid development of dermatology in both the UK and Japan was based on a rather similar social process. Helping the Japanese to think in English, was the aim of San Francisco dermatologists who set up the Pacific Skin Research Club, with an informal atmosphere in which to encourage their presentations. In Britain, we had the Dowling Club, and in Japan there was the Sky Club. Every young dermatologist, and many older ones, used to join the most senior London dermatologist Geoffrey Dowling at the *George Inn* near Guy's Hospital, London, to discuss dermatology once a month. It then became a travelling club, and was a huge influence in developing uninhibited discussion about dermatology between all age groups. The elder dermatologist Toshiaki Yasuda did exactly the same for the young Japanese. Toshiaki and his wife Hisako, a fine painter of watercolours, were exceptional hosts, and it was a pleasure to entertain them in Oxford on two occasions: once when Japanese dermatologists were the official guests of the BAD, and again as guests of the President, Darrell Wilkinson, when he and Toshiaki Yasuda were members of the International Committee of Dermatology which was also hosted in Oxford.

In 1981, on the occasion of being made Honorary Member of the Sky Club, the Japanese equivalent of the Dowling Club, I visited a small chalet where we spent one weekend. All the young ones, especially those that had been in England, were speaking in English the whole weekend and discussing freely with Toshiaki Yasuda and the two principal guests – myself and guest speaker Professor Takatsuki. The Sky Club and the Pacific Skin Research Club were a marvellous opportunity to enjoy each other's company and to socialise round the topic of dermatology. I also later visited leading microcirculation departments in Japan on several occasions, and there was a rather similar club focusing on microcirculation chaired and sponsored by the Professor of Internal Medicine, Masaharu Tsuchiya, Dean at Keio University.

Many British dermatologists have experienced hospitality in Japan that has been unique in its generosity and cultural interest, and they had this opportunity at the World Congress of Dermatology in Tokyo (1982) of which the President was Atsushi Kukita, who was always a leader in forging international relationships. At least 80 British dermatologists attended, many with their wives, at a time when there were only about 250 dermatologists in the UK, and there was a memorable meeting of the Pacific Skin Research Club in Hakone after that event.

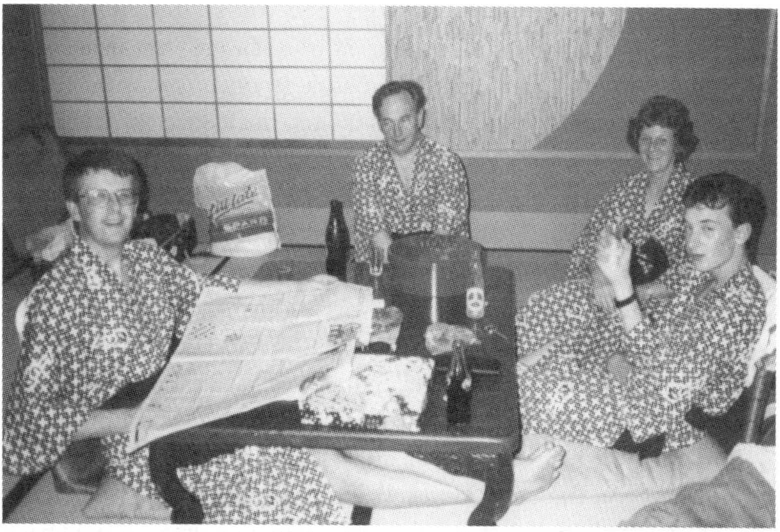

Adopting a Japanese way of life with my family and Peter Mortimer (far left)

I have lost count of the number of visits made to Japan – mostly for microcirculation, lymphatics, biorheology or dermatology, but remember some of the social events better than the dermatological content, and I have recorded the relationship of British to Japanese dermatology in *The Japanese Journal of Dermatology*.[2]

Perhaps our most exciting time was our first visit with my entire family at the 30th Anniversary Reception of Masakatzu Izaki of the Iwate Medical School in 1985, but the 1989 World Congress of Microcirculation, attended with Peter Mortimer, was another magnificent event. Peter Mortimer is a well-dressed Englishman with lace-up shoes – a huge disadvantage when trying to visit, shoeless, as many Japanese homes, shrines and temples as possible in one afternoon. My favourite visit was to Shoso Yamamoto at Shimane Medical University, who later became Professor and Chairman at Hiroshima University. Often we made our visits a holiday with our children and friends such as Peter Mortimer.

Japanese names were difficult to assimilate for British dermatologists, but it helped keeping a notebook to remind identification features such as 'wears glasses', 'grey with big stomach', 'small, bald', etc. In spite of my dyslexia, I seemed to have less of a problem with musical-sounding Japanese names than with European names.

One exceptional visit was a retirement party given for my benefit in Japan. This very special ceremony put on for my retirement in 1997 was well attended by many Japanese who had visited the UK over the passage of time. One was reminded not only of the similarities between our two countries, but also the cultural differences. Kiyoshi Nishioka once invited me to a wedding in his department, and he and his wife, he being Head of Department, acted as the hosts in this event in a very formal ceremony in which the parents of the bride and groom seemed to take rather less of a part. The retirement event also had some characteristic elements of Japanese culture, while I later welcomed to my house in Oxford a large formal Japanese doll in a large glass case, which had been purchased by the dermatologists for that occasion. If one goes into any home of a retired dermatologist in Japan, one finds a similar doll, similarly proudly displayed; to do it justice I had to find new space to provide it with adequate display.

It is now many years since the Japanese have been free thinkers, leading the field of investigative dermatology. Because of their industriousness and dedication to their job, they thoroughly deserve to be in this position. Fortunately, their parties – particularly their second and, even more, their whisky-based third parties at any official evening's entertainment – have not diminished in proportion to the seriousness of their dermatology. One can have more simple fun at a Japanese party than anywhere else, but that impression may be something to do with the liberal doses of *Sun Tory* (whisky). British dermatologists sometimes get caught by surprise and show little talent when asked to sing at these events. Ronnie Marks, Professor of Dermatology of the Welsh School of Medicine, was a frequent visitor to Japan, and I once helped him out at a 'second' party in Tokyo – at which he was unexpectedly invited to sing – by providing some biochemistry rhymes composed by Hans Krebs (a colleague at Green College, Oxford, and a Nobel Prize winner) to the tune of *Men of Harlech*, the well-known Welsh marching song.

Compared with the hospitality of the Japanese, British hospitality has not been good. The first meal I gave Kiyoshi Nishioka in 1971 was bacon and eggs in a Lisle Street pub in Leicester Square, and I left him to look for a room to live in. Later that week, he was found doing the most inexpert house painting, and filling up what he described as 'closing the gaps' to prevent the winter draughts. Later, he moved into an apartment in Blackheath, and was viewed all over the world on TV when it became apparent he was a neighbour of a Great Train Robber.

The International Foundation of Dermatology Adopted by the ICD

In 1984, following Darrell Wilkinson's presentation of his proposal, the International Committee of Dermatology (ICD) elected a sub-committee to discuss dermatology in the developing world and the setting up of the International Foundation for Dermatology. It was chaired by Darrell Wilkinson, and included ICD members Al Kopf (USA), Stuart Maddin (Canada), Braun Falco (Germany), Nils Thyrresson (Denmark) and Jean Civatte (France). How to fund this was a concern from the beginning. Darrell and I began to work on fund-raising from British dermatologists and, at the same time, the setting up of a bank account introduced the need to develop a legal status for the new organisation which would be international. One problem addressed by the sub-committee was that, until the concept of a foundation was approved by 51% of the delegates, it would not be possible to fund-raise in the name of the International Committee of Dermatology. It was an issue that exposed the need for a new funding structure for the ICD.

There was at this time a realisation that the International Society of Dermatology (ISD) which was a member of the International League of Dermatology Societies (ILDS), and therefore overseen by the International Committee of Dermatology (ICD) was *de facto* doing some of these jobs in the developing world. It was founded in 1965 as a society focusing on the tropical, geographic and ecological aspects of dermatology. Letters were exchanged in 1985 about the future roles of the two organisations. It was agreed that the ICD would have World Congresses and that the ISD would brand their congresses as being international. I made a proposal to have a regional meeting of the ISD in Oxford devoted to 'Dermatology in the Developing World'. A very successful meeting followed, held jointly with the American Society of Pathology. Colin McDougall prepared and donated sets of slides on leprosy and held a workshop. Leprosy, filariasis and leishmaniasis, as well as diabetes, had full sessions. There were public health sessions, such as a breakfast workshop on how to make posters that would not be misinterpreted by people from the developing world.[3] We had dinner in the Long Library at Blenheim Palace where we awarded Ma Haide,[4] the founder of the Nanjing Institute of Dermatology – and, under Mao, the controller of syphilis, fungus infections of the heads of children and leprosy throughout China – with a lifetime achievement certificate, and also had a barbecue at our home. One follow-up of this event was my appointment as President of the ISD.

In 1987, Darrell Wilkinson produced a one-page document outlining the role of an International Foundation of Dermatology, and in order to reassure the International Committee that it could be funded, he drafted an approach to National Societies. He raised a few hundred pounds from friends so he could say money was in the bank but did not declare how little.

As the time of the 1997 World Congress in Berlin approached, the British Association of Dermatology was asked by the ILDS to put forward two names for the election process for the International Committee, but that the voting delegate, also named the International Secretary, a role I then held, should not be one of these. Much shuffling of names and titles took place till finally three names were on the final list for election. Terence Ryan (Oxford), Professor Rona Mackie (Glasgow) and Professor Malcolm Greaves (London). I wrote to the Secretary of the BAD, asking for clarification of the processes but agreeing that Darrell Wilkinson had been an ideal candidate on a previous occasion, instead of myself as the BAD's nominee. A letter from the Secretary of the BAD, Martin Black, dated 19th February 1987, described his attempt to understand the processes that had been gone through from the time of my role as a delegate at the Munich Congress in 1969 to nomination for the International Committee in Mexico in 1982. It was clear that the ICD could by-pass national proposals.

There was now some anxiety by the sub-committee of the ICD about how much the future International Foundation could be a legal entity. There was also some private anxiety, of Darrell Wilkinson especially, that, if not elected, how would my long involvement and expertise be used. Not yet a professor, feeling much inferior to the other professorial nominees, ultimately I was elected to the ICD and appointed to the new foundation.

We met about every nine months – and this was at a time when the entertainment of the Committee could be extraordinarily extravagant. Some of the visits were site visits for future congresses or eventually the Congress itself, with the inevitable showing off of the city chosen. The partners included my wife Anne, and our host's wives hosted her extravagantly too. After a few such sessions, including the Vienna Opera seated in the Archduke's box watching Pavarotti in *L'elisir d'amore*, we decided that the purpose of the congresses included fund-raising for the developing world and that a dampener on extravagance was justified.

The International Congress committee meetings were stressful. Although there were some very good friends, I had to manage some people who were not sympathetic with what we were trying to achieve and others who were critical. It was pointed out that The International Committee of Dermatology (ICD) was appointed originally to serve dermatologists and did so through the International League of their Societies (ILDS). Of course the money provided for that purpose was for their education at World Congresses, and working with the WHO to produce an acceptable classification of skin diseases as well as an essential drug list. Darrell Wilkinson had thought of the IFD as solving the problems of patients in a resource poor world. When I was helping to develop the IFD aiming for healthy skin for all and later skin care for all, I did much that caused great anxiety to the ICD. Skin care was in my view not just for skin diseases and it was needed not just in Tanzania. Repeatedly during my time as a director and for a while as Chairman, I brought expansion into fields that were difficult to pay for and were not on an agreed agenda. I saw a need for nurses, traditional health practitioners, village doctors in west China and for wound healing, as well as therapies including yoga and herbals. I was fortunate that one of my interests unfamiliar to most dermatologists, leprosy, brought in substantial funds

Over the next 20 years, the foreseen problems of funding, legality and the role of London as a base in the future continued to be debated. I was a generator of policy for ten years, Chairman for five, and then immediate past Chairman and later co-opted as representing a sub-committee on leprosy. The WHO slogan, 'Health for All', was a stimulus to a later organ-specific slogan of 'Healthy Skin for All'. This was prepared by me (1991) under a contract set up by Francisco Kerdel Vegas, now an ambassador at UNESCO, between UNESCO and the International Foundation for Dermatology (IFD), initially using the heading UNIDERM. It

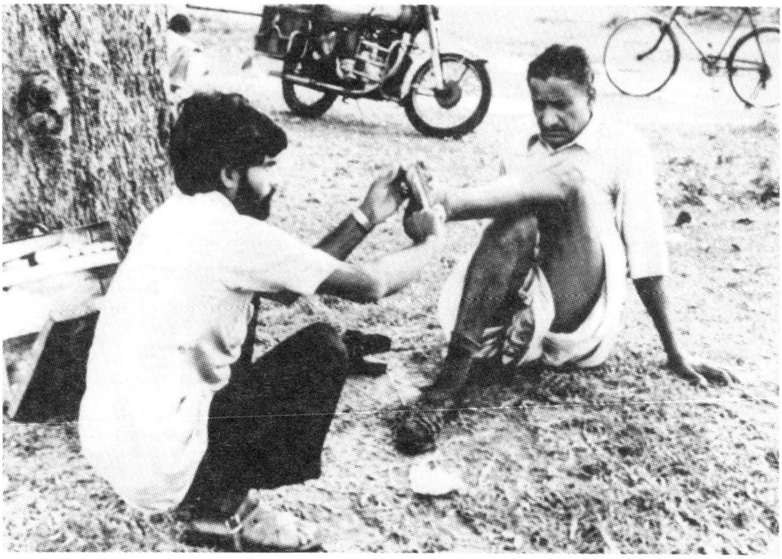

Frontispiece for Healthy Skin for All (UNIDERM), showing that anyone who cares for the skin should have access (bicycles), knowledge (previous dermatology training) and equipment (box of essential drugs and devices)

was an ambitious concept, detailing the missions of the IFD, accompanied by a budget that led WHO to respond with a letter:

> *We identify completely with its aims and objectives. Indeed, we could not fail to be impressed by such a comprehensive statement of commitment to the needs of the developing world by a globally representative medical body. If its ambitions are realised, its impact will be exemplary.*

In its first five years, the IFD was congratulated by WHO for its help in developing a revised 'Essential Drugs List' and 'The Model Prescribing Information for Drugs used in Skin Diseases'. Stuart Maddin from Vancouver was the energetic leader from the IFD that persistently fed WHO with advice on pharmaceuticals. It required an almost weekly exchange of letters over several years. The report to the IFD by Stuart Maddin in May 1994 succinctly tells of the role of the Training Centre in Tanzania (see Chapter

10) in setting up a pharmaceuticals programme. It also found experts to advise on Adverse Drug Reactions. It has distributed much information about therapy at many levels. It has encouraged the Rotary Clubs of Vancouver to provide two self-contained pharmaceutical compounding units in Tanzania. It has encouraged the provision of bulk supply of basic chemicals. It has campaigned and investigated ineffective remedies, and sought to make the provision of the most often used traditional therapies both safe and effective, and at low cost. It has contributed to the ethics of prescribing and sought to upgrade the skills of dispensers. Rod Hay from the UK has long been a main contributor to this field. I realised that even a partial achievement would have considerable benefits for humanity by emphasising the funding required should be for disseminating knowledge that we already have, most of which is low-technology. I emphasised that the knowledge must be distributed to the nursing profession as much as to the medical profession, and that its ultimate recipient is the patient via a knowledgeable carer. The focus is a caring society. The technology is locally available, sustainable and low-cost. Morbidity control of leprosy and lymphatic filariasis were two branches of tropical dermatology on which I placed most emphasis, especially on the nursing profession utilising low-cost low-technology self-help interventions.

As described in www.leprosyhistory.org, the 'Terence Ryan personal collection' describes my first visits to leprosaria, including, in the 1970s, the Medical Research Council centres in Kuala Lumpur, Fiji, Uganda and Pretoria and San Paulo – as well as Carville in Louisiana, a major teaching centre for leprosy, 77 miles from New Orleans.

In 1987, I became Honorary Medical Adviser to the oldest British charity in this field, the St Francis Leprosy Guild. It was a Catholic charity, raising funds mostly from the Catholic Church. On their behalf, although Protestant, I visited many Leprosaria around the world and also introduced the topic to medical students, some of whom would travel with me, while many were funded to make visits themselves. Because the Regional Dermatology Training

Centre in Tanzania was a WHO collaborating centre in this field, the Guild became one of its most generous financial supporters, and a nearby Tanzanian Leprosarium also was well supported and became our local centre for education in the field of leprosy.

In June 1997, I was a member of the Seventh Advisory Panel of WHO on Multi-drug Therapy, meeting in Geneva, and representing the International League of Dermatologic Societies through which the elimination of leprosy was planned. I was insufficiently expert to understand all the data presented but insisted that WHO experts on quality of life were given a hearing. When the IFD was initiated, quality of life studies were in their infancy. Few specialties have made a greater contribution to the language of quality of life in which Andrew Findlay of Cardiff has led the field. The curriculum of the IFD includes a full understanding of issues of stigma, and it has initiated a programme of income-generation for the disfigured and those disabled as a result of skin disease. Leprosy has been regarded as the prototype of disfigurement and consequent stigma.

During the following years, international leprosy congresses were visited in India, Brazil and China. At the one held in Orlando, Florida, religious organisations were equally divided between those who on no account would visit nearby *Disneyland* and those, mostly nuns, who wouldn't miss it.

The ISD has also held conferences and workshops on the role of women and of children as recipients of discrimination due to skin disease, but also as providers of care. As President of the ISD, I organised in Turkey with Professor Turkan Saylan of Istanbul and Maria Duran from Bogota, Colombia, the first congress on Women in Dermatology. The ISD followed this up by appointing a Maria Duran sub-committee on Women in Dermatology.

In recognition that a thanking system is an essential requirement for any organisation recruiting voluntary effort, and following on the practice of the ISD, the parent body of the IFD (the ICD/ILDS) set up an award-giving system, initially at my suggestion. It was a pleasure recognising and thanking people in public who had made a great contribution through their very hard work.

By the end of this period, the 1990s, the IFD had evolved priorities, and we knew in which direction we were trying to move dermatology.

Control of common skin diseases and STI that fall within the top five reasons for attending health centres:

- Early diagnosis of leprosy HIV/AIDS and skin cancer. Early management of infections leading to systemic disease such as scabies with streptococcal impetigo resulting in glomerulonephritis.
- Better management of disfigurement, scarring, itch and pain, thereby creating well-being and patient satisfaction, including the 'look good – feel good' factor.
- Data collection and epidemiology for long-term disease control and planning of interventions.
- Promotion of the principles of accident prevention, First Aid, and wound healing.
- Appropriate prescribing and management of medicines, and control of roadside sellers and inappropriate prescribing.

On reaching retirement in 1997, there was more to dermatology for me than the seeing of patients individually and naming thousands of skin diseases in Latin. I thought skin care was a better focus, based on restoring skin function. It could cover wounds, burns, lymphoedema and tropical diseases such as leprosy and lymphatic filariasis (LF). As an expert on morbidity control of both leprosy and lymphatic filariasis, common and disabling diseases affecting millions, the Department in Oxford has led leprosy research and pioneered approaches to causes of extreme swelling of limbs and genitalia. The population with limb swelling caused by highly prevalent conditions, such as cancer and its treatment, immobility of varied aetiology, the mosquito-borne parasite filaria and chronic inflammation due to many factors, all benefit from a common approach to self-help management. Furthermore, the care given to the swollen foot has much in common with the minimal care required in other diseases, such as leprosy or the diabetic foot. As populations age, so leg swelling increases and about 2% of the elderly have swollen legs, largely due to immobility. There are WHO collaborations for the elimination of LF and leprosy. Our objective is to make such care common knowledge and practice, thereby making all affected persons self-sufficient.

There is already in existence an organisation, 'International Lymphoedema Framework', that has the knowledge of the skin condition and its management, and the experience of delivering this knowledge by the training of populations in self-help low technology. It was initiated in the UK and had become international and focused on patient-led management, using all systems of health care. Although 'lymphoedema' is in its title, its basic care is any swelling. There is an alliance to manage all such skin failure against a background of poverty, climate change, mobile populations, emerging disease and neglected tropical disease. The International Skin Care Nursing Group and the International Foundation for Dermatology are partners that have played a role in lymphoedema management in 'The Global Alliance for the Elimination of Lymphatic Filariasis'.

Looking for My Forefathers in India

Because my father was born in India, it became a mission to look for landmarks of the family at Ootacamund in the cool Nilgiri hills of South India. A year later my cousin Vanya Orr took her mother to do the same. She went back a year later and decided to explore ways to help the community.

It was possible to visit the local library and see pictures of houses my great great grandfather had bought and records of his activities in the Masonic Lodge. We removed prolific weeds from several Ryan grave stones and saw that many infants were born in the 1840s but died within two years. We found the home in which my father was born in 1902 and visited the forestry centre in which his father worked.

I returned to Ooti with family or friends on several occasions to visit Vanya who first restored the family homes in Dodabetta, where they had run a Cinchona plantation and established a herbal plantation from which perfumes were made. She returned later and set up 'Friends of the Earth', a horticultural teaching establishment with luxurious growth from which she laid on instruction for farmers and local tribal women. She also managed to reduce litter in Ooti and especially plastic bags. She encouraged the opening of blocked elephant trails and restoration of natural indigenous forests.[5]

Temperature Control and Fuel from Waste: Topics of Global Importance

In 1987, Hugh Molloy from Sydney arrived in the Oxford Department. He strongly believed that overheating due to duvets caused skin diseases. We linked him up with Janssen's sleep laboratory and looked at sleep when subjects were heated or cooled. At about the same time, Eric Lamont-Gregory, an American and a highly intelligent variant of a confidence trickster, joined the Department of Dermatology. This was because I had been an internal examiner, with Professor David Morley from the Institute of Child Health, of his Oxford MSc at Green College. The college was in despair because Gregory never left an address and his viva had been fixed for a date suiting David Morley who was also often overseas in Turkey, China and Egypt. Eric had studied the so-called 'kangaroo method' of keeping a baby warm by close contact with the mother under a blanket wrap and traditional swaddling of the newborn versus the use of the hospital incubator. The one was simple, low-cost and effective in maintaining body temperature – the other, usually an expensive gift to hospitals from international donors that is usually poorly maintained and it becomes dangerous high technology in the developing world scenario. We passed him and were impressed. David Morley wrote to Eric, 'I learned a lot from reading your dissertation and thesis' – and he wanted him to pursue his studies and encouraged me to support him in the Oxford Department of Dermatology. Letters from David Morley in November 1988 to Lady Limerick, Patron of The Society for Prevention of Sudden Infant Death Syndrome were strongly supportive of Eric's ideas on cheap, reliable and unbreakable thermometers. It was in accord with my interests.

During the next ten years, Eric was attached to the Oxford Department of Dermatology. He had been supervised by a neonatal physiologist, Peter Rolfe and, too late, I discovered disputes about financing and ownership of ideas that were disturbing both Green College and the university. In fact, Eric was paid retrospectively out of funds given to Peter Rolfe, as a grant from WHO, but somehow the university fees for his MSc were not paid. In order for the MSc to go through after our enthusiastic examination, we had to access the WHO contract in order to get the university to reduce the fees to a university employee rate which at first had been the case in Rolfe's department. When Peter Rolfe moved to Keele, and because the university wound up his department, Eric was left unemployed and, indeed, no contract could be found even though Peter Rolfe had offered him a position, in writing, in 1985, and he was designated an overseas student. There was also much correspondence disputing ownership of equipment by Peter donated by WHO for part-use by Eric but also used by others over several years. When he registered as a student, he was employed on the Whitley scale for Biochemists and Physicists, partly to avoid the heavy expenses which overseas students pay, but also to satisfy WHO as they cannot on their statutes pay for the education of students. He worked in Turkey for three months on a WHO inter-regional study of ways to achieve thermal control of babies. The funding went direct to Dr Rolfe's department who received quite large amounts from WHO to distribute as he pleased. In 1985, he offered Eric the position of Visiting Research Fellow in the Bio-engineering Unit, University Department of Paediatrics at the John Radcliffe. It was to work on appropriate technology for thermal control of newborns and the evaluation of devices in the developing world. When Rolfe's department was folded up by the Oxford Health Authority in 1987, money for DPhil status was owed to Green College. Eric over-emphasised his ownership of equipment owned by the department. On the basis of correspondence with admirers, inclusive of Save the Children, the Institute of Child Health Technology at Low Cost (TALC), Overseas Development Administration (ODA) and WHO, my department took a chance of reimbursement and covered his debts, believing his actual student status to be incorrect.

While this was going on, there was another investigator of body temperature measurement of newborns in deep trouble. She was Bridget O'Connell, who had been suspended for work on keeping newborns warm, including crossing swords with nursing staff for keeping windows open in winter. It took four years for her suspension to be lifted and rated by the Public Accounts Committee as the biggest scandal in the entire history of the NHS. Eric arranged for her to support his work during this time, and it added to the heat of some of the controversy he managed to create in Oxford. Bridget was very grateful that we were supportive of herself and the studies she had been criticised for.

Eric was someone who never had enough money and was always in debt. He was served notice by the university for being in arrears with his rent of a flat in Banbury Road. Throughout 1990-91 the Department of Dermatology reluctantly bailed him out for his unpaid accommodation expenses. In July 1990, he was appointed as Oxford City Council nominee on the General Board of the Thames Business Advice Centre! He was a great story-teller and there were many who were entranced by what he had to say, while others – mostly women – did not believe him from the time of their first contact. He had many tales about his previous jobs, which included exploits in Israel as a CIA agent.

A strong point was that all his considerable energy was spent on the most worthwhile projects for the developing world. He read extensively, he worked long hours and had wonderful ideas. We worked together on low-cost insulating screens (baby cloches for which Eric had achieved part-ownership of the patents with *Baby Cloche Care* of High Wycombe) to protect the newborn from the cold. Many months were spent designing skin-surface thermometers, some of which were successfully tested in the developing world. The first of these was a liquid crystal device, often distributed as a toy and not usually very accurate. We improved it by adding insulation on one side, and by 1990 it was distributed by *Co-op*. Eric was to get 25p per thermometer. One trial in the developing world seemed to show its value but the paediatrician David Harvey could not 'make it work'. A letter from the Foundation for the Study of Infants Death quoted Dr Peter Fleming, who said that parents should feel their baby, check whether he or she was sweating, and use their common sense. Eric encouraged the makers to sell it to prevent cot death, but their claims that cot death was due to overheating led to a letter of rebuke from the Advertising Agency for which they had to apologise to the Agency and to me for careless wording. In fact, we were basing our views on studies by Nicoll and Davies that found many babies who had died were over-clothed and therefore at risk of overheating.

The spring of 1990 produced a number of letters banning Eric from the John Radcliffe and from the Radcliffe Infirmary. A second thermometer was an ingenious device which, according to Eric, used *NASA* technology and required a somewhat fiddly process to make the prototypes. It was tested mostly on babies in the Horton General Hospital, Banbury. James Ryan, my son, was involved, working many late hours helping with this. The Oxford Venture Capital Department, *Isis Innovation* and *Zeal Holdings Ltd.*, also spent many hours on negotiating an agreement on production. A memo from them on our royalty of £10.20 for the end of 1992 read: 'We have not, alas, got off to a fantastic start….' They were horrified when the *General Practitioner* of October 1992 carried an article condemning the device. It was Dr Peter Fleming who stated that he would not touch the device with a barge-pole. He pointed out that the association between overwrapping and sudden death was not proven to be an effect of high temperature and that the thermometer would go off on most days and worry parents unnecessarily. Though agreeing with some of the criticisms, Dr David Morley was more helpful and enthusiastic about the trials. Eric also involved Bridget O'Connell. There was an odd dinner party organised by Eric but paid for by me at which Bridget and a few others had to listen to me supporting Eric's plans, but Eric himself was not in convincing mode. Eric always needed editing and, as a consequence, when he appeared on *Horizon* or *Tomorrow's World* (7th February 1991), he came over very well. *AIR Shield Vickers* considered licensing the baby cloche and other technologies as early as 1989. Eric did some studies in Rotterdam and Cincinnati, but seemed to fall out with his colleagues there.

It was at this time that he was in contact with Dr Richard Guidotti in WHO, and Eric wrote a document for WHO on heat shields. One of the problems with Eric was doing tests without ethical approval, while another was that, in general, he was not liked by the neonatal nursing teams. On 24th April 1990, Paul Johnson, the Consultant Clinical Physiologist, wrote: 'Eric is a law unto himself. He has little goodwill in the JRH from his earlier exploits. My impression is that he works in bursts in many directions at once so that any one group of collaborators has a difficult time.' Typical memos from Richard Jones, the Business Manager in the Dermatology Department, showed total expenditure on our Dunhill Medical Trust account of £13,395 owed by Eric. Fortunately, I was on the District Research Committee and was able to persuade some money to come the way of the Department. However, there are several letters on file requesting reports on Eric's research which were difficult to write and were never on time.Fund-seeking took me with Eric to some unusual meetings with some venture capitalists.

People with money are not comfortable people to deal with but they were better than me at seeing through Eric. One of Eric's partial champions was the physiologist Ilkka Valimaki from Turku in Finland and the contact took me to Turku as a visiting professor. He and I were co-authors of one of Eric's few presentations at a European congress. Eric was surprisingly lacking in confidence at such events. Studies on the Finnish habit of overheating of babies in saunas interested me considerably. As mentioned above, the issue of overheating had a diversion into overheating and sleeplessness led by the Australian dermatologist Hugh Molloy, who believed that duvets caused overheating and took up this interest with Eric and did sleep studies with the psychiatrist Greg Storrs and with Dr Idzikowski at Janssen's. Neither had previously considered that overheating was relevant to sleep. The studies were full of interest but incomplete because of small numbers of subjects willing to be wired up for all-night tests. The results were therefore largely unpublishable. In

Australia, Hugh had an interested lay audience through the media and popular publications. It was also at this time that Eric diverted the project into a 'hand-held fertility thermometer' for measuring the rise of temperature that occurs mid-cycle with ovulation.

Eric tended to take advantage of any contacts I had, and for a while would turn up in Guatemala when I was there, with letters from various ambassadors praising his initiative. He used evidence of a brief relationship with WHO to introduce himself. While in Guatemala, he developed his interest in safe cooking and various heating devices that were economical. He tried to get *Isis Innovation* to take up a 'insulated biodegradable food packaging box'. There was a period when we looked at safe needles and their disposal in the face of the Aids epidemic but, after taking out a patent and prolonged negotiation between *ISIS Innovation* and *Becton Dickinson*, it was abandoned as impracticable in December 1991.

Our last prolonged study was on making charcoal out of garbage. Eric had a large network of supporters who always ended up as walking wounded. They included most members of my Department, my son James, Maureen Forest, the Chief Librarian of the Hospital, engineers and kitchen staff and, not least, myself. A memo to Eric from the Department's Nurse Manager, Janice Cameron, dated 27th May 1993, read: 'I understand that you have the vacuum cleaner belonging to the Renwick Vickers Ward. Despite requests from the ward staff for its return, you have not done so. Would you please return the vacuum cleaner to the ward immediately.' We requisitioned the disused greenhouse of the Young Disabled of Ritchie House to develop charcoal burners. The Churchill Hospital engineers were involved in briquetting on a disused ward but the charcoal dust was walked all over the hospital and the cleaners threatened to strike. One of the issues, as we learned from a study in Northampton, especially applying to sewage as a source of fuel, was the expense of drying waste before converting it to charcoal and then, when it was mostly a dry dust, the cost of briquetting it. The briquetting required mixing it with adhesives and the kitchen staff offered their mixers when we were seeking to take advantage of the glue on disposed hospital envelopes until the mixers became stuck. We took out patents on this and that with *ISIS Innovation*, the new university support system, but it failed terribly. My department probably spent £60,000 and I am still owed by Eric another £16,000 and have the IOUs to prove it. When we moved from the Slade to the Churchill, some large terracotta vases at the main entrance disappeared and were seen in Eric's garden. I simply 'stole' them back again and he never commented on it.

Some of the work Eric did required international visits or at least a car for local visits. There would be urgent garage bills, and on one occasion, when he was very late for catching a flight, there was a Heathrow fine because he thought it would be cheaper to park on a double yellow line for a few days outside a terminal than to pay for parking.

After he had left, the charity Fuel Initiatives Resources Strategies and Technologies (FIRST) which was headed by Maureen Forrest, the hospital's Chief Librarian, and which had been created to support Eric's charcoal interests, decided to continue to explore waste-to-fuel objectives but had to discontinue relationships with Eric and sort out ownership of some of his projects and equipment. He had moved to bigger equipment and had brought in county environmental and waste disposal advisors. He had borrowed and ruined some of the equipment on the farms of local landowners. He had set waste on fire in large containers and involved the fire brigade to control giant charcoal burners. No technology seemed to survive very long.

The lawyer Geoff Haley, who had been involved with the projects of the International Foundation of Dermatology, was brought on board as a trustee to make sure we were safe from Eric's destructive powers. Eric had contacts here and there where he expected to be employed, including briquetting in Addis Ababa and on the estate in Kenya of best-selling author on Africa, Kuki Gallman. She was keen to have links with Green College while her daughter was studying in Oxford. Anne and I had a delightful brief visit to her estate and saw Eric's abandoned prototype which she had tried to use for making charcoal out of a prolific weed on her estate. We met several of the characters featuring in her biographical accounts.

The contacts Eric made with the United Nations Environment Programme were of especial interest as they related to smoke pollution from cooking in various densely populated refugee camps. It was studies from South Africa that alerted us to the need to have a receptacle for waste and to find ways to convert its contents to fuel. There were respiratory diseases; there was surrounding destruction of trees for firewood. Women were raped as they walked further from the camps to gather firewood. Eric's solution was smokeless fuel such as charcoal from prevalent bush weed, coffee and sugar cane residue. I suggested they paid him in two parts with a small carrot and later reimbursed his salary. He moved from the university department of Geography to Engineering and all were short visits. I wrote in support of some, to be paid only on completion to concentrate his mind, which is better at thinking up projects than actually carrying them out. The University Estates Office, seeking to locate him, wrote: 'He has recently left one of our properties without returning his keys or completing any end-of-tenancy requirements.' Earlier, in 1991, *Isis Innovation* tried to get excessive telephone bills paid by one company that Eric was telephoning from the Department of Dermatology.

For a while, we looked at the Oxford and Vale of White Horse District Council and were horrified at how much wood was being sent to landfill. Rotting wood is a breeding ground for disease, while incinerated wood is damaging to the environment. Christian Lambrects of UNEP encouraged local district councils to match UNEP's grants to FIRST. Roderick Nicholson of Oxfordshire's *Nicholsons Nurseries* thought charcoal dust would be better mixed into compost. He was very supportive and helpfully tried out Eric's retorts. His family thought him mad to do so as they were clearly not efficient, and in the UK there was the cost of salaries for those filling and emptying the retort. Eric would frequently be doing this at 3.00am. My son James and Eric worked on this problem on several sites, sometimes creating fires big enough to call in the fire brigade. We were not the only ones interested, and it led to visits to sewage farms in Northampton on behalf of FIRST where they were drying sewage and then generating electricity by burning it.

Eventually, when the NHS began to see the need for its hospitals to convert waste (and clinical waste especially) to energy, it brought us nearer home and into the Dermatology Department. In 1995, we wrote on the topic to *The Lancet* and found some supporters, but this also brought an angry response from OXFAM for being too simplistic. We briefly found another eccentric in the form of Victor Buchanan of *The White Swan* in Pickering, North Yorkshire, who set up the company *Bioflame* to install burners in Central America to power the coffee business.

When I last saw Eric in 2005, the tales continued. This time it was about being a much-valued employee of Colin Powell on a job in Afghanistan! FIRST had now made the training centre in Tanzania its principal interest and was examining disposal of local waste sufficient to fuel the Kilimanjaro Christian Medical Centre. The nearby city of Moshi was twinned with Tübingen who had a green mayor, and interest in our project thus moved briefly to Germany. In 2002, the Oxford hospitals appointed a waste manager to address the yearly expenditure of almost one million pounds sterling on waste disposal. Each ward in the hospital was producing 28 sacks of clinical waste monthly and one sack of domestic waste daily. The project lived on for another decade.

In Tanzania, we tried unsuccessfully to create a metering system to record electricity usage throughout the day for six months, and as the field advanced and many nations were investing in waste to fuel expertise, it was clear that the World Bank would fund the project if we could get accurate data. Excellent data was collected by a medical student on the availability of waste, but the hospital engineers failed to get the necessary information on energy requirements. Finally, as the trustees aged, we gave up and folded up the charity FIRST.

Notes on Chapter 7

1) *The UK as a host to young Japanese.* At a slightly later date, following Drs Aoki and Nishioka, such visitors included Fumio Kaneko, Takeji Nishikawa, Masamitsu Ichihashi, Shojiro Nakagawa,

Takashi Miura, Ichiro Katayama and Takashi Harada – while Takashi Hashimoto worked with Professor Marks in Wales, and Shoso Yamamoto joined Malcolm Greaves and Sam in Newcastle, and later most established departments developed contacts in Japan. In Oxford, I was joined by Mikio Masuzawa (1983-85), Yasuhiro Horiuchi (1985-87) and Hiroshi Kakinuma (1989-91), but there were other important contacts to make. At the time of Mikio's visit to Oxford, Crown Prince Akihito was receiving tuition there for one year, and at one Oxford social event I encouraged Mikio to stroll up to him and have a chat. The Crown Prince was surprised but pleased: it could not have happened in Tokyo. The closest any of us got to him in Japan was at the official opening of the World Congress in 1982.

The Annual Meeting of the 52nd East Japan Dermatological Society, at which I spoke about adipose tissue in 1988 and introduced the paintings of Rubens, coincided with an exhibition of the influence of Japanese art on European art; and on another occasion, I accompanied an exhibition of the Pre-Raphaelite movement from the Ashmolean Museum in Oxford to one of the major stores in Tokyo. There was the 8th Annual Meeting of the Japanese Society for Psoriasis Research in 1992, at which Shigeo Nishiyama was a wonderful host. No doubt, the dermatology was good, but the *nouvelle cuisine* which combined exquisite French and Japanese food presentation was even more memorable. Fumio Kaneko was the attentive guide and, later, host on two occasions in Fukushima.

2) *The Pacific Skin Research Club.* In 1968, Bill Reed introduced me to Bill Epstein and the Japanese Kimie Fukuyama, leading investigators into the science of the skin in San Francisco. They set up the Pacific Skin Research Club to develop a relationship between the USA and young Japanese dermatologists. It had its first meeting in Japan at Morioka (1978), hosted by Masakatsu Izaki and his son. Fibrinolysis of the skin was the principal topic, and having published on this, I was invited to become a member of the club. and at its third meeting in 1973, it met in San Francisco. British dermatologists, Anne and Martin Black, were working on the west

coast of America at that time, so attended this inaugural event. There was later another wonderful meeting in Hanamaki in 1986, which several British dermatologists attended.

Makoto Seiji and Drs Aiba and Ohkochi arranged for tuition in making my own wooden Ko-Ke-Shi doll at the foot of Mount Zao in 1981. That same year, there were the wonderful Kobe steaks when hosted by Yutaka Mishima and Masamitsu Ichihasahi. There were also two memorable visits to Hokkaido University School of Medicine at Sapporo, hosted by Yusho Muira in 1981 and by Akira Ohkawara several years later. On the first occasion, we stayed at a hotel housing the competitors of a Sumo Wrestling competition – the only time I have felt small in Japan.

The Pacific Skin Research Club has met in the UK on three occasions – the latest in 1998 when there were 16 Japanese visitors; the previous occasion was immediately before the World Congress in Berlin in 1987. That was in Oxford when it was exceptionally cold, and our main concern was to provide enough woollen pullovers. Thanks to Cotswold sheep, we actually provided something like 30 little woollen sheep on the table at the main banquet as a souvenir of their visit, and were able to give them a warm reception at our home in Oxfordshire.

3) Linney, B. and Ryan, T.J. (1988), 'Visual Communication for Health and Development', in *International Journal of Dermatology* 27.

4) Ma Haide was born as George Hatem in the Lebanon. He trained in Buffalo, USA, and specialised in syphilis. He decided to study this disease where it was most common among the seafarers of Shanghai. He was eventually appointed by Chairman Mao to control this disease in China. Later he wished to control leprosy in China and established the Institute of Dermatology in Nanjing from which to do this. He visited Oxford to hear of some of the latest advances.

5) She had become involved in initiating a programme of restitution for the village there, setting up a Women's Organisation to find a new way forward after the cinchona plantation was closed. It was the first specifically organic production of medicinal hers in South India. Essential oils were distilled and a collection of

indigenous Medicinal Plants of the Nilgiris gathered in an effort to document and re-establish that Traditional Knowledge amongst the village women. They were among the first group to start composting town rubbish and dealing with the plastics problem in Ooty. She returned later and set up The Earth Trust which continued developing Primary Health Care in more than a hundred villages. It was also training and marketing organic/biodynamic vegetables with the farmers as well as the schoolchildren in those communities. Documenting indigenous herbs of remote tribal communities living in the forests and training village health workers was an important part of their activities.

8: Community Service in Oxfordshire

Eric Haines, the male nurse in the Department of Dermatology responsible for inpatients, but also for male sexually transmitted disease, gave lectures to the St John Ambulance Brigade. He asked the young, newly appointed registrar to the Department of Dermatology to give one or two lectures. Not long out of the Royal Army Medical Corps, where having learned about nuclear attack, I talked to a handful of St John Ambulance Brigade members about what they should do if they were the sole survivors of a nuclear attack on Oxford. The lecture was over-long and the advice given overwhelming, and they only just survived the incident!

The St John Ambulance Division was in St Ebbe's, long known to be the least privileged part of Oxford and, when a year later, they asked me to be their Divisional Surgeon, refusal was not an option. Not a particularly good lecturer, it was with St John Ambulance that I learned to stand on both feet and to talk without being extremely nervous, and to speak without notes.

In the week of Churchill's death, there was a call from the headquarters of St John Ambulance in London requesting that the Oxford Division should provide First Aid for Churchill's funeral – since he was to be buried at Bladon, a village less than ten miles from Oxford. The Divisional Surgeon was asked to take on this responsibility, and required a uniform – which the Division paid for. The hat was a problem because of a big head, but it arrived just in time. An account of this event is published in the *International Journal of Dermatology* and in *Green College Review*.[1]

After requisitioning a house in Bladon to act as a local hospital, the expected screaming wounded were divided from minor casualties by hanging a blanket from the ceiling in the garage. On the road between Hanborough railway station and Bladon, there were 2,000 police, 600 civil defence ladies making soup, and numerous Boy Scouts and Girl Guides. The main event had been in London watched on TV and Lady Churchill asked that the Bladon funeral should be private. It was very cold and no-one turned up to watch the event in Bladon. There were no additional onlookers and consequently not one casualty.

It took me a long time to work out the relationship between the St John Ambulance Brigade and its Association, London Headquarters and County Headquarters, and who the County Surgeon, County Commissioner, County Commander and County President exactly were. They seemed extremely important people, and over the years I became each one of these.

There was much to do as Divisional Surgeon arranging an annual calendar of events. I gradually learned how to train people for competitions, and how to make artificial wounds out of plasticine. The favourite was a burn consisting of a background of lipstick, a blob of Vaseline covered by a torn piece of tissue paper, covered in Collodian glue with a scattering of ashes. An unusual exercise was placing some of the Brigade members as casualties on top of a gasometer and getting them to be rescued by the Fire Brigade, and then treated by the Territorial Army led by the GP Patrick Lawrence. I spent two hours making up Eric Haines with an artificial neck inclusive of rashers of bacon, so that he could have a tracheotomy. It took me quite a long time to learn that realism required staging accidents that were appropriate to the setting. Being gored by a bull was hardly likely in an indoor setting! Being able to act was even more important. The charity called Casualties Union acquired skilled actors and gradually fulfilled training needs.

One of the most interesting First Aid events was the provision of the medical services for the annual St Giles' Fair – dealing with stab wounds, drug addiction, hypoglycaemic comas and much else. We probably saved the Casualty Department of the John Radcliffe some extra work.

It became an increasingly noisy event. In the early 1950s, it still included the Fat Lady and a boxing tent. The Fat Lady would not be a rarity in the attendance in 2016. Walking round her, one did not know whether to remain silent, thank her or congratulate her. On one occasion in the First Aid Tent, there was an elderly lady with a headache because of the noise. She had been to the fair for 80 years and remembered her father's single violin accompaniment on a penny-a-dance floor.

Gradual promotion from a Divisional Surgeon, to County Surgeon, Commissioner and County Commander followed, taking on a larger number of Divisions over a fairly extensive area of Oxfordshire. Some Divisions were trained to quite a high standard, so that they sailed through county competitions, and even through regional competitions, to get to the Grand Finals in London. One cadet even obtained the Grand Prior Prize, being the best cadet of the year partly trained with private tutorials at home at our home at *Abbey Willows*. He appeared many years later as a physician attending an opera at Glyndebourne. My experience through competitions was such that I became an examiner at several levels in the St John Ambulance Brigade, and also for some of the national industrial competitions, like the Coal Miners and the Gas Board.

Staging the annual competition, particularly if it was a regional one, was probably one of the most difficult exercises that anyone ever had to do. It depended on so many people. There were the casualties, there were the sets, there were the judges, there were the teas and there was the distinguished presenter of prizes. The worst occasion was when the Dorset Police, who were well-known to be the best of the teams in the country, were the victims of a lapse of security, and their marking sheets were spirited away. I had to announce to the presenter of prizes, the Lord Lieutenant, that part of the competition was invalid, and it caused huge controversy; the Commissioner of the day – a Wing Commander – felt that the incident had been handled poorly.

Eventually, as the youngest Commissioner in the UK, there were many other interesting experiences. Organising the medical services for the largest illegal pop concert, at Watchfield near Swindon, went on for two weeks. Planning was shared with the Health Authority. Organising the medical services for the evacuation from Cyprus was another significant event. Hundreds of people arrived only in their bathing suits to a rather cold Brize Norton, and over several days had to be looked after, fed and provided with clothing and much else. On several occasions, a national ambulance strike meant that St John Ambulance was in charge of an emergency service with the Red Cross. On first joining St John Ambulance at St Ebbe's in Oxford, it automatically put me onto the Oxford Ambulance Committee because at that time, in the 1960s, the St John Ambulance Brigade was actually in charge of the ambulance service.

One annual anxiety was the Annual Report, and the wish to show that the numbers were not continuing to dwindle. Each year, over the 20 years spent in the Brigade, there was a gradual loss of members in Divisions – actually, probably less in Oxfordshire than in many other counties. The demands for attendance at sporting events, and the demands for a regular commitment, became increasingly difficult to meet, with me quite often volunteering for the Speedway or football ground. Some of the very old had to be gently squeezed out of the system because they were actually unsafe in the event of an accident. Our home in Middle Barton was on land adjacent to the local female squire, Mrs Fleming, the national judge of Arab horses She had regular horse shows and her elderly chauffeur did the First Aid in St John's uniform without ever attending a revision course. After a mild protest from me, Mrs Fleming, tipped off by a Lady Dashwood that someone had moved into her village intending to set up a St John Ambulance Division, rang in fury but retreated when told that she was speaking to the Oxfordshire Head of St John Ambulance, and an invitation followed for Anne and me to a rather formal dinner in her very cold baronial hall. The other guest was the Master of Hounds and we were largely ignored.

A glance at the Minutes of the Council of June 1978 showed the strength of the back-up provided by Tim Collins (of the Tusmore Estate and head of the Guardian Exchange) in the Chair, two retired senior surgeons, Ronald Macbeth and Tim Till in charge of the provision of First Aid courses, and the Countess of Macclesfield giving support from her castle.

How to maintain numbers was a continuing problem. Some of the cadet programmes were boring: too many regulations and too much drill, and the expense of the uniform. These were balanced by some exciting duties at summer camps, and fulfilment of a desire to help people. Telling stories about the origin of St John Ambulance activities at the time of the Crusades and ceremonial enrolments in churches appealed short-term. I appointed, as my deputy, Mr Knott from the Wantage Division who, compared with me, thrived on regulations.

One event which, in my lifetime of meeting challenges, was probably the most important was the creation of an Enterprise Group. A group of about eight instructors was identified in the age group between 20 and 30. It included some doctors, a senior nurse, two school teachers, a welfare officer and my St John Ambulance secretary – and they were told that they would get whatever they needed to finance a programme that was exciting for teenagers. The programme included some wonderful outward bound-type events.

On one occasion, I was using my dermatology and leprosy contacts in Turkey, namely Professor Turkan Saylan, a leader in women's rights and head dermatologist, to help organise demonstrations of First Aid in the University of Istanbul. A group of 21 teenagers, who had never before left Oxfordshire, took a three-day train trip to Istanbul. It was not an easy journey: there was an attempt to put drugs in their haversacks, and there were difficulties with the police in Bulgaria. In Istanbul, the boys stayed in an emptied dermatology ward and the girls in the Florence Nightingale School of Nursing. We visited the Florence Nightingale Museum and the British cemeteries, and took a coach to Ephesus. We carried out tests of sunscreens for Stiefel Laboratories on the patio of Professor Turkan overlooking the Bosphorus. We slept on straw beds in hostels, and every one of us developed quite severe diarrhoea and vomiting, but the demonstrations of First Aid in the open air to 250 medical students went down well.

In the year of the Queen's Jubilee, we had a camp in Malta, and there were 100 of us marching through the centre of Valletta to the cathedral. On two occasions, as I was an advisor to the Dead Sea

Hostels, treating skin diseases in Israel, I took small groups to the Eye Hospital in Jerusalem, and arranged such exercises as decorating the paediatric ward. All these adventures were supported by my secretary, Sally Hardacre, by Elizabeth Stewart, a nursing officer, by Tony Macey, a GP in Princes Risborough. and by the Chairman of our St John's Council, Tim Collins.

The theme 'lay participation' (see Appendix 2) replaced 'voluntary help' in lectures given to the St John Ambulance annual conferences, and even to Richard Doll, Regius Professor of Medicine at Green College, who said he found it exciting! There is a biological need to help others; much can be preached about altruism. There must always be a supporting award system – medals, badges and certificates being publicly presented. In the end, sustaining the enterprise group was too difficult, and I sought advice from Brian Hulse, Treasurer of the Area Health Authority, and John Spencer, its Senior Administrator. They undertook a review of St John activities and suggested that St John should expand the field of community welfare linked with the Red Cross, but this was too big an undertaking. One of the points much discussed was whether we should train the public to give more voluntary support in hospitals. Mostly, we thought support was needed more in the form of professional services in the community. One consequence of this idea was the development of a toenail-cutting service. We also reckoned that, for every professional, one needed at least five volunteers on the list in support.

As Commissioner and Commander of St John Ambulance, I was leader of the voluntary paramedical services, and from there was elected to be part of the War Committee. This was a small committee composed of the Area Health Authority Medical Officer, Alec Gatherer, and me, and we met regularly to discuss how to plan for nuclear attack, particularly if and when Upper Heyford, the American air base, was threatened. Alec and I had a bunker under a house in Woodeaton, about five miles north-east of Oxford, a little like Churchill's bunker in war-time London.

As Commissioner of St John Ambulance, the voluntary organisations elected me onto the Community Health Council when these were first set up, and for four years thereby I learned the views of the consumer and worked closely with such people as Jean Robinson of the National Patient's Association, and Robert Elmore. For a while, I was in charge of the Primary Care Committee and, amongst other things, did a survey of rural transport and the needs of health centres, a precursor of contemporary 'Link' schemes. The Community Health Councils were set up throughout the UK to convert criticism of the NHS from litigation to work for improvements in the National Health Service. The appointment of an NHS and university medical consultant was probably not part of the plan. My appointment was unique.

In later years, travel for dermatology meant stopping off in places like Singapore, Australia and Fiji – and by prior appointment, I would play some role as a St John Ambulance Brigade visitor. In Australia, one experienced the gradual change from a volunteer St John Ambulance Brigade to a full-time professional one, and all the difficulties with trade unions and the loss of volunteers. In Fiji, there was the opportunity to go on a little boat for the annual tour of some of the smaller islands, for which St John Ambulance provided the only medical service.

Eventually, it was impossible to keep an eye on the Brigade in Oxfordshire at the same time as so much overseas travel for dermatology, so I resigned, having over the years collected The Order of St John and the Commander of St John, and eventually become a Knight of the Order of St John at an investiture at St James's Palace. At the investiture, I was accompanied by many of the senior supporters of charities located in many parts of the UK, and we all had to dress up as knights – a clothing ceremony which, had it been recorded on film, would have rivalled *Dad's Army* in entertainment .

Life with St John was very much like life with the Home Guard, and as Commissioner I had much sympathy with the TV show's character Mainwaring. I learned many skills, including First Aid, and used them in instructing Oxford's medical students, its university explorers, and eventually at the Royal Geographical Society's courses in London for explorers where Oxford personalities, Bent

Juel Jensen and, later, David Warrell, were in charge of preparing those who were to go on expensive and elaborate exercises. They expected to be bitten by exotic snakes and stung by spiders but that was very rare. My job was to tell them that the commonest accident befalling an expedition could be blamed on careless driving and poorly maintained vehicles.

The people one collaborated with in St John were always admirable. It was fun to work with the police and the ambulance brigades, and to go on duty at sporting events such as the Speedway, or to the theatre. The most difficult event at the New Theatre (later

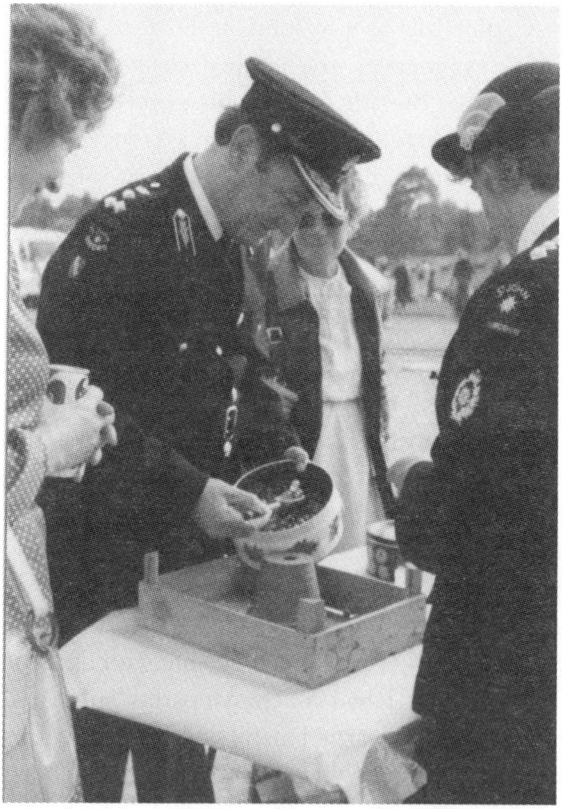

Officiating as head of St John Ambulance in Oxfordshire at one of its many public occasions

the Apollo) was the visit of the Bay City Rollers – dealing with squealing adolescent girls developing all kinds of hysterical signs.

Apart from the competitions, there were also the ceremonial occasions. Many was the time I would perform in the churches of Oxford at an initiation ceremony for cadets, but the really big parades in Christ Church Cathedral were more of a headache. They required months of planning, and with the senior hierarchy of the Brigade in attendance as well as the local Lord Lieutenant and many others, there were sometimes difficult last-minute decisions to be made. One of these was when the dons of Christ Church decided very much at the last moment that they didn't want a parade disturbing their afternoon nap. There was no way at this stage the parade could be stopped. I had to put on an act in the Bursar's office as though about to have a nervous breakdown. It was realistic enough to get the Christ Church Fellows to reverse their decision.

The St John Ambulance Band, based in Banbury, was something to be very proud of. At its best, it occupied almost 100 youngsters, and they performed at such events as the Last Post at Mons. On several occasions, they performed in the fields outside my house, before international meetings. On one occasion, the International Committee of Dermatology met under Darrell Wilkinson at Studley Priory, and the band put on a performance which was greatly enjoyed.

The story of the Brigade was, of course, preceded by the story of the Knights of St John and the Hospitallers in Jerusalem. It is a fascinating story, and on their return from the Crusades, they played a part in the life of the city of Oxford. The sense of history which the Brigade instilled in its members, and especially when thinking back to the days of Richard 'Coeur de Lion', Henry I and Henry II – it is fun to explore those origins, as they were, after all, born in Beaumont Palace, within yards of Worcester College in Beaumont Street, Oxford. There was one occasion when we came across a letter from the Order that had been based in Kidlington: they were requesting the monks of Osney to allow them to say Mass. The letter was sent to the headquarters of the diocese in Lincoln, and thence to Rome. It took two years of long distance travel before permission was given. One year, there was great excitement when we discovered an old window in the cellars of a pub in Kidlington which appeared to be the window of that original priory. It is now displayed in the St John Ambulance Headquarters in Kidlington.

One of my roles when in charge of a charity such as St John Ambulance was finding the money to buy ambulances, build new HQs or to support cadet camps. One such camp landed me with the receipt of illegal funds (see Chapter 7).

This was one of the best experiences I have enjoyed, because attempting to find ways for encouraging the young to commit themselves to voluntary effort is clearly highly desirable. The theme I developed for the Enterprise Unit never completely took off, but it took me to some high places delivering speeches on behalf of St John Ambulance.

Resignation from being head for Oxfordshire was necessary when dermatological activities became international, though I remained on the Council of The Order of St John in Oxford until 2007.

Having the skills to resuscitate, I always stopped for road accidents as well as on flights, attending to deaths on two occasions and twice being called on behalf of race horses. On some long journeys, they were carried at the back of the plane. Once it was just that an attendant wanting to swap seats to be nearer her horse. On another occasion, a young female attendant had been told to transfuse saline if her horse began to sweat. All I had to do was to open the bottle which she was failing to do. When she passed a needle through the large jugular vein in the neck, I helped her to adjust it but then wondered whether I was insured for such an activity and gave up. The horse survived.

Once, whilst on a hovercraft to Belgium with an American colleague, Professor Barnhill, the front windows blew in and there were many cuts. The unfortunate aspect of the event was that it was very cold and wet, and the return journey to Ramsgate was slow. There were no blankets so the casualties included several with hypothermia. The event was reported in *The Times*.

I have always been keen to manage hypothermia ever since sharing space in the Radcliffe Infirmary with an investigator, Keating, of the deaths when *HMS Lusitania* sank. My teaching saved an explorer who fell down a snow-covered mountain in South America as he had learned to use a thermal blanket successfully.

Combining community service in Oxfordshire with global approaches for dermatology had some benefits for both. Teaching at the training centre in Tanzania could mean breaking down barriers with a class of students from up to twelve African nations. Mixing up a team of eight to treat one of the class modelling a spinal injury was a good way of doing this. It was something learned at Stoke Mandeville from doctors treating paraplegics. The basic rudiments of care and gentleness are worth teaching to any class, even if it is an attendance expecting instruction about the skin.

Note on Chapter 8

1) Ryan, T.J. (1995), 'Caring for the wounded at Churchill's funeral', in *International Journal of Dermatology* 34: 665.

9: GREEN TEMPLETON COLLEGE: FELLOW, VICE-WARDEN AND EMERITUS

On receipt in 1979 of the invitation from Richard Doll to join the second appointed group of Fellows at the new Green College, I said yes with some enthusiasm. We met in St Anthony's and a year later moved into the college.

The appointment meant playing a part in the development of a very important building, the Observatory. Founded in 1772, linked with the idea of measuring longitude by sending Captain Cook to the South Seas, it was built first by Henry Keene and completed by James Wyatt who copied the Greek Tower of the Winds. It is recognised as very beautiful and has a well recorded astronomical history. It has measured the weather each day of its life, and continues to do so as part of the long-term European records. The Observatory is named after an important physician whose legacy was used to fund its building, and its history is linked to the accurate determination of longitude as a result of which the yard and meter became accurate units of measurement, no small contribution to science. What is insufficiently recognised is its contribution to medicine. The Regius Professor Henry Acland called upon its meteorological skills during the mid-nineteenth century to shed light on Oxford's Cholera epidemic. Much is made of the London observation that cholera is spread by water but little is made of the equally important fact – emphasised by the Observatory – that it is not spread through the air.

In the early 1930s, the Observatory functions moved to South Africa. It was then purchased for the Radcliffe Infirmary by Lord Nuffield, who believed (as did Farquher Buzzard, the Regius Professor of that time) that the future practitioners of medicine and surgery would increasingly need somewhere to do research.

Earlier chapters of this autobiography emphasised that 'humanities' in Oxford took complete preference over the 'sciences'. The purchase of this observatory was the beginning of a transformation, culminating ultimately in Oxford's world leadership in scientific medicine. Nuffield first thought it would house clinical research but clinicians considered the building impracticable for inpatient care. Eventually it became the Nuffield Institute of Medical Research. This Institute founded Neonatology and Cineradiology – two branches of medicine of no immediate interest to the physicians of what was then a small county hospital. Lord Nuffield followed this up by founding the Academic Centre of Clinical Medicine but then World War II broke out, and within two weeks it became a standard clinical medical school, accepting students from the London hospitals which had previously taken Oxford students for their clinical training. After the war, when I entered the Medical School, one of the first books I was given to read from my tutor's library was by the Spanish surgeon Joseph Trueta, who used the Observatory to study the vascular response of the kidneys to crush injury. The Observatory was the only place a clinician could find the facilities to do such research, and Trueta was not the only clinician to visit it.

Even in 1953, when I was president of the medical students, our journal, *The Medical School Gazette*, was a main publisher of a debate about the future. As a custodian of sports, social events and pantomimes, as well as being well satisfied with our teachers and not yet too focused on their scientific research, my notes on the debate at that time suggest we were happy just to be good clinicians, and to leave the science advancement to the then distinguished groups in the pre-clinical laboratories and the Institute in the Radcliffe Observatory. There were budding Nobel Prize winners in both. I had no expectations of being a researcher until several more years were to pass (Appendix 1).

Knowing the 'Tower of the Winds' when it was the Nuffield Institute of Medical Research, I wrote about that Institute in the book *Tower of the Winds*.[1] It is an important tale of excellent medical research into the two specialities: foetal physiology and cine radiology. Over a 40-year period, the foetal studies were on pregnant sheep which had to be encouraged up the stairs into the main laboratory. Much of the technology developed was later of great value to cardio-vascular research and cine-radiology, the first on any internal organ that moved, which was to lay the foundation for many of the technologies now underlying cardiac and intestinal investigative studies. It generated some unusual stories, such as the keeping of a Cayman crocodile in a bath by the radiologists to study swallowing while some believed it was there to prevent the neonatal experts from taking the space; and studies on the sword swallower from St Giles' Fair, requiring a secretary to stand on three volumes and pass the sword while his arms were kept out of the way. Some of those who worked in the Observatory during that period were disappointed that in an effort to make it readable by the lay person, the book published by Green College describing the Observatory in a chapter by Loudon and me, had too little detail on the scientific advances made therein. George Cherry, while in the Dermatology Department, collaborated on some vascular studies on wound repair, using Cineradiology.

Later, when I was on the Medicine Board, the decision made after the retirement of the Director Geoffrey Dawes[2] was a difficult one: to keep the Institute going was too expensive, and the remaining workers were redistributed. This was after 40 years of outstanding research which for a long time was the only site of the new scientific look to Oxford medicine.

Besides the Tower of the Winds, the Observer's house, linked with the Observatory in the 1950s, 60s and 70s, was the home of the student body of Osler House, and for several years we used what is now the Principal's office. When Green College was founded, there was a student rebellion, supported by some of their senior staff. Shifting the students up to the John Radcliffe was not a comfortable process but it was part of the new look of the Medical School. Green College was to be a stimulus to the other Oxford colleges to take more seriously the training of their medical students, while preserving some of the characteristics of the university approach to teaching such as the tutorial system and the excellent dining.

The jobs handed to me included setting up, with the surgeon Mannie Lee, an exhibition of paintings by Louis Turpin, the Rye flower painter, as the first use of the gallery which the Art committee developed for the college. Other jobs were to help to set up the Common Room Committee and the Music Society. The Doll's piano had belonged to a pupil of Clara Schumann. There was also the task of buying a billiard table. Because many people were giving the college wall decorations we did not really want, I suggested we had an Art and Décor Committee to help us to refuse some items. Joan Doll was on it, and as she had largely been responsible for the college décor, she was a dominant opinion. Anne and I admired Sir Richard and Lady Doll, but with the latter's very strong personality, such respect included an element of fear.[3]

Later, when it was decided that the Warden's wife should always fill this role, it was Betty Walton who should have succeeded her. Richard wrote and asked for Joan to stay on and, rather daringly, I wrote and said no.

For the 200th anniversary of the Observatory it was my job to celebrate the event with a noon mark designed by the well-known sundial maker, Christopher Daniel. It was a celebration of observations on the sun.

The college put aside £10,000 to buy 750 pieces of cutlery, silver-plated and crested. In the vaults of London, only £2,000 was spent, and it was fun organising a competition for a silver centrepiece for a dining room table. Rod Kelly from Norfolk designed an octagonal bowl on the theme of the Greek winds. It was to win many prizes.

When the college began to receive requests for donations to the Ashmolean, the Natural History Museum and various Oxford charities, I launched a Charities Committee to raise money for that specific purpose and for the college hardship fund.

Richard Doll invited as an Honorary Fellow the American Lawrence P. Bachmann with Bettina, his wife, with whom we became great friends; we invited Bettina onto the Charity Committee. Larry, as he was known to us all, was born 12th December 1911 in Los Angeles. He began his career as a student of English Literature and

Psychology at the University of Southern California, and obtained his BA in 1932. He was attracted by medicine but diverted to psychiatry under the supervision of Dr Aaron J. Rosanoff, whose writings for the US Army Medical Corps in World War I and from the very large New York State Mental Institute included the first study of monozygotic twins in the aetiology of schizophrenia. Larry was with him during his development of insulin shock therapy.

During World War II, Larry was a Lt Colonel in the USAAF, and wrote a book from the USAAF Aero Medical Research Laboratories entitled *Physiological Aspects of Flying*, and a cartoon book for less educated airmen, *Your Body in Flight.* From 1942 to 1945, he acted as an overseas correspondent and consultant psychologist to the Air Force in the Pacific Region, China, India and Burma. Much of his later years were spent to Oxford's benefit as he was on the Vice-Chancellor's Appeals and Income Generating Committee. He brought film and theatre celebrities to St Catherine's College which made him an Honorary Fellow. As a good tennis player and member of The All-England Tennis Club, he helped Oxford University to upgrade its tennis and was awarded for this by the university.

Always a keen writer, Larry wrote and worked on the filming of the TV soap, *Dr Kildare*, studying hospital practice and people, and making many lifelong friends who later achieved great distinction. This entry into the film business, beginning in Hollywood, 1933-35, and employment with MGM, 1936-42, also introduced him to the Hollywood environment and film friends.[4]

At the end of World War II, he was appointed to the State Department in Berlin, and as European Director for MGM, had much to do with the restoration of the German film industry. He then spent a decade in London as an executive film producer with Paramount, making such films as *The Village of the Damned* and the Agatha Christie series with Margaret Rutherford as Miss Marple, as well as a *BBC* film series, in 39 parts, *Zero One.* His last film *Whose Life Is It Anyway?* (1982) was with Tom Conti, but he continued to be interested in the education of the public in science and worked on the script of *The Double Helix.*

Larry was introduced to Green College by Sir Richard Doll in 1982, and it became his greatest love. He was disappointed that they valued him rather less than St Catherine's. But he brought in his friends, such as the script writer, John Briley of *Gandhi* and *Cry Freedom*, and organised previews for the college. He reintroduced Hitchcock's *Rear Window* specially for the college after years of only limited distribution. He married the millionairess Bettina Hart, and took pride in her hobby of purchasing neglected historic houses and modernising them. The *Daily Telegraph* wrote of Villa Rosetta, the King of Rome's residence in Umbria 'in shocking pinks, bright orange and sludge green' with stagey props. These houses included one of the oldest in the Île de la Cité in Paris, and the Manor House in Great Haseley, near Oxford. Bettina's design for London Bridge was short-listed in the competition won by Lord Foster. She and Larry were MGM people and this could have been a problem when elected to membership of Green College's fund-raising committee. There was an alarming plan for fund-raising at Green College that included her designs for conversion of the college gardens into a one-night MGM-like set which had to be tactfully declined. They wanted to spend $100,000 to raise much more. The procedure was to convert the college into a Hollywood film set and invite top media people. We had doubts whether they would accept.

When Larry eventually decided to retire to the MGM nursing home, he left his library to Green College. He did not make it clear that he had also told Sothebys to take the best books, and family members to take others. Finally, I was given two hours to take what I thought would be worth having. Lord Walton had just moved out of the Osler Library at Norham Gardens, and I measured the shelves and guessed I needed 700 books. I was only out by ten books. I took those concerning post-war American and German history plus much on the media. After three years in the Osler Library, they are now deposited with the Reuter Foundation.

Bettina died two years before Larry in a palatial MGM nursing suite in Hollywood, but Larry was critical of this MGM's well-endowed old peoples home in which she lived because he missed Oxford's intellectual stimulus. He had however begun a script to film the home's inhabitants 50 years or so after their peak performances.

We had many good times with the Bachmanns and a very enjoyable few days in their 'King of Italy House' in Italy. It too had lost some of its eighteenth century character through being given décor more attuned to a Hollywood film set.

After the retirement of the founding Warden, John Walton was appointed.[5] He could not join us for a year, so Trevor Hughes was acting Warden, He was a distinguished neuropathologist, and as an historian, he wrote a biography of the first neurologist, Thomas Willis. He has also written his own autobiography.

In 1984, Green College was five years old and many new projects needed funding. As President of the successful World Microcirculation Congress held in Oxford, some profits could be given to the college. The Japanese contingent to the Congress was large and was led by a microcirculation friend of mine, Professor Tsuchiya Dean of Keio University.

There appeared on the scene Dr Mike Natori, a short young man with a pointed beard, who claimed to be in a position to negotiate a transfer of large funds from Japan to the college. His personal contacts were with the Chairman of the Japan Shipbuilding Industry Foundation. This company wished to establish in Oxford a centre concerned with the consequences of unemployment, work practices, social and health matters. Green College was seen as a potential partner. Within a few weeks, Dr Natori came forward with another potential partner: the *Mitsubishi* conglomerate. I wrote to ask Professor Tsuchiya to confirm the credentials of Dr Natori, since some in Oxford University, including a Japanese colleague in the Department of Dermatology, Dr Mikio Masuzawa, wondered whether Dr Natori was all he claimed. Prof Tsuchiya replied: 'He is one of the most reliable Japanese in England.' During October 1984, it was proposed to transfer to Green College $200,000 for a 1985 symposium on 'stable employment and healthy life'. John Walton wrote to find out more from the Registrar of Oxford University, a message which crossed with one from me, expressing slight anxiety. He added a footnote: 'We are treading very warily.'

Dr Yuziro Shinoda, President of the Japan Shipbuilding Industry Foundation wrote, saying $100,000 was committed and that both he and Chairman Sasagawa would attend. Natori now proposed a new institute and fellowship at Green College, funded up to £1.5 million.

The Warden wrote on 9th November 1984 to Dr Shinoda about the proposed symposium, now entitled 'Employment in a Changing Society'. He added a PS, stating that the Vice-Chancellor had shown him a letter sent by Dr Shinoda to Dr Natori, stating that he should be aware that all overseas projects were managed by the son of Mr Sasagawa, and that support was determined by a committee and were subject to government approval. 'The part I wish you to especially understand is that our personal friendship has no relevance to this Foundation. Therefore I expect you to take upmost care in all your dealings with this Foundation.'

The Warden, now John Walton, then requested clarification from Dr Shinoda and received a letter in reply from the Japan Shipbuilding Industry Foundation dated 22nd November, denying that Dr Shinoda had written any letter or made any commitment for a symposium. Dr Natori then visited the Bank of Yokohama in London and invited the Presidents and Senior Executives to the Symposium in an invitation apparently from the Warden of Green College.

On 30th November, Dr Natori asked me to give him three weeks to sort out the confusion 'which is a consequence of the Japanese social system, a totally different cultural system'. He wrote, or purported to write, to Mr Sasagawa, saying that he should write to the Warden of Green College with a commitment or risk being reported to the Japanese Minister of Transportation – his reputation would be hurt in Britain and in the United States.

On 4th December, Professor Tsuchiya wrote: 'I am very sorry to say that he has proved to be dangerous person and actually has become notorious as an impostor in Japan in the past.'

Dr Natori's last letter in January 1984 declared that 'opponents of Professor Tsuchiya are questioning his handling of funding for the next world congress, and that there is no commitment by Japanese Government to support Professor Tsuchiya. I feel

Professor Tsuchiya is too emotional and chicken in many ways'. So that was the end of that fund-raising exercise.

After retirement as Warden, John Walton – now Lord Walton – as an admirer of Sir William Osler,[6] focused on upgrading the home of the Oslers at 13 Norham Gardens. He used Osler's library as his office and, with his wife Betty, had a first-floor flat there. He created the 'Friends of 13 Norham Gardens', on which the historian Alastair Robb-Smith and I served and then began the fund-raising necessary for refurbishment by obtaining donations, especially from the UK, USA and Japan. He handed over the Friends to me to make more of the story of the 'Open Arms' household of Sir William Osler, and to arrange archiving of the files collected by Robb-Smith, which Rosemary Fitzherbert Jones later carefully annotated. I learned that there was international enthusiasm for hearing more about the history of Oxford in the twentieth century. With the help of the Royal College of Physicians and many friends, it was possible to furnish the ground floor with furniture that had once been in 13 Norham Gardens. In 2017, I arranged a loan of a chest belonging to Paul Revere, the American patriot which had been in the hall as a belonging of Grace Osler, a descendant of Paul Revere. Eventually the library was filled with sufficient appropriate books to be called 'Public Health before and after William Osler'.

One of the pleasures of being a member of Green College was Betty Walton's support of musical activities. Depending on the year's admissions, there would sometimes be a great choir and at other times great soloists.

The third warden was Sir Crispin Tickell, Ambassador to the United Nations, who appointed me his Vice-Warden. We hoped that his profile would make Green College better known. Once he got used to calling himself Warden of Green College in his very many public speeches, he probably did do that. It meant, however, that he was very often absent so the Vice-Warden was kept very busy. I enjoyed making him attend to college needs, including answering a letter of complaint from a woman who objected to condom dispensers in the toilets. Crispin wanted a distinguished advisory board. For a while, Princess Anne would sit on discussions about the future of education. There were several visits from Parliament and the ambassadors of the Court of St James. Mrs Thatcher was one visitor. One problem was that the main rooms for meeting visitors, such as the dining room in the Observatory, had appalling acoustics.

Eventually his successor had to be found, and it was my job as Vice-Warden to do that. It was a very interesting exercise with 60 applicants and six short-listed. Eventually, we chose the head of the British Council, Sir John Hanson.

Coming to retirement age and with the college approaching its 25th year, I offered to begin to set up a college alumni association, and at the same time to look at the need of a medical faculty alumni association. It then became common knowledge that the Oxford Medical Graduates Club (OMGC), chaired by John Ledingham, was thinking of folding up. It was set up in the nineteenth century for medical students to join after their BA degree, when they went to London hospitals and wanted to revisit Oxford in a medical capacity. Most students in 1990 were now staying on at the John Radcliffe Infirmary.

At that time, it was noted that Oxford's Medical Faculty had no alumni – possibly the only medical school without an alumni association. It was the business needs of the graduates of the Said Business School which broke the college opposition to the concept of faculty alumni. Most important of all was the need of the New Sciences Division to answer the question: 'Where are all the people you have been associated with and what are they now doing?' This fitted in with the desires of several of us to commit history to writing before it is forgotten, and perhaps set up a system which rewards a few people that have done well, unknown to those who taught them. Some inspiration came to me from being a professor at Oxford Brookes University where alumni activity seemed more in evidence, but especially from experiencing monthly the pressures, enthusiasm and fund-raising ethos of Jefferson Medical College in Philadelphia which keeps its adjunct professors in touch – so totally different from Oxford. All Jefferson's faculty – past present and possibly future – receive a colourful alumni magazine which does not let them forget that they are wonderful people. Even the parents of potential students are not ignored by some establishments in the USA. Many, even across the Atlantic, receive the minutes of faculty meetings.

My researches into what was known of past students with successful careers took me to the Oxford Development Office, where it was shocking to find that, in the year of celebrating the new millennium, they had almost no knowledge of the history of the contributions of Oxford medical graduates. Robb-Smith had written about female medical graduates. A rather feeble attempt to encourage legacies by the Development Office included alumni of the seventeenth century, and they had on their list the deceased Nobel Prize winner Dorothy Hodgkin. They had not registered Richard Doll or William Osler, but were celebrating Edwina Currie, a not very popular MP, and Rowan Atkinson, a comedian.

Pursuing the idea of faculty alumni, one found that the Music School had something similar for playing string quartets together. There was also a Bridge alumni, independent of the colleges. Most significant of all, the new Business School wanted to keep in touch with its alumni. John Ledingham and I therefore set up the Oxford Medical Alumni (OMA). My intention was that it should focus on celebrating its past members, whilst hoping that this would, in time, bring in legacies. Chairmen should not be in post for too long, so Jim Holt, a physician, took over from me after three years, and he handed over to Derek Jewell, a gastroenterologist, who handed over to Peggy Frith, who handed over to John Morris, the first chairman from the university science laboratories. Colleges kept in touch with their students but faculties did not. The OMGC was one of the few faculty links with past members, but by 2000, as most students now stayed on at Oxford to learn their clinical medicine, it was becoming obsolete. Even its Treasurer was 100 years old. The stimulus of finding that there was a lack of personal reminiscences about the last 50 years, and little celebration of graduates of that same period, encouraged a few of us to seek a remedy. There were some very important omissions. Thus the Nuffield Institute of Medicine's contributions to understanding how the foetus survived birth and all aspects of cine radiology were uncelebrated and unknown. Eric Sidebottom focused on the history of the William Dunn School of Pathology, and has described the role of the pathologist Ritchie in founding his specialty. The *Oxford Medical School Gazette* has been encouraged to record more of Oxford's recent medical history. Two voluntary curators of 13 Norham Gardens, Max Blythe and David Cranston, have written biographies of significant Oxford alumni.[7]

There was clearly a need to celebrate achievement and to do much more about advocacy. Staying with an obstetrician friend who lived in a fine house in Melton, Suffolk, I strolled across the road to the church and found a plaque commemorating the deaths in the trenches of two of the sons of Sir Archibald Garrod who succeeded Osler as Regius Professor of Medicine, and soon after these were followed by the death of another son. Following this up, it was clear that my friend's house was the unmarked home of this famous Regius Professor. My former wine tasting colleague, Norman Heatley,[7] who brought so much technical expertise to the Oxford penicillin story, was born and left for university from an unmarked house nearby in Suffolk at a time when Sir Archibald could have discussed the young man's career with his locally celebrated father. It is these small pieces of history that Oxford had missed out on by not having an alumni system that was keen to record, advocate and award, or sometimes to rebuke. Until recently, Oxford, unlike London, has not done much to place blue plaques on the buildings in which its famous scientists have lived. I arranged for a blue plaque to be placed on the birthplace of Norman Heatley in Suffolk. Later, the urology surgeon, David Cranston, and Eric Sidebottom wrote his biography.

While John Hanson was Warden of Green College, he looked carefully at 13 Norham Gardens which the college rented. It was the first Victorian house to be built in Norham Gardens, and some very famous medical names had lived there: John Conybeare, Sir William Osler, Sir George Pickering, Sir Richard Doll and Lord Walton. It was currently owned by the university and housed the Reuter Foundation and the Newcomers Club. My wife Anne chaired the latter which aimed at looking after the partners of visiting academics. Eventually, the Newcomers Club was moved by the university to the Graduates Club, and Green College was in 1983 introduced to John McGovern, a past President of The American Osler Society, a philanthropist, to help it to refurbish parts of the house urgently needing attention.

The extraordinary metamorphosis of the Science Area and the Clinical School into a single Sciences Division was also about to take place.

Oxford Medical Alumni (OMA) was launched largely by me, with John Ledingham as President and Eric Sidebottom as Secretary. We began by organising reunions in Oxford and New York. In the latter we were helped by Professor Donald Chambers, an Honorary Visiting Fellow who combined running a big biochemistry, molecular biology and immunopathology department in Chicago with being an active supporter of the Oxford Medical School and of Green College, as well as being an admirer of Sir William Osler. His support included an informal initiating of the link between Green College and Templeton College and setting into motion the donation from the USA of a million dollars to buy 13 Norham Gardens and create an Osler McGovern Centre, as well as forging a collaboration between Green College, the University of Illinois and the New York Academy of Sciences[8] to celebrate the 40th anniversary of the discovery of the double helix. For several years the College Handbook acknowledged this link with Illinois as especially providing some of its most valued students. Donald Chambers also has an unusual perspective of history that causes him always to celebrate Thanksgiving Day in Oxford. In my earlier days, we had some common scientific interests, as well as sharing some heretical views on the links between Green College and the rest of the world. The link with the Americas remains one of Oxford's principal stimuli; it is well over a century old, and if we develop our alumni link, it can be based not on the need to progress together but focus a little more on nostalgia.

Does anyone want to be kept in touch with the Faculty of Medicine or its amalgam of the centre of excellences from South

Parks Road and the hospitals? It should be remembered that few of the clinical faculty are appointed to colleges, so that contact by alumni with Oxford by Oxonian medics cannot be relied upon. OMA welcomes all who have researched or taught in its hospitals, but a reliance on college attachments can be for only a minority.

Having been given the interest of 13 Norham Gardens, it was necessary to work to make more of it. In 2015, we invited the American Osler Society and the Japanese Osler Society to spend a week in Oxford. With the help of Dr John Ward (a much admired Abingdon Family Practitioner and member of both the London Osler Club and American Osler Society) and his wife Ruth, we set up a very special week of Osler celebrations.

Most of the time that my wife and I were active at Green College we were living in Iffley Village, in a fine glass-fronted double-storey house, overlooking a garden designed by Katherine Shock. It had an area of sunken garden from a swimming bath we did not want. Even though it was quite small, it had mystery walks. There was a marvellous Japanese azalea surrounded by Zen-like pebbles and several sculptures by the Thompsons of north Oxfordshire. It was often rated the best garden in the annual Open Day, but I cheated and only opened it on the day if it was looking good, rather than advertising it in advance and risking failure.

In retirement I kept an interest in preserving, through Green Templeton's ownership of the Radcliffe Observatory and 13 Norham Gardens, Oxford's Institutional Memory of the transformation that made it a world leader of the medical sciences, with great advances in clinical research starting in the observatory with the Nuffield Institute of Medical Research. In 13 Norham Gardens there lived William Osler telling the world how the best practice of medicine requires the best possible attitude; George Pickering influencing medical education and preaching one of Oxford's oldest adages, 'Manners Maketh Man'; Richard Doll explaining how epidemiology reveals the causes of disease; and John Walton in the House of Lords adding to Hansard hundreds of speeches on creating the legal basis of the ethics of modern medicine. Keeping my office in 13 Norham Gardens with the help of many organisations interested in its history, I have made it an exciting place to visit for those interested in the history of medicine.

Notes on Chapter 9

1) Loudon, I. and Burley, J.T. (2005), 'The Observatory and the Nuffield Institute for Medical Research' in *The Tower of the Winds: A Biography of an Observatory*. Published by Green College (2005), 134-44.

2) Obituary (1998) Geoffrey Sharman Dawes, 1918-96 by Sir Graham Liggins. Biog. Mems. Fell. Roy. Soc. Lond., 44, 109-25.

3) Keating, Conrad (2009), *Smoking Kills: The Revolutionary Life of Richard Doll*. Oxford, Signal Books Ltd.

4) Larry Bachmann wrote six novels and several of these were published in English, French and German, while several were made into films: *Death in the Doll's House* (1943), *The Kiss of Death* (1950), *The Valley of the Kings* (1956), *The Lorelei* (1957), *The Bitter Lake* (1958), *Letters of Joseph Nokato* (1971). *The Ultimate Act* (1972). These were generally well reviewed in the USA and UK.

Best Sellers reviewed *The Bitter Lake* as follows: 'Superb! The author brings to his craft elements of suspense, character, growth, good writing. He is to be congratulated and the book is highly recommended. He writes with a deep understanding which argues for a long life with us as a fine writer.'

5) Walton, John (1993), *The Spice of Life*. Royal Society of Medicine.

6) Bliss, M. (1999) *William Osler: A Life in Medicine*. Oxford University Press.

7) Cranston, David (2017), *William Osler and His Legacy to Medicine*. Bicester, Words by Design.

Cranston, David, and Sidebottom, Eric (2016), *Penicillin and the Legacy of Norman Heatley*, Bicester, Words by Design.

Cranston, David (2015), *John Radcliffe and His Legacy to Oxford*. Bicester, Words by Design.

Blythe, Max (2017), *Pioneering Physician: The Life of Charles Fletcher*. Bicester, Words by Design.

8) Don Chambers conceived, organised and chaired a 'landmark meeting' for the New York Academy of Sciences in conjunction with Oxford and UIC, celebrating the 40th anniversary of the elucidation of the double helical structure of DNA, the proceedings of which were published in 1995 by the New York Academy of Sciences Press: *DNA, the Double Helix, Perspective and Prospective at Forty Years*, edited by D.A. Chambers.

10: Dermatology's Public Health Agenda: Africa, Guatemala and China

British Dermatology – A Service under Threat

Throughout my career, the ability of a dermatologist to provide a service that the public needs has been curtailed by lack of finance. While I was a junior in the service, Darrell Wilkinson, the Amersham dermatologist, was arguing for more time to be made available so that every patient could have a consultation of adequate length.

It was not until I was appointed in 1992 as President of the British Association of Dermatology that it became my job to do something about the fact that the service was getting worse rather than better. During that year, my contributions included preparing a position document,[1] boosting the dermatology nursing profession, controlling the habit of GPs seeking advice from retired dermatologists who were not keeping up-to-date, and building and displaying a model dermatology building. It was necessary to maintain full commitment to an assault against the ever-present affliction of skin disease and the stigma with which it is so closely associated. About 10% of consultations in general practice are skin-related, but three quarters of skin conditions, diseases or trauma are not seen by a doctor. In any week, 3% of the population will have a skin complaint, and those so affected are mostly children or the elderly. In the year of my presidency, 33% of 800 practice nurses were seeing up to ten patients per week, and only 7% had the knowledge to deal with them. The tale for pharmacists was somewhat more troublesome.

The UK's record of long waiting lists and short consultation times was and still is dismal. The Ministry of Health tends to believe that the nation's skin disease needs only a small specialty. The size of the problem – the increase in skin malignancies as the population over 70 greatly increases, the control of common skin diseases such as eczema, acne and psoriasis by increasingly difficult-to-manage therapies, and a recognition that to look good is a part of well-being contributing to health – all demand improvements in the service.

Medical schools give insufficient time to the teaching of dermatology, and most family practitioners have had no training for what is the commonest organ they are consulted about. The ratio of dermatologist to patient in the UK bears no comparison with most European countries, and many cities in the USA have more dermatologists than the whole of the UK.

In my year as President of the British Association of Dermatology, I had to deal with an increase in the demand of family practitioners for dermatologists to leave their hospital practice and visit the community. This, of course, meant longer hospital waiting lists, less teaching of medical students and less supervision and encouragement of trainees. My diatribe publicising the problem continued: 'Serious diseases remain undiagnosed for an unacceptable length of time, and severe discomfort is left untreated, harmless and common skin lesions are treated inappropriately, expensively, and with risk of preventable side effects.' The government was not sympathetic, and on top of demands that dermatologists should do more outreach clinics, they were expecting them to be on call over the weekends for general medical emergencies. It would leave little time for the reading that dermatologists are usually good at in order to keep up-to-date with pathophysiology and new interventions.

Three priorities of my presidency were to demonstrate the role of the skin in *achieving*, the need of anyone whose skin is *failing*, and how to make the available service *caring*. It was my job to emphasise that there were many successes to celebrate, such as acne research in Leeds, melanoma studies in Scotland, pharmacology at the Institute of Dermatology in London, much sowing of seeds for advances in wound healing, and in the understanding of molecular biology and genetics. There were new buildings and 15 chairs of dermatology.

DERMATOLOGY - A SERVICE UNDER THREAT

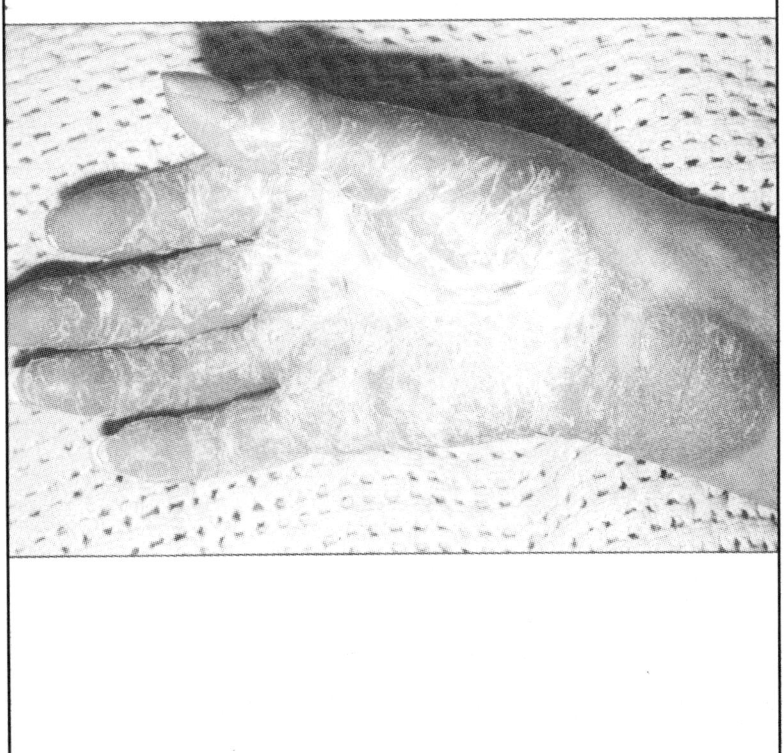

A position document for the
British Association of Dermatologists

The front cover I produced for public examination to explain the many difficulties besetting the Profession of Dermatology during 1992, the year that I was President of the British Association of Dermatology

The aims were that anyone with a skin problem should have access to expertise, and the provision of more education at all levels, as well as more funding of research.

The International Foundation of Dermatology in Africa

The great step forward having been taken by the International Committee of Dermatology (ICD) in 1987 by creating the International Foundation for Dermatology (IFD), it was ambitious then to carry out its list of objectives. These were based on a case of need, much influenced by three workshops on Dermatology in Basic Health Services, organised by Henning Grossmann, in Berlin 1987, in Mexico in 1993, and by myself in Oxford in 1988.

In the first five years of the IFD, its parent body, the ICD, initiated official relations with WHO, helped by work done on the 'Essential Drugs List', and by the UNESCO document UNIDERM prepared in 1991, which described what needed to be done if a

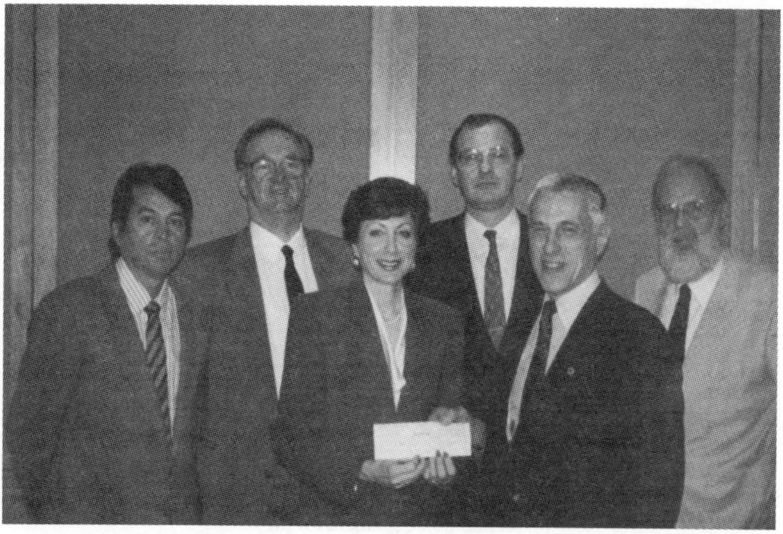

Henning Grossman (far right), first Director of the Regional Dermatology Training Centre in Tanzania; Erwin Blandon, Chairman of the Training Centre in Guatemala (far left); and Al Kopf, Chairman of the International Foundation of Dermatology while he receives a donation of £10,000 from each of two members of the pharmaceutical industry.

public health agenda were to be developed by dermatologists.[2] Within five years, the Board of the IFD was able to announce that almost all the proposals had been initiated. Most credit must go to the Chairman of the IFD, Al Kopf, and the directors of the training centres, Henning Grossmann and Erwin Blandon.

During the first 20 years of the IFD, what is described below was in fact achieved, under a new heading widely adopted from the WHO programme named 'Healthy Skin for All'.

Members of the International League of Dermatological Societies have produced valuable data and publications on the interventions required, but these have relied on a few individuals and have not been adopted by all dermatologists.

Tanzania

At the first sessions of the IFD, it was decided to focus first on Africa – a continent with, in our view, the greatest needs. Visits to embassies in London organised by the dermatologist Francisco Kerdel Vegas, as Ambassador from Venezuela, resulted in the choice of Tanzania for a site visit. There were a number of reasons for this. It was easy to travel to, had a high level of literacy, the much-admired German dermatologist Henning Grossmann was based there, and one of Africa's few skilled dermatologists, Aaron Massawe, a Tanzanian, was keen to act as host. The achievements in Africa which followed our initiative included building a training centre (overlooked by Mount Kilimanjaro in northern Tanzania) complete with outpatient and treatment facilities, teaching rooms and faculty offices. There is a comfortable hostel for 28 students, three blocks of married accommodation for faculty, and a substantial dermatology ward. There is a centre for persons affected by albinism and a block for pathology. There has been curriculum development, and after a decade, its evaluation. It is a pan-African programme to provide more than twelve English-speaking nations with dermatology practitioners, programme organisers, advisers to governments and to universities, as well as contributions to leadership of national programmes such as HIV/AIDS and leprosy.

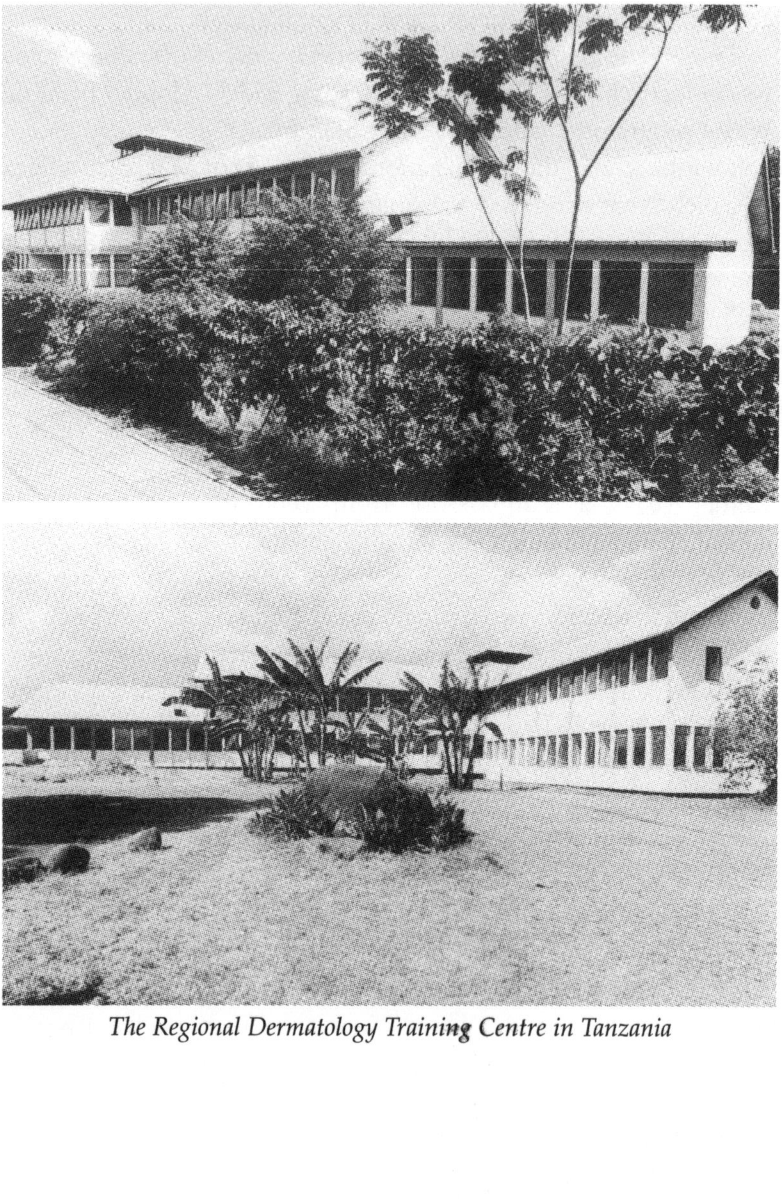

The Regional Dermatology Training Centre in Tanzania

For someone such as myself, not expert at fund-raising, this was a difficult exercise. From the beginning, we had to raise stipends for students, enabling – by the time this autobiography is read – about 300 students to receive training for a two-year period. Much of this was raised from national dermatology associations, but industry, leprosy charities and some government programmes were successfully petitioned.

Even before the International Foundation for Dermatology was founded, Darrell Wilkinson discussed the need to have some initial funds. He set up a bank account and appealed to friends. We raised £1,600 in the UK before the project was launched. Fund-raising was an issue even at the first board meeting in Berlin, at which Al Kopf (USA) was elected Chairman, Stuart Maddin as Secretary, and Hans Rorsman (Norway) as Treasurer.

On 15th December 1987, Al Kopf wrote to all members of the International Committee, asking for donations to cover the cost ($3,000) of incorporation in the state of Illinois, with submission of documents to make the IFD tax-exempt, and to set up book-keeping with Dermatology Services Inc., an organisation servicing the American Academy of Dermatology based in the USA. The members of the committee paid up, but since they all paid for their own travel and that of their wives to board meetings, several believed they were already paying enough. Indeed, most of the numerous overseas trips, often made with Anne, were self-funded. Some ICD members from poorer countries or from behind the Iron Curtain were not allowed by their governments to pay up. Richard Blake of *Hamilton Laboratories* in Australia (husband of a bridesmaid at our wedding) made the first donation from industry. *Beechams* responded to Stuart Maddin (Canada) with a grant of $20,000, while Al Kligman donated $7,500. Helped by Francisco Kerdel Vegas, as ambassador to UNESCO, I obtained a grant from that organisation of $25,000 in 1991. The fly laboratory for larva therapy of septic wounds was financed by John Church, the High Wycombe orthopaedic surgeon.

There were efforts year after year to make the centre self-supporting and sufficiently financed by the government of

Tanzania and the University of Tumaini in northern Tanzania. Money came in from many directions and sometimes purchased and delivered goods on the way. My department in Oxford was one route, and the Regional Dermatology Training Centres (RDTCs) often received both goods and money direct. Al Kopf insisted that all purchases and receipts were made known to him, and preferred no other route be used than through the American bank, something that did not suit the German funding agency of Henning Grossmann, nor the St Francis Leprosy organisations, nor the BAD, three of the most substantial donors. Many of the scholarships were paid directly to the RDTC. Some sums went into the International League of Dermatology Societies (ILDS) account. Often we were spending before promises materialised. Some of the biggest promises, such as the 61 million Lira from the Italian Rotary in the year 2000, hardly materialised at all. LEPRA in 1989 promised £10,000 per annum for three years but had to withdraw in the second and third year because of their financial difficulties.

Al Kopf and Stuart Maddin were unrestrained askers for money. None of us received as good a response as our expectations. Board meetings were difficult because successive treasurers questioned the competence of myself and Stuart Maddin, the Secretary-General of the IFD. We were driving a programme before being assured of its finance and effectiveness. Several of the Board did little work for the IFD, and did not pay much attention to the volumes of information that we sent to them. Of the various Presidents of the ILDS with whom I worked, Klaus Wolff from Austria was the most generous in thanks to those who worked hard for the project. By 1996 we had raised $1,780,134.

A fund-raising letter was prepared for National Societies but, as explained by Takeji Nishikawa on behalf of the Japanese national societies who were already contributing substantial dues to the ICD/ILDS, further dues needed much explanation and persuasion. Klaus Wolff, as President of the ILDS starting this initiative, secured donations from the Austrian Society of Dermatology. The British Association of Dermatology and the American Academy of

Dermatology followed suit, and Al Kopf obtained a recurring grant from the American Dermatology Association. Expenses included legal fees for an elaborate but unsuccessful attempt, employing the lawyer Geoff Haley, to get money out of the European Commission and for curriculum development workshops in Nairobi and Tanzania. Money had to be raised for buildings for which at least $460,000 was budgeted in 1990. Nine pharmaceutical industries contributed but none gave more than $10,000 for buildings and scholarships. My own Dermatology Department in Oxford and Al Kopf's office at New York University, and in his private practice on the top floor of the Empire State Building, paid for postage and secretarial help which was not a small amount. Writing, publishing and distributing 16,000 copies of *Healthy Skin for All* cost the Oxford department £20,000. This was not NHS money but research funds earned from multiple sources. It had been envisaged that the home nation of each student would provide the funding for scholarships which were needed for each of a two-year training period. Initially, the East Central African Commonwealth Community and the German government provided scholarships, but by the second intake it became necessary to find other sponsors. Some paid up in advance for two years, some for much longer.

Al Kopf set up a $500 club to pay for the Training Centre. By 1997, it had produced $20,000 but this was insufficient funding and therefore Al Kopf founded the $1,000 Club, appealing to his many friends to add $1,000 each to the Endowment Fund.

In 2002, the Tanzanian Head of Nursing of the main hospital asked for a new minibus to assist training in villages for education on the topic of Female Genital Mutilation. Anne, my wife, was given this job and succeeded in raising the money.

In 2000 I wrote once again to every national dermatology society, requesting $7,000 per annum as a scholarship. Each student thus supported was identified and was encouraged to write a letter of thanks. 20,000 individual leaflets about the IFD were distributed to as many dermatologists as possible. A few, like Gunther Burg in Switzerland, worked very hard and effectively on fund-raising. He provided a telemedicine link between Switzerland and Tanzania for histopathology. Jose Mascaro (Spain) and, later, Benvenuto Giannotti (Italy) held fund-raising seminars in Athens and Florence at which all ICD members spoke. Michael Waugh of the International Union for Sexually Transmitted Infections also provided much support, especially through finding salaries for teachers in the field. The British Association of Dermatology was very supportive, providing substantial funding for faculty. Barbara Leppard, a British dermatologist of inestimable value as a teacher, organised a 'James Fund' to part-cover her salary at the RDTC, where she was an exceptionally fine teacher. However, after a few years she developed an irregular heart beat which we had to get treated in Nairobi. When it recurred several times, I made the difficult decision that she should return to the UK.

The Herzog Foundation in the USA, through its chairman Peter Bentley, was the largest donor. Because he was a donor to their departments in the USA, only John Strauss and Steve Katz who headed these departments were allowed to negotiate with him. His gifts were of $150,000 for furnishings, $112,000 for a road between the RDTC and the doctors' compound, and eventually the gift of $600,000 for the Endowment Fund which was made up to a million dollars by a surplus from the World Congress of Dermatology in Paris. The RDTC was designated in 1998 a WHO-Collaborating Centre for Dermatology, Sexually Transmitted Infections and Leprosy, and its students needed leprosy experience as they were examined on this topic. My role became that of raising funds from leprosy sources. As adviser to the St Francis Leprosy Guild, a Catholic charity founded in the late nineteenth century, I received great support, including a *Land Rover*, our first vehicle in Tanzania, which was still on the road 20 years later. Some years the Guild donated £40,000, and rarely less than £15,000. Within the first ten years of the IFD, they donated $300,000, being at that time the largest donor. Money given to the Upendo Leprosy Home at nearby Arusha was of benefit to the RDTC as a teaching centre. The IFD Board never fully understood that several other of my partnerships were also routes into finance or gifts in kind. Some of these collaborations appealed to major donors to the IFD. Gerry Bodeker, Chairman of Global Initiatives for Traditional Systems of Health, was one of these. Money provided for collaboration with traditional healers was hardly understood by the Board of the ICD. Henning Grossmann hoped they would recognise the value of Traditional Health Systems by arranging a visit to their nearest major centre, but he did not succeed in gaining the ICD's sympathy. By western standards, their practice was neither evidence-based nor germ-free, but it was first on call in a country with few biomedically trained health service providers.

In 1993 we had paid out $90,000 for the new programme in Guatemala. The Student Hostel was completed at a cost of $267,703. There had been a hiccough of $11,600 for damaged tiles, theft and legal fees.

The ICD/ILDS had to develop its own financial security and eventually was itself able to inject larger sums of money, viz: $50,000 annually into the IFD. It also negotiated that the World Congresses would benefit the IFD by injecting surpluses into the IFD endowment fund every five years.

The burden of fund-raising was much discussed. Both Constantine Orfanos (Berlin) and Robin Marks (Melbourne) took their roles as Treasurer of the ILDS very seriously, and were cautious and critical. There would be risks in appointing a fund-raiser and it could not be afforded. One was appointed but immediately disappeared off the scene. Many hours were spent on appeal documents and often visits to other countries to make the best contacts.

There were attempts to involve the overseas departments of other governments, such as the UK's Overseas Development Association (ODA) and the Israeli and Japanese equivalents, the Italian Ministry of Foreign Affairs and the Tuscan Regional Council, DANIDA in Denmark and the Canadian equivalent in Quebec. Al Kopf and Stuart Maddin also approached the International Development Research Centre (IDRC). Al Kopf corresponded with the Secretary of Health and Human Services and the head of the National Institute of Health (NIH) in the USA.

My unsuccessful application to the European Commission involved visits to Brussels with the IFD lawyer. In 1991, I tried the Africa Grants Centre of Comic Relief. Henning Grossmann, Al Kopf and I all had to contribute to the filling of vast forms for these attempts, and often it was too difficult to meet deadlines, especially for Henning in Tanzania. Henning was more successful with the German Foundation for International Development.

Rotary Clubs in North America were helpful as donors to the Upendo Leprosy Home and to the compounding facilities for tropical skin applications at the RDTC in Africa, and in Guatemala, as a steering committee. I was awarded a Paul Harris title by the Arusha Rotary.

Over the years, there were visits to and hosting of many African embassies, but while enthusiasm for the RDTC was clearly stated, especially at the annual advisory board meeting chaired by a government minister, the government of Tanzania was slow to provide their promised funds.

Every year at the RDTC there is a graduates' reunion, with the hosting of visiting lecturers and other visitors on safari, often organised by a later President of the ISD, Coleman Jacobson. His intention was to provide funds by charging extra on a safari, but not

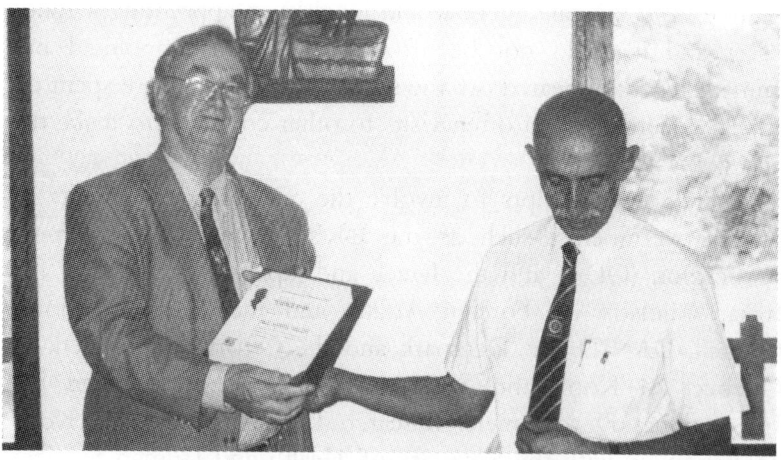

Receiving the Paul Harris Award from the President of Moshi, Tanzania Rotary

all visitors realised that they were drinking the profits at the large evening social events. As the millennium approached, we became more successful at fund-raising

Barbara Leppard earned for the IFD $300,000 by doing a trial of the antifungal Lamisil for *Janssen* while I was a Paul Janssen Fellow, but much of the work negotiating this was done by Stuart Maddin, who also negotiated $40,000 dollars from the Merck Foundation. Huge gifts in kind were negotiated, especially from *Stiefel* whose container of topical pharmaceuticals lasted ten years. After the Stiefel family had sold up, Barbara Stiefel also paid several hundred thousand dollars for a much-needed dermatology ward.

This is a tale of huge investment, and a great deal of energy put into helping and funding but, sadly, often with ultimately disappointing benefit to the IFD.

Albinism

The profession of dermatology has met the rise in the prevalence of skin cancer with vigorous campaigns of prevention, early detection, and improved therapy. Many of the IFD Board members, such as Robin Marks from Australia, have played a global role in significantly raising standards of skin protection from the sun, as predicted in the early documents of the IFD.

One programme of special significance in Africa which has achieved generous funding has been the programme for persons affected by albinism in Tanzania. This is an especially vulnerable group benefiting from a programme of education, sun protection and early therapy of malignancy in the skin. At the beginning, there were some very destructive facial cancers, but 15 years later, with a programme for about 600 people affected by albinism, it now detects much fewer immediately life-threatening cancers. Due to deficiency of pigment in the retina and in the cochlea, people thus affected have poor eyesight and, to a lesser degree, poor hearing – as shown in a study by Oxford medical students. Initially, Barbara Leppard from the UK, Donald Lookingbill and James Nordlund, both from the USA, helped to set up a programme of early diagnosis, treatment of pre-cancerous lesions and negotiation with the education department to provide more effective teaching. Fund-raising was successful and included an awareness article in the UK *Sunday Times* colour supplement. By far the most horrifying problem was the murder of infants by witch-doctors for body parts believed to have medicinal properties. Since 2006, 96 have been murdered and a further 69 attacked, while Tanzania has more than 16,000 people with albinism living in fear. The governments of East African nations have a multifaceted plan to manage this. In 2017, bald-headed men in Tanzania and Malawi were also murdered for their body parts.

Any report from the RDTC in Moshi will mention Henning Grossmann, the German dermatologist with a passion for Africa and for island ecology. Behind great men are so often great women. His wife Herma Grossmann was one such. She was in Africa even before Henning, and her specialty was Occupational Therapy (OT). She founded and ran the OT at the Kilimanjaro Christian Medical Centre, but later became an influence on occupational practice and teaching throughout the developing world. She initiated income-generating activities by rehabilitative intervention through OT and received international awards for her pioneering work.

If anyone thinks of OT for patients affected by skin disease is making raffia baskets and papier maché pots, and weaving linen, then they have not experienced its role in the twenty-first century. No longer do patients make such unmarketable items, but the aim is rather income-generation by selling goods needed by the community in which they live. It is an accepted fact that meaningful activities are needed to support mental health and well-being. The OT at the RDTC took up the challenge of supporting clients, such as patients affected with albinism or xeroderma pigmentosum, or those disabled by leprosy or lymphatic filariasis. Not only are OTs in a position to assess disability and ability, but they are good at matching abilities to the needs of the community.

While in Tanzania, the OT for the Department of Dermatology at first focused on leprosy, but it now also provides a more comprehensive service for clients with disabling skin diseases.

The OT at the RDTC trains patients affected by albinism in activities of daily living, providing protective devices and adaptations against the sun and mechanical damage, which can occur – e.g. during cooking, washing, cleaning or farming. The overall management goal is then to facilitate productivity and greater self-reliance by food production, keeping livestock, tailoring/shoemaking and other essentials.

The RDTC initiated vocational training in cooperation with the Rehabilitation Centre at the Young Women's Christian Association in Moshi, Tanzania, in the areas of tailoring, shoemaking, and producing solar cooking devices and small orthopaedic aids. In both workshops, people affected by albinism are working indoors and it is planned that they train their peers to enable them to establish income-generating activities in their own communities.

Today, the heading under which rehabilitation is carried out is 'Income Generation' and 'Self-Reliance'. It has become a necessary branch in the management of disabling skin diseases, helping to make those once rejected more accepted in their family and community.

The OT at the RDTC is therefore facing great challenges in developing creative and innovative therapeutic approaches for clients affected by disabling skin disease – by increasing and distributing widely the number of people trained to teach income-generating activities. People with impairments living in isolated communities will have greater opportunity to receive training in a number of skills of value to their neighbours.

The IFD in Tanzania opted to teach allied health professionals rather than MDs. Entering the field of public health has a very different focus on populations and human behaviour. Some MDs were taught as faculty but, having spent much money and energy on African doctors from Tanzania and Ghana, training them partly in the UK as well as in Africa, some sadly failed to reach our expectations or left us for private practice.

Mali

The French members of the International Committee were envious of the activities in English-speaking East Africa. One member, Prof Thivolet from Lyons, was very angry when I sought help for our work in Mali from their rival Bordeaux dermatologists because of their experience in the developing world. They were not members of the IFD or ICD, and I was ticked off by the President, John Strauss, for such lack of tact.

A pilot study of the diagnosis and management of common skin disease in Bamako, the capital of Mali, found scabies was treated as pyoderma with expensive antibiotics such as rifampicin, taken from the leprosy elimination programme, and that impetigo and fungal infections were common – but also that both were being treated with inappropriate and expensive antibiotics. We sought help from Antoine Mahé, a French government medical employee from Senegal, and he selected the young Osmane Faye in Bamako to run a programme, and we had to handle tactfully more senior persons looking to be appointed head of the programme. A teaching programme of one-day courses for a large sample of Health Centre staff in Bamako and one rural location was set up. The IFD sent me to support the programme. It was the week of the African football cup but we managed to have posters all over the place and TV time to encourage people to visit the health centres. I stayed in an American hostel which even had its milk flown in each day from Paris. Later, Rod Hay took over supervision of the programme. The study was fully written up and evaluated, and has received much attention and publicity at WHO.[3] It demonstrated that diagnosis which differentiated scabies, impetigo and fungus infections could be improved and inefficient prescribing could be reduced. However, its effect on the health of populations was not very marked because of low use of the health centres. In Mali, as in most of Africa, traditional health practitioners are first on call and very numerous.

Guatemala

In 1990, the Board member of the IFD, Francisco Kerdel Vegas from Venezuela and Ambassador to the Court of St James in the UK, received a letter from Erwin Blandon, Ambassador for Guatemala, expressing an interest in an RDTC for Guatemala. He had trained in Adelaide as a surgeon with an interest in cancer. He was appointed Ambassador when his brother-in-law was appointed President of Guatemala, and while in London, he took the London University Diploma of Dermatology.

In October 1990, there were letters of support from Francisco Kerdel Vegas and the President of Guatemala, and from the Guatemalan Minister of Health, as well as letters of support and interest from Guatemala City dermatologists, Hernandez-Pere and Eduardo Silva Lizama.

In December 1990, Andrew Fogarty, an Oxford medical student, was funded to visit Dr Cordero, a dermatologist in Guatemala City, to analyse 11,301 outpatient visits and to initiate data on the case of need.

On 6th-7th December 1990, I made a site visit to Guatemala with Al Kopf, Stuart Maddin, Francisco Kerdel Vegas, David Ramsay and Erwin Blandon. There were discussions with the President's office, the President's wife and the Minister of Health. We met with two groups of 'rival' dermatologists and made a site visit to proposed locations for an RDTC. Deep in the countryside, there was one small hospital filled with survivors of a massacre the previous night, caused

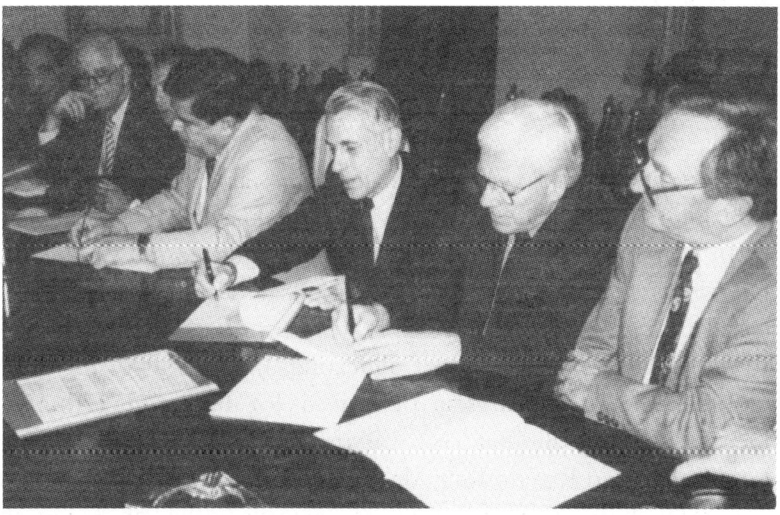

Al Kopf and Stuart Maddin with the Minister of Health signing an agreement between the IFD and Guatemala in 1990

by no good reason other than lack of discipline of a small number of soldiers. Our intention was to help the rural deprived, but as help to such people was seen as supporting communists, it was clearly important to have government approval to work in such a rural area. A site at a hospital in Chimaltenango, where there were empty buildings previously built by American plastic surgeons for their short-term projects on cleft palates, was selected.

In December 1990, I enlisted the help of Manuel Saravia, General Manager of *Squibb Pharmaceuticals*, Guatemala City, to give us some insight into local politics, and the help of lawyer, Geoff Haley of *Theodore Goddard*, London, to prepare a preliminary contract between the government of Guatemala and the IFD.

Orlando Canizares, the American dermatologist with the greatest interest in tropical medicine, then wrote, suggesting a focus on skin hygiene and public health with nurses as the main recipients.

It became clear that Dr Carlos Cordero of the Institute of Dermatology, Guatemala, and Dr Silva Lizama of the Association of Dermatologists, had differing agendas, and so Manuel Saravia advised me that the Guatemala City Rotary Club should act as a steering committee.

In March 1991, Kenneth Stuart, Chairman of the Commonwealth Caribbean Medical Research Council, gave his written support. The President's wife and sister of Erwin Blandon arranged the furnishing of buildings in Chimaltenango, but there were continuing rival views and uncertainties about the government allowing use of hospital buildings in Chimaltenango.

In March 1991, I visited Venezuela and enlisted the support of Dr Clovis Lombardi of the Pan-American Health Organisation based in Venezuela. In July 1991, we went ahead and appointed Erwin Blandon as Director, allocating him $15,000 for four months, and a vehicle was purchased for him. On 12th-15th December 1991, another visit was made with Al Kopf, Henning Grossmann and Ramon Ruiz Maldonado from Mexico to include a meeting with the steering committee and visits to the Pan-American

Health Organisation, Erwin Blandon's offices, and also to Dr Cordero at the Guatemala City Institute of Dermatology.

On 16th May 1992, there was an inaugural course for nurses in Chimaltenango, and we had an opportunity to report on this to Central American ambassadors in New York at the United Nations.

In February 1993, there was a transfer to the RDTC of the library from the now late Orlando Canizares, and this was immediately followed by the transfer of office equipment from the late Dr Gilbert Schiff. The offices were opened and a curriculum for nurses was planned. The Steering Committee was active and helpful. To meet the concept that training centres should be regional we made an overture to neighbouring countries, Salvador and Nicaragua concerning the regional role of the Guatemalan RDTC.

There was good progress at first but one year later, on 11th March 1994, we received news about the RDTC at Chimaltenango from Ramon Ruiz-Maldonado, the ICD member from Mexico, reporting lack of support from dermatologists and from the government. He suggested moving the RDTC to Guatemala City. As urban activities were not our aim, my opinion was that a move to the capital was against the IFD's objectives for rural development and would excite rivalry amongst the dermatologists.

In May, we had to agree on partial usage of the RDTC building in preparation for a cholera epidemic. By June 1994, we had held four courses for nurses, and there had been an expansion of outpatient attendance in Chimaltenango.

In May, the ICD met in Sydney where disquiet was expressed about Guatemala. I gave a full report and obtained letters of approval from the President and Secretary of the ICD, John Strauss and Ramon Maldonado. They asked that the Colombian member Maria Duran visit the RDTC in September, and there were further letters of disquiet because she reported on the rival groups of dermatologists and lack of support for Erwin Blandon in Guatemala.

In October 1994, Al Kopf outlined a plan for the next few months for the termination of the contract with the IFD to be on

1st March 1996. However, on 1st December 1994, he reported on another site visit that 122 nurses had received training, and that there was improved collaboration amongst dermatologists. Even so, on 14th February 1995, Al Kopf informed Erwin Blandon that his contract would terminate on 1st March 1996, and he sent a letter to the Ministry of Health, informing it that, although there had been achievements, we planned to terminate the contract.

Shortly after this, a co-ordinating committee of Guatemalan dermatologists was set up by Maria Duran and Ramon Maldonado, emphasising liaison rather than a directive role. But correspondence from Erwin Blandon in May 1995 stated no cooperation was likely. There followed news from Ramon of the refusal of dermatologists in Guatemala to play a role on a co-ordinating committee.

My purpose at that time was to present the Guatemalan RDTC as a success,[4] and to plan for Spanish-speaking Nurse Rebecca Penzer from my department in Oxford to do an evaluation based on the opinion of the 258 nurses that had been trained. She reported strong support for the teaching of the Training Centre. Importantly, there had not been a decline in the private practice of the dermatologists. Figures of 5,000 extra referrals to the private practice of dermatologists were obtained, resulting from increased confidence of the nurses in their diagnostic skills.

On 18th August 1996, the Guatemala Ministry of Health considered doing its own evaluation, and Jose Mascaro, the Board member from Spain, corresponded with them but they did not respond. Erwin Blandon requested a further grant but this was not approved at an IFD Board meeting in Athens. The Guatemalan project was closed down.

China

In the 1950s and 1960s, my girlfriend was sister to an Oxford friend, Jo Penney, whose family was run by an Edinburgh 'Nanny' named Ducky. Ducky saw my potential and took me to be vetted at a weekly Edinburgh Nanny meeting. Present were Nanny MacDonald, Nanny Fraser, Nanny MacIntosh and several other named 'Nannies'. Then, one day, she said we should go and meet

Aunt Frances who had not been made fully welcome by the family because she was a communist. She had twice been married to Norman Bethune, the Canadian surgeon beloved of Mao (and by all Chinese), and after whom several Chinese hospitals and universities are named. He died from sepsis whilst surgeon to the Revolutionary Army. Frances had several books signed by him. I took one to China and gave it to Professor Xiu, Director of the Institute of Microcirculation. She presented it to the women of China in the Great Hall of the People, saying that she noted it was about a woman and adding, "Any woman that Norman Bethune was interested in I would like to emulate." The book was *Madam Bovary* by Flaubert. I feared for my head!

Because leprosy has long been a principal interest of the Department of Dermatology in Oxford, for many years there have been links with the American-trained Lebanese Ma Haide,[5] the first Director of the Institute of Dermatology of the Chinese Academy of Sciences, Peking Union of Medical Sciences. He aimed to eliminate leprosy from China. Whilst Chairman of the International Foundation for Dermatology and Honorary President of the International Society for Dermatology, I nurtured these links.

Ma Haide, when visiting my home, received a classic novel, Hardy's *Jude the Obscure,* signed by Norman Bethune. Dr Li Huan-Ying, who was responsible at the Nanjing Institute of Dermatology for syphilis control, also stayed at our home in Oxford and was later, with me, on the seventh WHO (1997) Expert Committee on Leprosy, which revised Multi-Drug Therapy Guidelines.

In 2000, I led an 'Ambassador' travel club delegation of 30 dermatologists to China, including Henning Grossmann and Michael Waugh, President of the International Union of Sexually Transmitted Infections. Dr Anne Laumann, a dermatologist from Chicago, was also a member of the delegation. Her husband was co-author of a paper on the rise of chlamydial infection in China, later published in JAMA (2003) from Nanjing. Rebecca Penzer, a nurse from the Department of Dermatology in Oxford, also joined the group. Professor Prunieras and his wife from Paris were with us as well. On this tour, a lecture by me in the Department of Dermatology in Xian alerted a young Iranian dermatology trainee, Javad Hosseini, to the objectives of the IFD. Fluent in several languages, he acted as interpreter during that visit. He followed this up a year later with a request for an RDTC at Xian. I set up a steering committee for discussions within China, and asked Dr Hosseini to act as Secretary.

In 2001, Dr Gilbert Shia, who had been a Chinese GP trainee in the Oxford Department of Dermatology, organised a visit to Shanghai from the UK for people interested in Chinese traditional medicine. He asked me to lecture on his course; it was an opportunity to visit both Xian and Nanjing with my wife Anne. Chinese interest in the IFD/RDTC was considerable after my presentation of the criteria for establishing an RDTC, which included the need for government and national dermatology support. A proposal from Javad Hosseini and from Nanjing was presented to the Board of the IFD and remained on its agenda, while further information was gathered. The IFD committee emphasised that Africa was its priority, and that no funding was available for other substantial projects. I aimed to collect data that would convince and recruit donors of the need for such an intervention, but was conscious that the IFD Committee was not on my side.

The Institute of Dermatology in Nanjing has, since its inception by Ma Haide, had a responsibility for National Leprosy and STD control. It provided leadership in education. It was the co-ordinator of international relationships. It was the only centre in China with a networking role throughout the whole country. It published the leading journals for Chinese dermatology. It distributed newsletters for leprosy and STD. It was the recipient for HIV/AIDS funding from the USA. It had the only Institute of Dermatology in China.

Immediately before the visit to Nanjing in 2003, accompanied by Dr Javad Hosseini and Oxford colleagues Dr Gerard Bodeker and Dr Gilbert Shia, I visited branches of the Academy of Medical Sciences in Beijing. I had previously been appointed an Honorary Professor at its Institute of Microcirculation in Beijing and at the Institute of Dermatology in Nanjing. The Director of the Institute of Microcirculation, Professor Xiu, had previously been Vice-Chancellor of the Academy, and for many years had been a Member of Parliament. She had attended the 1984 World Microcirculation Congress in Oxford. We also met at the China Academy of Traditional Chinese Medicine and at the Chinese Medical Association to discuss participation at the forthcoming International Congress of Dermatology, as well bringing the dermatology project to their attention.

The aim was to take skin care and its traditional partners, Sexually Transmitted Diseases (STDs) and leprosy, into the general health services in China. I wanted to take skin diseases and STD health care out of the almost exclusive domain of big urban centres, and make them more accessible to residents of smaller towns and rural areas. We had learned that, on the Old Silk Road, lorry drivers had replaced camels and had brought with them sexually transmitted infections, and that brothels were numerous. The focus was to be common problems and potential epidemics met by the 5.52 million village health workers and 1.32 million village doctors. A goal was poverty alleviation by the provision of correct diagnosis, preventative medicine and appropriate, sustainable and essential drugs or the use of

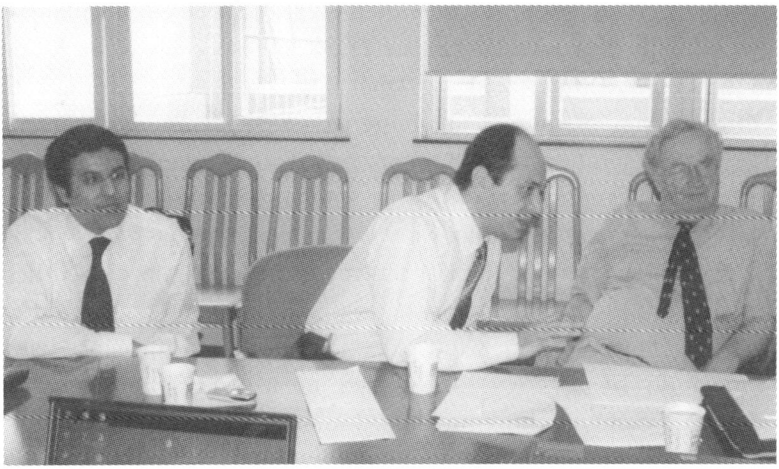

Preliminary discussions in Xi'an between Babar Vaqas (left), Javaad Hosseini (centre) and Terence Ryan

traditional medicine, available within half a mile – as recommended by World Bank Technical Paper No. 187 and by Gerard Bloom of the Institute of Development Studies, University of Sussex, Brighton, as well as strategic papers on STD and leprosy submitted by the Institute of Dermatology at a meeting with myself.

A preliminary report was prepared by an Oxford medical student, Mr Babar Vaqas, who spoke Urdu, the language of village doctors in the far west of China. He was funded by the Lord Mayor of London and the St Francis Leprosy Guild. His report was based on interviews of key personnel, heads of departments of major academic centres and regional hospitals in Nanjing and Xi'an, interviews with county hospital doctors in training, and with village doctors in representative locations – e.g. the extreme rural west of China and a rural site near Nanjing in the east, interviews with Chinese administrative departments interested in developing the project, and with international agencies already setting up programmes in rural areas for the retraining of village health workers.

These interviews were fully supported by photographs and, where appropriate, by video. Dr Javad Hosseini, the Secretary of the Steering Committee for this project, provided detailed support and translation skills as well as making all necessary contacts.

The need was greatest where there were some 56 ethnic minority groups with their own languages. These are especially to be found in the west of China, including Tibet. This I had gleaned at the 15th Anthropology Congress in Florence 2003, when hearing the Research Institution of Ethnology and Anthropology from China present an application to host the International Union of Anthropology and Ethnology.

It was proposed that a pilot scheme or model be developed first in Xin Jang Province, western China, which has 100 counties with 993 townships, previously termed 'communes'. This province has a population of 19,250,000 exposed to a rising prevalence of HIV/AIDS. Over the course of four years, four groups of 25 doctors would receive one year's training in Nanjing. During this time, the Masters Programme for Public Health Dermatology would be developed.

In fact, a four-tier system was proposed: Tier 1 – an RDTC based at Nanjing and supported by the ILDS, would aim to train through its internationally accredited Masters programme 10-20 programme managers. (Since neighbouring countries have similar needs, the designation 'international' referred to both its faculty and potentially its students.) These would be the trainers of Tier 2, the 2,961 doctors (Public Health Dermatologists) at county level, who would in turn receive a one-year course. It is these public health dermatologists who would train Tier 3 township doctors at a local level, and these would in turn provide Tier 4, the village doctors with Ministry of Health-accredited short courses. Such courses would be in response to both national and local needs for improved management of common skin diseases in the locality or in response to epidemics such as HIV/AIDS or a resurgence of leprosy.

The Institute of Dermatology in Nanjing had raised $4 million ($1,800,000 from the Chinese government) to build a new block of seven storeys, with a completion date of 2004. The RDTC was offered two floors at no cost to the IFD. This was the main reason I thought I could persuade the International Committee of Dermatology to take up this new programme.

The annual income of the Institute and its hospital stood at $8 million. The Institute could apply for further funds from the government to allow a greater National Public Health Programme and training (CME) of 85% of the workforce for HIV/AIDS work, beginning in 2004. 300,000 patients attended each year. The SARS epidemic had influenced the thinking of the government with respect to public health. Other factors were the threat of a resurgence of leprosy and the rapid increase in the size of the HIV/AIDS epidemic. The changing face of dermatology and increased life expectancy of the population was also recognised.

A delegation visited Beijing and Nanjing, 4th-6th November 2003. The agenda included visits to branches of the Chinese Academy of Medicine in Beijing and Nanjing for the discussion of leprosy, STD, dermatology and Chinese Traditional Medicine. Three weeks earlier, the Secretary of the steering committee, Dr Javad Hosseini, had visited Nanjing to prepare for the visit. I accompanied him for the

IFD, along with Dr Gerard Bodeker for Global Initiatives for Traditional Systems of Health, currently acting in various capacities for WHO and the Commonwealth, especially in Asia, and Dr Gilbert Shia, an Oxford-based advisor on Chinese Medicine and to the Guys Hospital Poisons Bureau, London, on Safety Issues and Traditional Medicine. With a population of over 1.3 billion, with one billion in neighbouring countries, and based on an estimate of one village doctor for every 1,000-2,000 persons, it was estimated that between 700,000 and 1,300,000 village doctors would require training. It was felt the model developed by the International Foundation of Dermatology in Mali might be used. The commonest skin problems were to be identified, and all health centre employees were to be given a one-day course on how to manage them – a programme similar to that in Mali.

Following preliminary discussions, it was estimated that, initially, 2,861 county hospital doctors could provide this training. Therefore, a decision needed to be made as to how best to organise the training of such county hospital doctors. It was suggested that Nanjing should co-ordinate such training, and that the public health dermatologists so trained, acting under the supervision of Nanjing, would determine local priorities and act as local programme organisers and trainers of county dermatologists in a one-year programme. The curriculum for the community dermatologist would cover dermatology, STDs, AIDS, leprosy, burns, data collection, teaching skills and the management of essential drugs and traditional medicine. Possibly only ten such persons could be responsible for the entire programme. Once trained, these could either be based at prestigious training schools or could be 'free range', setting up and recruiting even at the level of the county hospital, through which they would provide training. There are usually one western and one traditional hospital showing a degree of integration at all levels. Quality control would be through regular updating of the Programme Managers, and through external examinations and evaluation. The essential objective of upgrading the knowledge of the village doctors and the least qualified but more numerous village health workers would be the responsibility of townships.

I repeatedly emphasised that IFD programmes seek poverty alleviation, and that the Chinese system of supplementing doctors' salaries by taking a percentage from drugs prescribed, and favouring the prescription of more expensive 'western' drugs, was unacceptable. The response at Nanjing was that this was both recognised as a problem and seen as a challenge to be addressed over the coming years – as indeed it was by the supervision of excessive prescribing practice by a state drug administration and a Bureau of Price Control.

The need for setting in place a locally sensitive training opportunity for village doctors had become obvious to all since the rising prevalence of STD was believed to increase the likelihood for the spread of HIV/AIDS. By the year 2010, syphilis was as common as it had been when Ma Haide had successfully arranged to control it. There was anxiety about leprosy, with a rise in new cases, more children affected, a disability rate in new cases above 20%, delay in diagnosis averaging two years, case relapses, problems due to migration from rural to urban areas, and 47 counties with a prevalence of leprosy at more than one in ten thousand at the end of 2000. Many modern medicines are not available in rural areas, and availability of the alternative and cheaper Chinese traditional medicine had to be part of the plan.[6]

In the cities, Traditional Chinese Medicine (TCM) is integrated with western medicine. The best of it is bought up and exported by an alert international pharmaceutical industry, and Chinese ownership may be lost. What remains is affected by a preference for western drugs by the scientifically trained doctor. Market forces raise costs and a lack of evidence contributes to the downgrading of traditional medicine. (A hundred claims of the effectiveness of traditional medicine followed the SARS epidemic, and there were claims that more rapid recovery and fewer complications followed TCM prescribing.) The Oxford delegation, including myself, met with the founder of MEBO, a successful and widely used plant based remedy for burns. Evidenced-based trials are few, but one from Singapore suggested at least equivalence with standard therapy using silver sulfadiazine, and it was much cheaper.

The leading centre for traditional medicine in Beijing had a substantial WHO collaboration with four hospitals and one eye hospital in the city. There were 4,000 staff, including 800 professors. Somewhat lacking in advocacy of its achievements, they claimed to have a large database and much evidence from basic research. Western systems of diagnosis were increasingly integrated. The concept of 'sub-health', meaning predisposition and vulnerability which affected 50% of the population, was possibly better researched by epidemiological technology than in the West. Acupuncture had as many as 300 researchers currently employed on the investigation of meridians, pain mechanisms, electrophysiology and biochemistry. There was a large Chinese literature in which there was some proof of efficacy. In the library of the Institute of Dermatology, it was noted that 254 Chinese and foreign journals were taken, including 62 foreign titles. Eight titles were on dermatology and two on venereology. Very few of these were known in the West. The Global Initiatives for Traditional Systems of Health had Gerry Bodeker and myself as directors, being mostly concerned with the public health need for the identification, measurement and utilisation of Chinese Traditional Medicine (TCM).

The safety of TCM in China is well recognised, but its substantial exports, employing lesser-trained prescribers overseas, is less so. TCM studies include standardisation of horticulture and the processing of herbs, and the reduction of toxicity as well as quality control. More difficult was the policy of individual titration for prescribing that makes controlled trials so difficult to interpret. (For example, by the Cochrane Studies of traditional medicine in the management of dementia.)

Under the heading of poverty alleviation, TCM has a role to play as a provider of a low-cost, locally available and sustainable resource. It also has a potential for income-generation. For these reasons, approaches to the EU and to the World Bank were to be considered by Dr Gerard Bodeker. Everyone would be pleased if this huge establishment, devoted to Integrated Medicine, would publish more evidence of efficacy. The proposed Public Health

Dermatologist would need a reliable database and evidence on which to base lower-cost prescribing.

The central points of discussion regarding a traditional medicine component for the planned RDTC programme were outlined. There was a high level of interest in and commitment to the traditional medicine component of the China RDTC programme. A scientific basis for this and the production of standardised and safe medicines was possible and necessary. China's leading dermatological and TCM academic institutions had pledged their commitment to this, ensuring that the best possible start to the programme was in place, with clear guidelines for best clinical practice and training materials, and an agreed curriculum. Dr Gerard Bodeker had meetings at the Guananmen Hospital of the China Academy of Traditional Chinese Medicine in Beijing, and noted that there were a number of studies on the use of traditional medicine for HIV-related illness, including skin conditions. The Hospital Director offered participation on developing evidence-based protocols and institutional partnerships.

It was expected that funding of a provisional survey of the case of need at village level would follow the signing of a Memorandum of Understanding with the National Institute of Dermatology in Nanjing. The signing of such a memorandum took place at the Chinese Academy of Medicine in Beijing, overlooked by the President of the Academy. Because dermatology in China is focusing on a high-technology western model of care suitable for about one third of its population, there has been disappointing support for the public health needs of its 800 million village population. Alternative approaches, other than through dermatology, to deliver skin care, were needed at village level, focusing on absent skin – viz. burns, wounds, ulcers, full thickness blisters (especially where due to prevailing epidemics), leprosy, diabetes, HIV/AIDS, and drug reactions. There were several potential partners, including China's Centres for Disease Control (CDC).

The International Committee for Dermatology was never enthusiastic about this programme. I was very concerned about the well-being of Javad Hosseini, my employee and representative in

Nanjing. In spite of all the promises from the Chinese in Nanjing over a two-year period, he was given little support and none of the promised room for manoeuvre materialised. At one stage, they postulated that he was a spy from Iran. I paid several visits to attempt to trigger the programme. I brought Javad to an ICD meeting in London but he was not greeted with enthusiasm. To facilitate his negotiations on my behalf, I had allowed him to have a visiting card, indicating that he was representing the IFD. Although an essential tool in China, this card was crossly taken off him.

In September 2004, there was a final meeting in Nanjing chaired by my successor Professor Rod Hay. The plan was to go ahead with a pilot study of rural health needs, a pilot educational programme modelled on the Mali or Mexico programmes, a 'training the teacher' course aiming for a diploma in dermatological public health, and participation in the early HIV recognition project. Offices in the new building were agreed, The regional WHO representative would be invited onto an advisory board. The way forward for managing finance was agreed.

Not long after this, Javad reported that four senior personnel at the Institute in Nanjing had been sent to prison for diverting funds

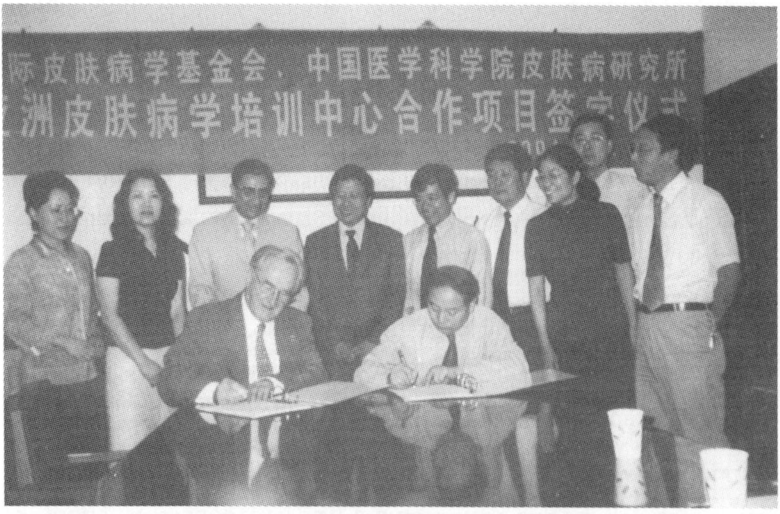
皮肤病学基金会，中国医学科学院皮肤病研究所
皮肤病学培训中心合作项目

Signing a memorandum of understanding between Nanjing's Department of Dermatology and The International Foundation of Dermatology

to themselves and for buying lasers to treat wrinkles in Shanghai. The IFD ceased to take an interest in the programme and Javad sought new employment with his Iranian embassy.

For the next few years, I tried to keep my personal involvement in Chinese affairs from folding up altogether. I had another contact in China: Jean Watson – the leading authority on occupational therapy for leprosy who had given a course at the RDTC in Tanzania and was now in China. In 2006, a delegation which included three podiatrists from Southampton, an Australian nurse, Tim Goodacre (the senior Plastic Surgeon in Oxford), Gail Todd (the Professor of Dermatology in Cape Town) and I worked for one week with Jean and her charity 'Project Grace' in Kunming, Yunnan, to evaluate the case of need and appropriate teaching materials. Jean introduced us to top-level and impressive hospital care and rehabilitation for burns, strokes and other neurological disabilities. She also took us to a leprosy village. There were many of these 'homes for the disabled'

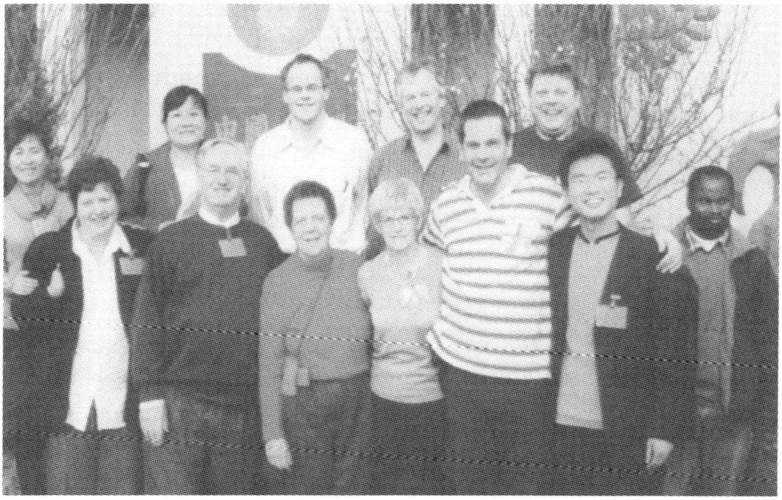

Visiting China. Front row: Professor Gail Todd (Cape Town), Jean Watson (central in jumper), Jan Ross (a senior nurse from Melbourne), a podiatrist (Southampton), a Chinese traditional practitioner, and a traditional practitioner from Mali.
Back row: a medical student, two podiatrists from Southampton and second from right Tim Goodacre, Senior Plastic Surgeon, Oxford.

in Yunnan. We saw a young man with much-delayed diagnosis of leprosy, even though his neuropathies had admitted him to hospital and his father was known to have the disease. In the villages, we saw how the Chinese government provided housing and food, but health care was lacking.

In Oxford, for some six years before I retired, we had set up, under George Cherry, the Wound Healing Foundation and regular tuition in laboratory techniques. The Chinese military sent us their best young burns surgeons for a year or more. Many years later, these are generals in charge of major city hospitals, and they have become part of an objective for improving skin care in China to be described in the next chapter.

Back at Oxford

While responsible for developing this major initiative in Africa, Guatemala and China, there was at the same time the experience of being appointed to some of Oxford's major committees and working for British dermatology as President of the British Association of Dermatology. The support of public health was to be found more in the hospitals of the National Health Service than in the science areas of Oxford University. The Faculty of Medicine was chaired only occasionally by someone who could guide it in its dealings with a parochial Hospital Board of Management carrying out the demands of the National Health Service. All the medics belonged to the faculty, and I chaired it in the late 1970s. I would discuss whether it was necessary to inform faculty members about anything, as often only a few would turn up to meetings. Some faculty chairmen said it was the thought that counted! It was run by an oligarchy reporting to a General Purposes Committee that reported in turn to a Medicine Board wearing gowns. I remained scarred by the experience of arriving at my first meeting of the Board in a pullover

The Medicine Board, when for a brief period in the 1990s I was Chairman, would receive requests from the UK's General Medical Council to teach in the medical school much that the scientists were little in sympathy with – for example, Alternative and

Complementary Medicine. On one occasion, when requested to introduce more social medicine, it evoked the response of throwing up of hands: 'Oh, not human behaviour!' The scientists wished to find new molecules rather than to disseminate knowledge already available to populations most needing it. Earlier, Sidney Truelove had introduced statistics to the hospital clinicians at the Radcliffe Infirmary, while later the Cochrane Centre and the Evidence-Based Medicine movement, growing out of Perinatal Mortality, found a home in north Oxford.

As described in Chapter 4, advocacy for some of the extraordinary creativity of the science area did not have the support of all the colleges. Scientific creativity was at first largely misunderstood behind the college walls. The High Tables for dining were attractive to short-term visitors, but were available to only limited numbers of an expanding faculty. As described in *Teach The Senators Wisdom* (Masterman, 1952), much was achieved by a mixture of the ambience of dreaming spires and the eccentricities of their top performers arguing for the preservation of traditions that appealed to the visitors, but sometimes infuriated the residents trying to introduce science to the arts.

Mrs Caroline Miles, as Chair of the Health Authority, describes in a small history of the Radcliffe Infirmary, a letter from Sir David Weatherall, in which he wrote:

> *What nobody seems to have understood is how Oxford has arisen, as a kind of county hospital to which has been cast the duties of a district general hospital, a major teaching centre, and more recently a major research centre.*

There have been times when the university failed the hospitals. Not supporting the intellectual development of the nursing profession was an example. The university and the hospitals benefited from Thatcherism and the opportunity to be entrepreneurial, but the university declined to award her for it.

One other organisation with which I was involved over many years was as a Trustee of the Oxford International Biomedical

Centre (OIBC), founded by the Oxford biochemist Charles Pasternak. Charles transferred to St George's Hospital, Tooting, and continued to run this organisation as an Oxford intervention, at first focusing on technology transfer and topics such as traditional herbal medicine, but eventually changing its focus to the teaching of science in schools. I benefited by many interesting discussions with other trustees, such as the editor of the journal *Nature* and Dame Anne McLaren, known for her development of the ethical issues surrounding *in vitro* fertilisation. Some of the trustees like myself favoured taking into schools applied science, and focusing on issues relevant to the needs of the developing world. Eventually, the burden of financing OIBC was better solved by linking Oxford's leadership in pure science and the hard facts of scientific progress in understanding the mechanisms of disease by teaching sessions to the young in the UK, rather than technology transfer from Oxford to a resource-poor world.

In 1997, discussions between the Chairman of the Global Initiative for Traditional Systems of Health, Gerry Bodeker, and myself were based on the fact that, in many parts of the world, at least half of the population were paying for Complementary and Alternative Medicine (CAM) for chronic illness, and that a study of atopic eczema, acne and psoriasis in Oxfordshire would shed light on such behaviour. It was well-known that adverse reactions occur from some interactions between complementary and orthodox medicines, and that most patients do not discuss with their doctor what medicine they are taking. More evidence had to be made public of the many benefits of CAM, while many leading scientists were convinced that there was little benefit. We were concerned that collecting evidence was often too expensive in the developing world, and that lack of evidence was not proof of ineffectiveness. Plans were made to join other groups to take this interest forward. In documents on healthy skin for all and on integrated medicine, we argued strongly for education of the practitioners of traditional, complementary and alternative medicine rather than their abolition. Eventually, as described in Chapter 11, most of my publications in this field were a collaboration in India. Bodeker and I, with other

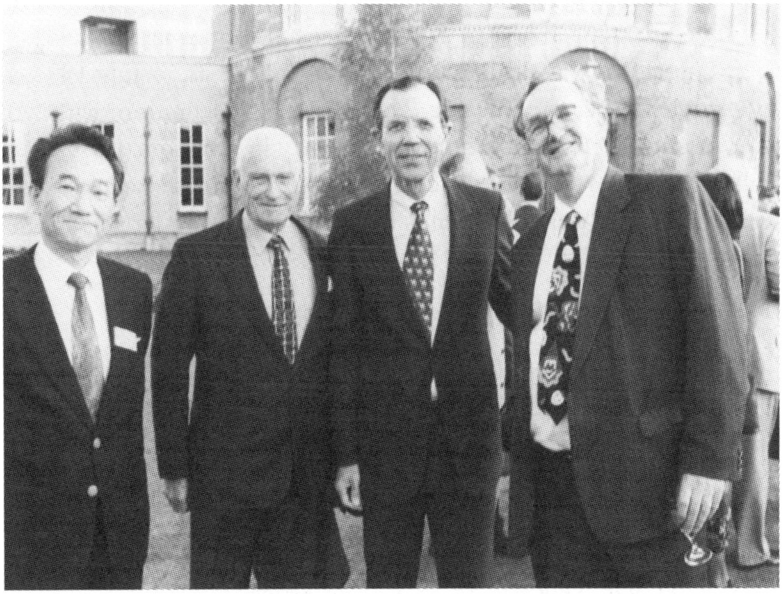

Outside the Radcliffe Observatory on the occasion of my retirement party. Left to right: Kyoshi Nishioka (Japan), Professor Charles Calnan (UK), Bill Green (Texas) and myself.

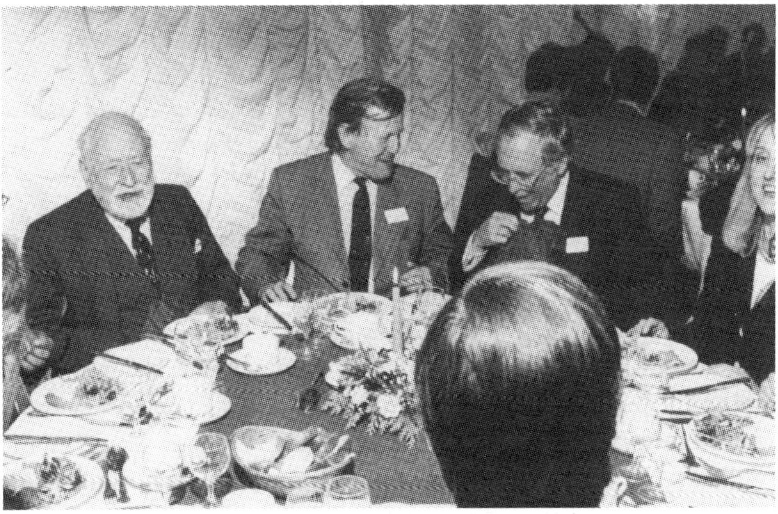

On the occasion of my retirment dinner. Left to right: Darrell Wilkinson, Rodney Dawber, John Wilkinson and Finella Wojnarowska.

trustees of Global Initiatives for Traditional Systems of Health, continued to publish and talk to Chinese authorities in the field.[6]

Eventually, it was time to retire from Oxford as, in July 1997, I had reached the age of 65. There was a celebration with an afternoon of lectures and an evening party in a marquee at Green College. Besides the presence of many previous trainees and colleagues, there were old friends from Belgium, Italy, Japan and the USA.

Notes on Chapter 10

1) 'A Service Under Threat' – a document prepared for the British Association of Dermatology when I was its President, 1992-93.

2) UNIDERM – a document prepared with UNESCO for the International Committee of Dermatology, eventually published as a booklet, *Healthy Skin for All*, and as an article for the *International Journal of Dermatology*.

3) Faye, O., Hay, R.J., Ryan, T.J., Keita, S., Traore, A.K., and Mahé, A. (2007), 'Impact of a short-term training of primary health care workers on basic dermatology to improve leprosy case detection', in *Leprosy Review* 78: 11-16.

WHO/FCH/CAH/05.12 – Discussion papers on Child Health. *Epidemiology of Management of Common Skin Diseases in Children in Developing Countries.*

4) Ryan, T.J. (1994), 'Nurses complete their training in Chimaltenango', in *International Journal of Dermatology* 33: 526-27.

5) Ryan, T.J. (1989) and Haide, Ma (1910-1988), 'A dermatologist to emulate', in *International Journal of Dermatology* 28: 41.

6) A list of essential, traditional dermatological medicines was a goal of the programme, and it was recognised that an evidence base would be needed for this. To this end, the Chinese Academy of Traditional Chinese Medicine offered access to its traditional medicine and dermatology database. The market-driven health economic system resulted in medicines being priced out of reach of the poor and of those most in need. Consequently, locally produced

traditional medicines might offer a viable and effective option in meeting dermatological need. They also offered the potential for generating local enterprises to produce these medicines and to market them more widely, introducing an income-generation component to the RDTC programme.

We were especially concerned for the 56 ethnic minority groups of China, the largest being the Tibetans. Their cultural traditions of medicine could assist in making the programme meaningful and hence enhance its effectiveness.

Many modern medicines are not available in rural areas, and the traditional medicine programme would ensure that known and effective medicines were available.

Training materials and curricula for RDTC trainers and health workers, as well as for communities and families, would need to be developed in the early stages of the programme. A start had to be made by establishing the partnership between the China Academy of Traditional Chinese Medicine in Beijing and the Nanjing Institute of Dermatology in producing a course on TCM and dermatology for the International Conference on Dermatology in May 2004. The Traditional Medicine Institute in Nanjing had a dermatology department, and this also would be involved in curriculum development for the RDTC programme. Clear guidelines for good clinical practice in TCM would be needed, and this would accompany the development of training materials and curricula.

From meetings that Gerry Bodeker had at the Guananmen Hospital of the China Academy of Traditional Chinese Medicine in Beijing, it emerged that the Academy was associated with a number of studies on traditional medicine and HIV-related illness, including HIV-related dermatological conditions. Hospital director, Dr Cui, had offered participation on developing curricula, medicines, institutional partnerships and an evidence base for this dimension of the programme.

From existing EU and World Bank connections, a network of prospective funders would be developed.

11: After Retirement: Lymphoedema, Community and Care

In 1997, after retirement from the Department of Dermatology in Oxford, I decided not to try and keep up with all aspects of dermatology but to retain some leadership in the field of the lymphatic system and the management of the swollen leg due to venous and lymphatic failure. There followed the advising of law firms on a number of their cases of lymphoedema following accidents. I flew to Ethiopia to observe podoconiosis, a condition affecting millions of agricultural workers in which limb swelling occurs in those who, walking barefoot, till an irritant soil. Decades earlier, in 1970, with a vascular laboratory in London, I was visited by Frederick Price who believed that silica in the soil in Ethiopia was paralysing cells in the dermis normally protecting the skin from such infections.[1]

This was not the only reason for visiting Ethiopia. In the capital Addis Ababa, there is a centre named ALERT which has trained many dermatologists throughout Africa, the UK and the USA to become experts in leprosy, so it was important to make a link with the WHO collaboration at the RDTC in Tanzania for Dermatology, Sexually Transmitted Infections and Leprosy. In Mekele in northern Ethiopia, the dermatologist Aldo Morrone from Rome had established an outreach dermatology programme which hosted an annual workshop. It was at one of these that a new international branch of Community Dermatology was launched with me as Chairman. Because Rome had become overloaded with immigrants from Africa, Aldo Morrone had established an annual conference and a centre for management of their many health problems. It was there that a workshop was held on behalf of the International

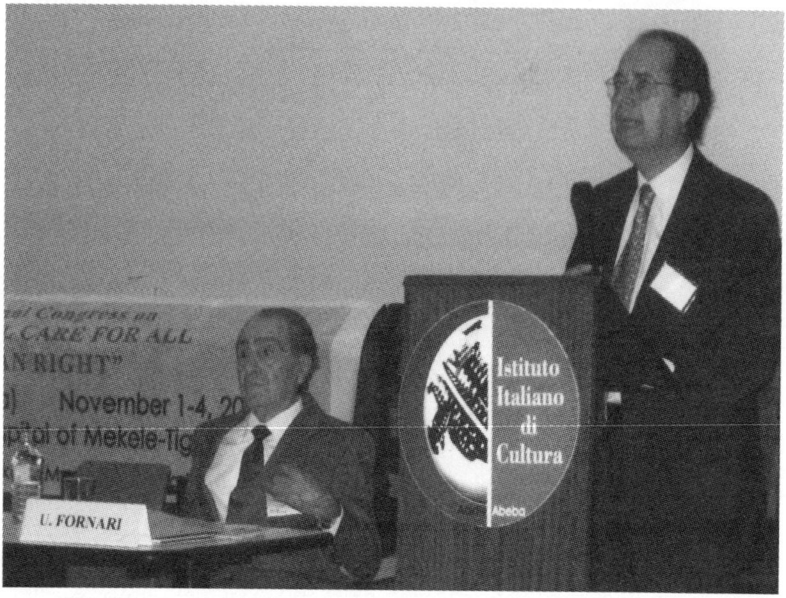

Aldo Morrone and his senior advisor Ugo Fornari at the launch of 'Dermatological Care for All' in Mekele, Ethiopia

Society of Dermatology to discuss interventions in the face of the migrant crisis.[2]

Moving into public health, several British dermatologists and nurses became expert in interventions for the control of limb swelling, requiring a solution to the great public health problem – elephantiasis due to filariasis. It was realised that treating entry points for bacteria such as between the toes or avoiding pinpricks and other inoculations was essential if recurrent inflammatory episodes were to be avoided.

There has been much discussion of the practice of prescribing long-term antibiotics to treat bacteria entering through the epidermis when treating entry points in this way did not always work. Studies in Brazil[3] and in India[4] pointed out that regular washing and emollients compared with daily penicillin, in controlled trials, proved that prescribing such antibiotics was not so often necessary when and if the skin was cared for by washing and emollients.

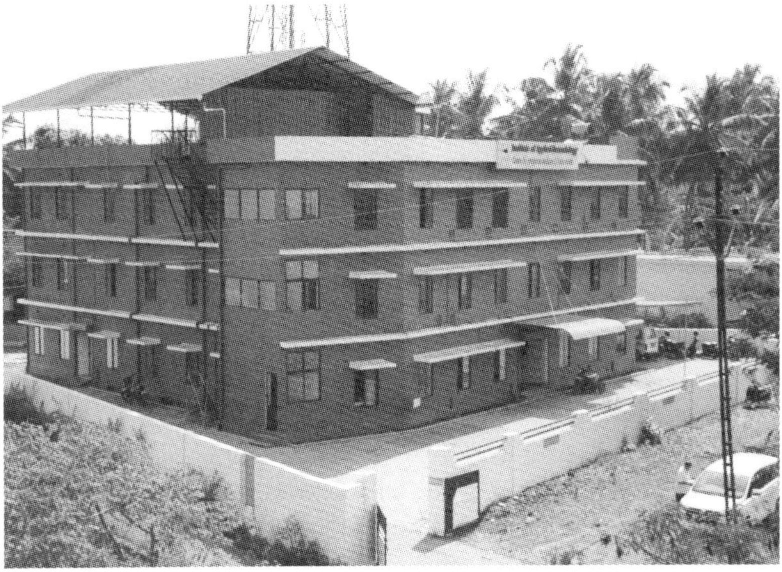

The Institute of Applied Dermatology in North Kerala, India, where I am Mentor for the Management of Lymphoedema

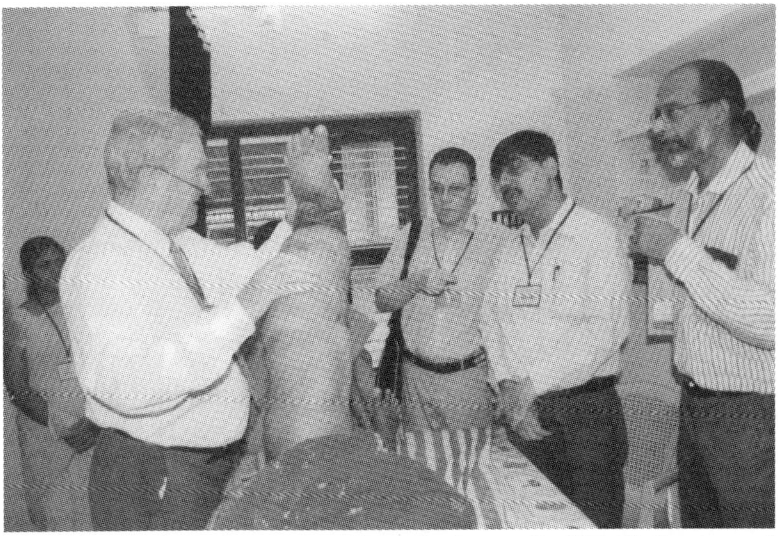

Steve Ersser and Prof M Ramam (in the background), All India Institute of Medical Sciences, New Delhi during a demonstration by myself

Prescribing to whole populations once a year two or three drugs that inhibit production of filaria was a WHO-led programme on the elimination of this disease. Those affected, although no longer able to transmit the filaria by the mosquito, are left with the lymphoedema also known as elephantiasis. In Tanzania, support of the programme's morbidity control had meant involving British nurses. Now in India, where there were millions of cases of limb and genital swelling due to the mosquito-borne parasite filaria, I was to become much more involved. Babar Vaqas, who was described in Chapter 10 as visiting village doctors in the far west of China in his final year as a medical student, wrote with me in 2003 *Lymphoedema: pathophysiology and management in resource-poor settings – relevance for lymphatic filariasis control programmes.*[5]

For the developing world, we wrote that lymphoedema had to be managed with whatever was available locally. Water for washing could contain anti-bacterials found in local herbal mixtures, and to promote lymphatic flow we suggested yoga might do the job. Dr Narahari, a dermatologist in Kerala and his wife, Dr Prasanna, took up this theme. He treated every patient with integrated

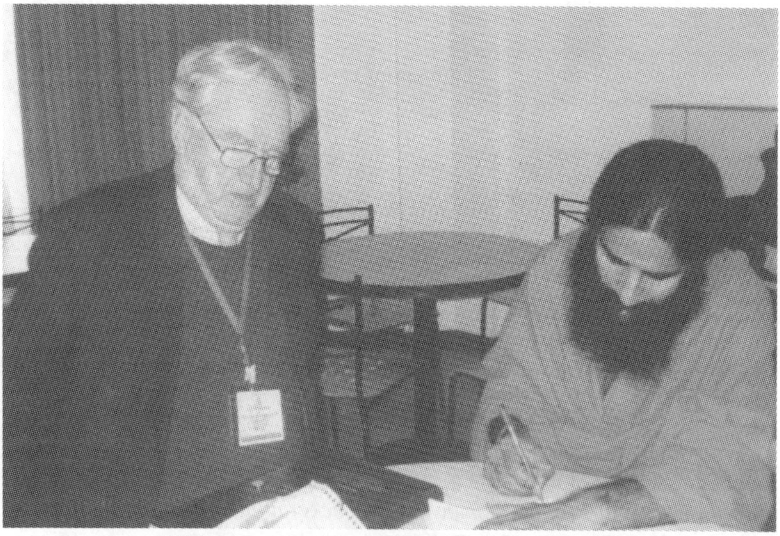

The Guru Ramdev and myself discussing the effect of yoga on the lymphatic system

medicine from local systems such as ayurveda and homeopathy. He took me on as mentor of a programme at the Institute of Applied Dermatology (IAD) in Kerala which had been initiated in 1999 as a charitable not-for-profit venture and eventually became internationally famous for its mostly low-cost and effective treatment of lymphoedema, even in remote outreach sites. With a small team of leaders from the IAD, most of the staff were locally recruited and trained, and medicinal resources were easily available in local markets.

An annual visit to the IAD has increased my experience of managing limb swelling, and has also helped to introduce the concept of integrated medicine in several publications.[6] I have encouraged members of the Narahari team to publicise their work at several international congresses, and arranged for many of the world's leaders in the field to visit the IAD. The practice of integrated medicine is essentially using biomedical knowledge of mechanisms learned in the past 50 years to help prove the efficacy of Indian systems of medicine first developed more than two thousand years ago. At the IAD, patients are seen by practitioners of biomedicine, homeopathy, and ayurveda. The results have been so good that there is support from the state of Kerala and the government of India. There are now several well-known international mentors. There is also a fine new building and 50 employees.

I visited the multi-billionaire guru of yoga in North India, named Ramdev, and found his well-financed research unit was unfamiliar with the lymphatic system, but a collaboration has refined our use of yoga. Essentially, it is about promoting the flow of tissue fluid into and along lymphatics by promoting tissue movement. All lymphatics drain into the large veins within the chest, and their emptying is helped by effective breathing which is also a function of yoga.

Plans to mentor the management of limb swelling in India and Ethiopia have led to collaborations that have included further research into the mechanisms underlying lymphoedema. A dermatological approach led to further studies of why skin care, and especially washing and moisturisers, are so helpful. It has long been realised that bacterial and soil irritant entry through the skin is reduced by such care of the skin. A little later, Paul Matts, a senior scientist of *Procter & Gamble*, and Claire Fuller, most recently Chair of the International Foundation of Dermatology, took up podoconiosis in Ethiopia as a mission. Using PUR, a water cleanser provided as an humanitarian gift by *Procter & Gamble*, they showed convincingly how effective washing and emollients could be. This led to studies of transepidermal water loss, and evidence that its control reduced the inflammatory response of the epidermis.[7]

From my early days of seeking to show how the epidermis controls its blood supply, through the days of the study of inhibitors of fibrinolysis through studies of the effects of mechanical forces, I have moved from studies which can be described as pure science into public health (see Appendix 1). The science most focused on in recent years is that the slightest injury to the epithelium affecting its barrier function makes it turn on a change in behaviour to a repair mode.[7, 8] In health and at rest, the epidermis is an organ almost without mitotic figures with a very slow turnover, mostly anaerobic or at the very least requiring little oxygen, and it is not manufacturing inflammatory cytokines and growth factors. After injury, its basal cells begin to divide and multiply in its upper layers; instead of being lifeless, they demand oxygen and the epidermis releases numerous stimulants to its blood vessels in the upper dermis, impairing fibrinolysis and encouraging fibrin deposition. White cells arrive on the scene, some of which demand 50 times more oxygen and secrete destructive agents such as elastases which destroy the elastic support of the lymphatics.

One of the commonest of skin diseases, especially in the young, atopic eczema, has led to intensive study of barrier function and treatment when the epidermis fails. There has also been extensive study of elderly skin which also has less effective barrier function, dries out and cracks. Such studies which relate to two important public health problems, on the one hand affecting up to 15% of children and, on the other hand, affecting the rapidly increasing population of the elderly, have identified control of trans-epidermal water loss (TEWL) as a prime function of the skin

(Rawlings and Matts, 2016). It has been proven to play a role in moisturisation, pliability and prevention of cracks in the surface and exfoliation. Too great water loss results in desiccation and exfoliation, such that the barrier becomes no longer effective.

With Paul Matts, a senior scientist at *Procter & Gamble*, we have emphasised that an underlying function of the skin depending on the epidermis is the control of transepidermal water loss. When this is not controlled, many inflammatory mediators are released, leading to increased blood vessel permeability, dermal swelling and overloading of the lymphatic drainage system. Washing and the use of moisturisers such as glycerine,[8] reduce transepidermal water loss, consequently switching off production of inflammatory mediators, and is a low-cost, low-technology intervention affordable in resource-poor regions.

While such activities were going on, a new interest was developing at WHO in Geneva. In various parts of the world, but especially in west Africa, a bacterial cause of large ulcers in young people was increasing in prevalence. Known as Buruli Ulcer, and caused by a bacteria which destroys subcutaneous adipose tissue, it is responsive to the antibiotics streptomycin and rifampicin. However, once the ulcer is formed, it requires more than antibiotics to prevent the healing process resulting in disfiguring scars. Help with the general principles of wound healing was requested from the USA wound healing expert, John MacDonald, and in due course, in 2010, a committee was formed at WHO to write a white paper entitled *Wound and Lymphoedema Management*. This included four chapters by me, and led to a book on the shelves of WHO.[9] The advice given included control of limb swelling. At the same time, a World Alliance for Wound and Lymphoedema Care (WAWLC) was launched.

In the UK, Christine Moffatt, a nurse well-known in the venous leg ulcer field, had published an article on the high prevalence of limb swelling in London, especially among the elderly.[10] Christine formed an organisation named the Lymphoedema Framework which soon became international and provided guidance on the management of limb swelling, and to which the IAD added a chapter. To develop more experience in resource poor countries in preparation for the WHO book, Christine and I went to Sierra Leone where we were the first to diagnose Buruli Ulcer. Christine also visited Kerala and became a mentor to the Institute of Applied Dermatology (IAD).

In the meantime, there were a number of dermatologists keen to develop a different approach to skin diseases and wound healing in the developing world, to be known as Community Dermatology. Community Dermatology has been practised by Gurmohan Singh of Benares Hindu University, Varanasi, with tribal peoples in India, and also by Roberto Estrada in Mexico and Aldo Morrone in Ethiopia. A long-established Community Dermatology programme involving diagnosis and management of common skin disease for a rural region inland from Acapulco in Mexico was initiated by Roberto Estrada. It has been much admired and was seen to be an example of what the IFD would hope to achieve. In 2002, a formal relationship between this programme, headed and developed by Dr Roberto Estrada, and the IFD was agreed.

Community Dermatology's formal manifestation as a society was suggested by both the German Luitgard Weist and the Indian Shyam Verma, a dermatologist from Gujarat in India and first editor of *The Indian Journal of Dermatology Online*. In 2009, the Task Force for Skin Care for All: Community Dermatology was launched in Berlin, with me as Chairman.[11] Colleagues Rod Hay and Roberto Estrada and I wrote that:

> *Community Dermatology embraces common skin diseases. It is inclusive of wounds and lymphoedema, and has long had neglected tropical diseases such as leprosy, the prototype of disfigurement, and its abuse as a major interest. It requires data on prevalence and human resources, though not exclusively. These may be isolated, peri-urban or mobile communities, often against a threatening background such as strife or climate change. Community Dermatology is a concept that extends the focus of care delivery from the individual patients who come to see the doctor about something wrong with the skin, to a proactive intervention to improve skin care and diseases that present with*

skin signs in the broader community in which they live. In this way, community dermatology is applicable in the richer countries as much as the poorer. So, for instance, holding pigmented mole clinics for Australian surfers or promoting sun-safe practices in Australian schools, are community dermatology. Essential to this is the idea that one uses all means of achieving this goal, and therefore those that involve other groups, e.g. burns care experts or providers of protective fashionable clothing are all manifestations of the same basic principle that, to achieve the best results, teams are usually multidisciplinary and sensitive to local practices and needs.

The task force for Skin Care for All, whose language is public health, manages failure of skin functions, as discussed in previous chapters, such as lost intact barrier function (water loss from evaporation or ulcer healing), thermoregulation (managing heat cold or flood), and sensory defects giving rise to itch, pain or numbness. In addition, the skin communicates as colour prejudice, love at first sight, or the look-good, feel-good factor. It is aware of the stigmatisation of the disfigured as with the person affected by leprosy in the Middle Ages, and being unwelcome because of disfigurement, viz. the one-eyed and one-legged Long John Silver of *Treasure Island* making kindness unlikely and participation all the more difficult. Thus a principal feature of the programme was the simplification of diagnosis, moving from learning up to 9,000, mostly Latin-based, diagnostic terms for skin diseases to just four failing functions of the skin.

A second feature of the programme is the widened workforce of human resources. It concerns all the professions caring for the skin, such as dermatologists, nurses, podiatrists, wound and burns specialists, lymphoedema experts, and those managing tropical diseases such a leprosy, leishmaniasis, Buruli ulcer, onchocerciasis, trachoma or yaws. The International Society of Dermatology, which was founded in 1965 to promote interest in skin diseases, and the influence of ecology and geography, especially in the tropics, has individual members and publishes the *International Journal of*

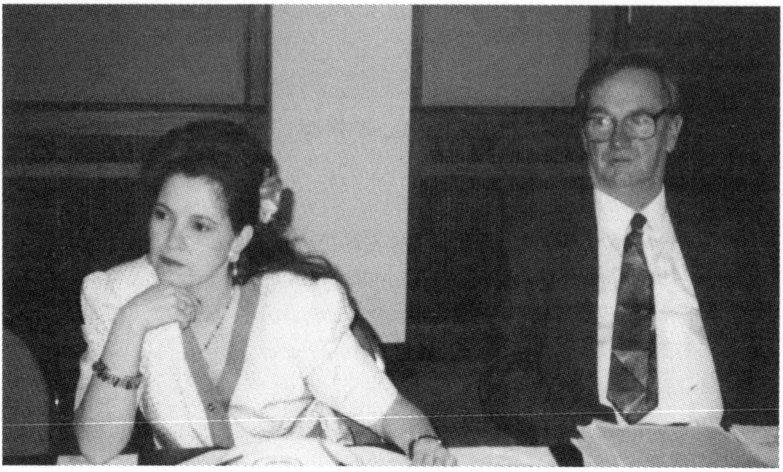

Seated with Maria Duran in Colombia, whose name was to be ever linked with that of the promotion of the needs of women, both patients and caring professionals

Dermatology. It has two sub-committees, Empowerment of Women, named after the Colombian Maria Duran who was a co-organiser of the initiating conference set up by me in Turkey,[12] and now Community Dermatology.

In the beginning, for the International Society of Dermatology, we prepared a CD celebrating 43 achievements of Community Dermatology, and we published some of these achievements in the May 2011 number of *International Journal of Dermatology*, and the website www.skincareforall.org was prepared with the help of the London College of Fashion. It showed capacity to benefit and advertise both good looks and considerable achievements in public health fields.

A few years ago, Paul Matts, the *Procter & Gamble* expert on the outer layers of the skin, and I as Honorary President of the International Society of Dermatology (ISD), sowed the seeds of a collaboration between the London College of Fashion and the ISD. 'Better Lives' is the title of a series of seminars organised by the London College of Fashion by focusing in part on body image and self-esteem. I had in earlier days written about the skin not just as the body's protective outer sleeve but as an organ presented to the public gaze as a coat of great beauty. Concern with the skin is influenced by fashion and hence by market forces which often determine the attitude of 'the eye of the beholder'. There is however the reality that 'a mass of naked figures does not move us to empathy but to disillusion and dismay'. So writes Kenneth Clarke (1956),[13] who adds that 'we are concerned by wrinkles, pouches and other small imperfections'. In his book *The Nude*, he writes of two different concepts of the human shell:

> *The balanced prosperous and confident nude versus the huddled and defenceless naked body. The one is a concept of the ancient Greeks that the spirit and the body are one, the other, that is characteristic of medieval Christianity, is that the body is an object of humiliation and shame to be rejected. Few are lucky enough to have a 'body beautiful' throughout life and it is not therefore a question of imitating a normal quality but a search for perfection. Perfection is impossible to obtain and, in the quest for it, there is inherent conflict in placing a value on good looks and equating this with admirable qualities of the spirit rather than the self-interest of narcissism.*

It is a conflict we must win by helping all to esteem their body image, fighting off phobias and bringing to the fore those admirable qualities of the spirit.

The International Foundation for Dermatology which, as described in the previous chapters, was founded by the ICD for the International League of Dermatological Societies to assist in the development of dermatology in underprivileged communities, became an immediate supporter of the new taskforce which in 2014 became a sub-committee of the ISD. As described in Chapter 9, many who were concerned about the burden of disease wherever there was poverty had previously called for a programme to be outlined with suggestions for bringing about Healthy Skin for All. The suggestions so made were enthusiastically embraced by WHO. Now we wished to shift the emphasis of Skin Care for All to main themes such as:

1) Skin care with low technology at low cost, viz. the use of water and emollients.
2) Skin protection from a threatening environment (climate change), focusing on protection from hazards such as heat, cold and flood, and learning to live with the hazards of climate change.
   Impairment of the skin has been underestimated as a handicap in a threatening environment. Turning to the public health problem of the hazards of climate, there have been several studies in Australia about protection from the sun. In Africa, the study of people affected by albinism and early diagnosis of skin cancer with low-cost therapies has made a great impact. The ISD and I agreed that this was just one example of the hazards of climate change which could be part of the Community Dermatology programme, and appointed the Scandinavian Louise Andersen and American Mark Davis to regularly update the society about protection from heat, irradiation, cold and flood.[14]
3) Management of absent skin, such as occurs with burns, pressure ulcers in the elderly and paraplegic, venous ulcers, diabetic foot ulcers. tropical ulcers and toxic epidermal necrolysis, which is often a severe drug reaction.
4) Integrated medicine, which is combining the best of biomedicine (also known as modern or western medicine) with the most useful of other systems of medical alternatives, complementary and traditional, as listed.
5) Making sure that the technology of care was backed by the desirable attitude of care.

Since my retirement, these themes have been developed, mostly by practising in Africa, India and China. Disorders such as lymphatic filariasis, leprosy, Buruli Ulcer and burns have taught us as much about best practice as working as a dermatologist in Oxford for 50 years. Quite often the revision of practice has been helped by the fresh minds of medical students and nurses. It began partly due to the influence of the International Skin Care Nursing Group which we had initiated in Oxford. Rebecca Penzer joined me and the dermatologist Laxmi Nair in Calicut to take up the concept in India. Dr Vineet Kaur had been with us in Oxford, working on the concept, and later on returned to Varanasi in India to give the topic the lead it needed. In Bangalore, the dermatologists, led by Professor Sacchidanand and Dr Neelima, launched a community dermatology programme for family practice that especially focused on hygiene.

Interest in leprosy took me to South America, to Sineccio Talhari in Manaus in the heart of the Amazon, and to a leprosy congress in Iguasso. I visited Francisco Kerdel Vegas in Venezuela, and was officially made an 'Amico of Venezuela'. Lymphatic filariasis took me to Recife and Guyana. At the latter, Tess Macpherson, Anne's daughter, once a family practitioner trainee in my department, was doing a DPhil on bacterial entry points in lymphoedema.

The International Foundation for Dermatology began in the late 1990s to seek other sites for regional dermatology training centres. My successor, Professor Roderick Hay, oversaw new centres in Cambodia and Patagonia, Argentina.

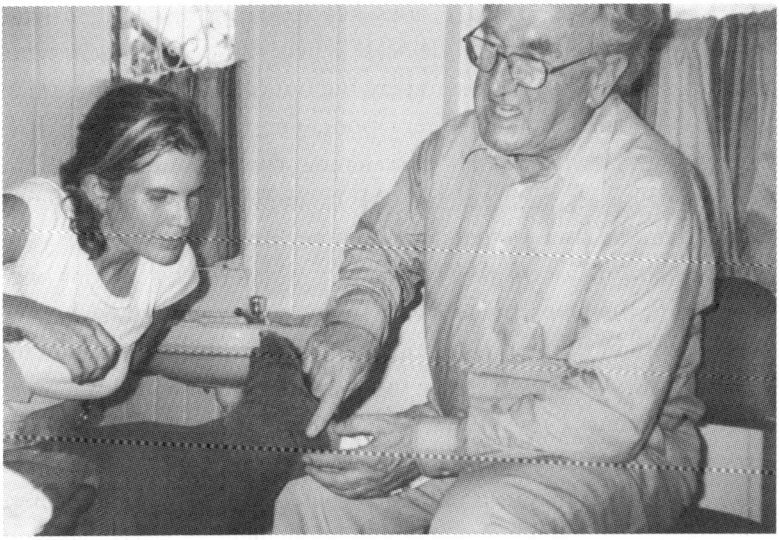

With Tess MacPherson in Guyana,
discussing bacteriological entry points in Lymphoedatous legs

One of the most recent initiatives involving Rod Hay has been a workshop in Atlanta to discuss collaboration with the Centres for Disease Control (CDC). It pointed a way forward for a valued collaboration, especially with scabies. In China, discussions have also been held with their CDC in Beijing and in Kunming. They admit their need for a collaboration to enhance early diagnosis and efficient prescribing. The Institute of Dermatology in Nanjing is a CDC partner.

Today, the factors that require an urgent reappraisal of Healthy Skin for All include:

- poverty;
- climate change;
- mobile and migrating populations;
- emerging diseases;
- neglected tropical diseases.

The functioning human being requires a healthy skin, but it is the skin of the face, genitalia, hand and foot that is most vulnerable. The range of skin diseases affecting these sites is large but the treatments are few because, for example, washing and emollients, movement and protection, are effective low-cost interventions for most diseases. To disseminate such knowledge does not require investment in large buildings or new drugs and devices. Where these are needed, other organisations will have a role to play, but our objective is education of a global population that is very poor, and often migrating, It is exposed to an increasingly threatening climate and affected by emerging diseases such as HIV/AIDS and diabetes, and suffering from common diseases that have been neglected.

The many major military hospitals in China run by persons once students in the Department of Dermatology in Oxford have given me an insight into a number of health problems outside my experience in Oxford.[15, 16] The high technology which allows those with 100% burns to survive with a new but imperfect skin has drawn my attention to what happens to such people if, without a limb or blind, they return home to where there is no family. There have been discussions also whether such high technology can be extended to two major epidemics in China, foot ulcers in the obese diabetic or pressure ulcers in the elderly. Of special concern in this huge country is the depopulated far west with its 56 ethnic groups. The military burns hospitals have begun to set up wound care units staffed by nurses, and the heads of these hospitals teach that which they experienced in Oxford, in its wound healing unit run by George Cherry. By giving support to this field of skin care, the Chinese Traumatology Society awarded me $1,000 with a certificate of appreciation in 2016.

When seeking to achieve best practice of medicine, a number of questions must be asked: Which system of medicine? Where practised, and by whom? How important is it that it should be evidence-based and scientifically valid? How important are the guidelines written by past role models, such as Hippocrates or Willam Osler? Is one seeking 'Health for All' or 'Care for All'?

Writing from Europe on best practice has evolved rapidly, based on discoveries over less than 200 years. While some discoveries such as the germ theory followed by germ control by antibiotics, have had a very large influence on practice, factors such as better housing, nutrition and sanitation have had an even greater affect on bacterial diseases such as cholera, tuberculosis and leprosy. Compared with the herbalist and the prescriber of heavy metals of 200 years ago, today's preparer of medicines, the pharmaceutical industry, is massive and hugely expensive.

Those who advocate that the patient should have a say in determining interventions to restore health are surprised and irritated by a patient's preference for alternative and complementary medicine, and by the fact that in much of the world the traditional health practitioner is first on call.

Some practitioners believe that the best way forward is to integrate the various systems of medicine. There are scientists who strongly oppose this, believing that the best of biomedicine is weakened by practices for which there is little scientific evidence. Integration meets contemporary impediments such as those observed in Sierra Leone where rapid deforestation was destroying the herbals with most therapeutic potential – actually, an antiseptic soap made from the bark of trees. New technologies such as the mobile phone can help us add to a practitioner's knowledge. Evidence-based medicine prefers that large numbers be studied in costly randomised blinded trials, although recognising that lack of evidence is not proof of ineffectiveness, and that the many who are excluded are probably examples for which evidence is most needed.

Over thousands of years, the sayings of role models have been valued. Thus there is value in the words of Hippocrates: 'Do no harm' and 'To cure sometimes, to relieve often, to comfort always.' Concepts of care find wisdom in the sayings of Confucius, Buddha, Jesus Christ and, more recently, William Osler or the Dalai Lama.

What is it one wants for the world? If it is the World Health Organisation's 'Health for All', surely that is Utopian and impossible to achieve.

'Care for All' might be aimed for in the knowledge that it might be achievable. But exactly what do we mean by 'care'? In the UK, there has been much attention to examples of lack of care. Whole hospitals have been accused of it. On analysing what lack of care means, definitions have included absence of compassion and kindness, or failure to preserve human dignity.

Aronson (2016), when discussing care,[17] writes:

> *Provision of care that is, as far as circumstances allow, respectful of and responsive to individual patient needs, values, priorities and preferences, striving to maximise the patient's well-being without simultaneously compromising the needs, values, priorities and preferences of others, achieved by collaboration among all of those involved.*

During my career, I have had two projects which caused me to doubt whether science can explain everything, and I have also doubted the common sense of some scientists who would discount all the value of alternative, complementary and traditional medicine.

A Dutch psychologist arrived at the Department of Dermatology in Oxford in 1967, stating that he was employed by the Catholic Church to examine difficult cases of stigmatism. He wanted us to give a bed to a Portuguese woman who at midday every Friday developed a wheal on her forehead in the shape of a cross that later bled. The Church had decided that she was not a saint and she had a brother who was making money displaying her on Fridays. He added communion bread to arum lilies, and she would smell the lilies and appear with the bread in her mouth. Coach-loads of people were visiting her and he had enough money to build an alternative church. The Archbishop of Lisbon was worried. The psychologist thought it was a chance to study mechanism as, often when stigmatists were regarded as holy, the Church disliked such investigation. It so happened I had a patient fully investigated year after year, who developed urticarial swellings which then bled whenever she was anxious. There were at that time several articles on the painful bruising syndrome and psychogenic purpura. All agreed that, however fully investigated, a scientific explanation could not be elicited, but emotion and sometimes the spiritual played an initiating role. Anxiety, bleeding and pain were linked.

While a medical student, I listened to a lecture on Indian fakirs, body-piercing and beds of nails. Later, in South Africa, I watched and photographed a Malay group perform to music a body-piercing ceremony in praise of Allah. Large pointed instruments pierced the face and a dagger fixed the cheek of one ‘performer’ to the floor. Another stuck a sword four inches into his abdomen above the liver and danced to the music. They suffered no pain and there was no bleeding. They had done it often before and there was no scarring. There was some skilled technology. Thus, having finely pointed instruments and pressing them slowly through pinched skin probably reduced initial damage to blood vessels. They knew some anatomy, such that instruments passing through the neck should enter and progress behind the main vessels, and that in the abdomen, they should pass above the liver and below the lungs.

When our children were in their early teens, we regularly met up with a neighbouring family for tennis and musical evenings They were sceptical of biomedicine but not of alternative medicine, such as osteopathy. One day, their eldest son developed spontaneous bruising of the skin and became a patient. I diagnosed Henoch

Scoenlein purpura, a well-known condition of childhood and one I was considered an expert on, which follows a sore throat and can damage the kidneys. My policy was bed rest and wait for it to get better spontaneously. It did not do so, and after a few weeks, I transferred him to the Professor of Paediatrics. He was placed on steroids by mouth and gradually the dose was increased without response. Eventually, a high level of 80mg per day was reached and he began to develop side-effects. His parents were not impressed. They called in their osteopath who said a bone of the spine was pressing on the nerves supplying the thymus, and he advised the steroids be stopped. He would manipulate the spine and correct the condition and said that the child would be better at home leading a normal life. Stopping steroids abruptly and discharging the child while still so ill was, in the view of us doctors, a bad thing to do, and there was no science of manipulation to influence immunology. The approach was considered dangerous and nonsensical.

We saw him the following week and he was completely well without any signs or symptoms. We had no explanation for this. A few years later, he developed, when recently married, inflammatory disease of the bowel and then cancer of the bowel with involvement of the liver from which he died. Managing this problem 20 years later, I would probably have called for the integration of both systems of medicine.

When the Department of Dermatology took on Gerry Bodeker and inaugurated the Global Initiatives of Traditional Systems of Health with him as Chairman, we studied the risks and also the benefits. George Cherry had visited Vietnam to examine their use of herbals or frog skin for burns during and after the Vietnam war. Gerard Bodeker was writing up the Vietnamese use of traditional medicine for the World Bank. A young traditional healer from Vietnam using herbals came to Oxford to study laboratory techniques with us, and ended up as Professor of Stem Cell Research in Singapore with a multi-million dollars' worth of patents. When working in Africa and India, I saw that Traditional Health Practitioners (THPs) outnumbered biomedical doctors and were clearly first on call. Of course, the placebo effect on the emotions and on the body's inflammatory responses is understood. When managing snake bites, THPs have used some bad practices such as scarification and tourniquets. These were also used in the UK within my lifetime. However, in managing fears that the snake could induce a state of shock, or managing the belief in evil spirits, the THPS were better than me. They could be taught better management of the bite, and they had mobile phones to photograph and identify the snake, and they could communicate with anti-venom centres.

I have learned in India that yoga and herbals can be an effective means of managing lymphoedema, and the Institute of Applied Dermatology in Kerala is a superb model for the use of systems still lacking in evidence and short on scientific proof. We are trying to remedy this, but some would have put a stop to our efforts before we could show that they were very helpful. When David Sackett, the guru of evidence-based medicine, came to Oxford, Gerard Bodeker and I met him in 2002 to discuss the difficulties of randomised controlled trials in resource poor regions. I was surprised when, on my retirement, he wrote:

> *Please know our affection and high regard for you. And please accept our thanks for making this place so much better through your brilliant dedication and hard work.*

During the years 2010-2020 the Institute of Applied Dermatology was able to provide substantial evidence that their integrated medical approach is effective. This led the Indian Government and the Bill and Melissa Gates Foundation to provide substantial support for taking the system into other States within India.

In recent years, I have become curator of the home in Oxford of William Osler. When a student at the Radcliffe Infirmary, I received teaching from three physicians, Hobson, Mallam, and Cooke, and one surgeon, Abernethy, who had, 40 years previously, attended ward rounds by William Osler and, much later, at Green College, one of the few females, Cecily Williams, would speak of a similar experience.

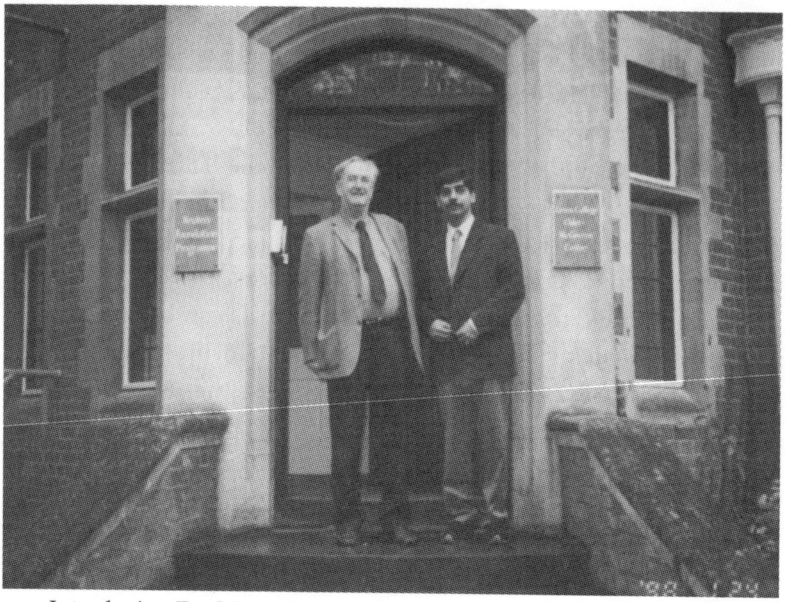

Introducing Dr S.R. Narahari from India to Osler's home in Oxford

The year 2019 is the centenary of the death of William Osler. A focus on his aphorisms helps to interpret the modern world. There is no better summary of the man than that by Richard Golden:[18]

> *William Osler is the quintessential physician of our time because of his literary legacy, scientific and clinical accomplishments, educational contributions, and influence on intra-professional relations. He had an extraordinary personality, a facile wit, a bibliophilic spirit, and a philosophy of life that permitted him to envision and achieve remarkable goals. Osler's humanism, which permeated all his activities, was the sine qua non of his particular claim to posterity. His continuing influence on succeeding generations is that of a role model (or hero in older parlance) that has often characterised as the 'Osler Tradition', a concept appropriately defined by Bryan (1994) as 'a virtuous approach to medicine and life as taught by and modelled after Osler.*

The life and philosophy of William Osler continues to serve as a standard of excellence and a model for the evolution of the profession and its practitioners.

Osler had a greater power of 'friendship'! This is what is meant by the 'attitude of care'. It is perhaps the major factor in determining the physician's contribution to 'Better Lives'. It is needed wherever medicine is practised and it can contribute healing properties. I am sure that some of the success of the programme in Kerala is because of counselling which is generous and friendly to patients who, because of their appearance and odour, have experienced isolation.

Osler's thoughts about science are worth noting:

> *With reason science never parts company, but with feeling, emotion, passion, what has she to do? They are not of her and owe her no allegiance. She may study, analyse and define; she cannot control them, and by no possibility can their ways be justified by her.*

It is a part-answer to the management of the frail elderly. Hospitals are overcrowded and should not house them for longer than acute medicine and surgery determines. My good friend, the Venezuelan Francisco Kerdel Vegas, writes in his old age in *Medical Paradoxes: Contradictions in Modern Medicine*[19] that:

> *Old people's homes do not solve the overall emotional problems of the old person – they are still strangers to one another – isolated and separated from their family.*

Francisco writes of therapeutic friendship contributing to the success of the medical act. Atul Gawande writes in the international bestseller, *Being Mortal*,[20] that more investment should be made into keeping the elderly at home. The alternatives of hospital, nursing home and care home do not meet the need for familiarity of environment and companions, and it is less easy to be friendly.

These are contemporary issues affecting all nations. I am involved with China and see it as a model that could, in time, strongly adopt friendliness as a principle and a country to become the leading model for 'Health for All'. Juan Tao et al (2015) of Shandong University wrote a letter to *The Lancet*, saying that doctors of Traditional Chinese Medicine would read Confucius to become more considerate people.[21] There is, they wrote, an insufficient reading culture, and that the humanities are needed to educate students 'to establish a more harmonious relationship between doctors and patients.'

The fact is that Confucian wisdom preceded Christ's, and in the eleventh century, China showed more evidence of civilisation than any other nation. Today it has had a thousand years of many of its peoples in poverty, and an absence of an attitude of care. It has a Chinese dream[22] of a *technically* great future to which it must add the *attitude of care.* If, as I suppose, it one day succeeds in nourishing and pleasing the world's most populated nation, with a genetic background of a capacity for kindness older than any other, then its present problems affecting the management of its legal system, and affecting so cruelly its wisest advisors of those who wish it to care for its animals, environment and ageing population, may make it tolerant to some wonderful people which at present it treats so cruelly.

William Osler would be pleased to see how his home at 13 Norham Gardens, Oxford, has in recent years been host to some important sowing of seeds on Chinese soil of the concept of care. It has also, through David Cranston,[23] assisted the Chinese Medical Association to inaugurate a Chinese Osler Society. We of course, hold copies of the neurosurgeon Harvey Cushing's two-volume autobiography of Osler, It is well-known, but I prefer the lesser-known *Consecratio Medici and other papers*, published in Boston in 1928 in which he discusses the relationship of science to the practice of medicine. He would not be surprised by the above stories. He wrote of science and of practice as capable of both good and bad effects, and would have favoured integration to find the best of both and elimination of the bad. Osler, he states, said that humanism should not exist without science, and science should not exist without humanity. Hippocrates said it in an earlier form: the love of humanity associated with love of his craft. Cushing emphasised that Osler's special form of integration was based on friendship – 'brotherly helpfulness' to fellow doctors and 'an extraordinary capacity for friendship which will always remain the characteristic which overshadows all'. Today, science of the mid-brain shows that everything which is intellectual and probably pathophysiological also passes through the emotional centre where lies the attitude of care, compassion and indeed friendship. Perhaps the excess activity of the emotional centre of the stigmatist, and the control of emotion of the body-piercer, or perhaps too the friendliness of my neighbour's osteopath, compared with the scientific approach of the professor of paediatrics, found different pathways in the mid-brain.

ACTAsia (an acronym for Act, Compassion, Together) is a ten-year-old NGO that seeks to promote, throughout Asia, kindness and respect for humans, animals and the environment, recognising that all forms of life are interrelated and therefore interdependent.

On 7th April 2016, in Birmingham, UK, ACTAsia won the Ceva Animal Welfare Awards Charity Team of the Year Award for its outstanding contribution to animal welfare and education, and the team's tireless efforts to encourage social progress in China.

The Principal of Green Templeton College (formerly Green College), in an email, invited help to entertain officers of ACTAsia, together with 14 young employees of the cosmoceutical agency that provides major funding for this NGO. After chairing a pre-lunch meeting at which the common interests of the NGO and the college were discussed and finding that their programme in China, which focused on educational objectives, matched my interests in China, I arranged, on 4th November 2016, a follow-up meeting with Pei Feng Su, the Founder and Executive Director of ACTAsia, and Joy Leney, Chairman of the Advisory Board of Directors at 13 Norham Gardens.

Until her retirement, Joy Leney was the International Projects Director for the World Society for the Protection of Animals (WSPA), and Pei Feng Su was part of the Projects team. In 2004,

Pei Feng Su left the employment of WSPA and set up ACTAsia. This resulted in the focus on China and its fur trade.

The objective became an Introduction of Care and Compassion through the education of children, something which would benefit not just animals but humans and the environment. Although small administratively, it has had several powerful supporters such as the ballet dancer Sylvie Guilem and the late Princess Elizabeth de Croy.

Present at the first meeting at Green Templeton College, Oxford, in 2016 was KK, the young and very successful Chief Executive Officer of the cosmetic firm *Cassiey*, which employs more than 800,000 young people in China and is a major funder of ACTAsia.

The mission of ACTAsia is that Asian cultures should evolve into caring societies, respecting all forms of life. It is registered as a non-profit organisation in UK, Australia and the Netherlands, and it has representatives in China and Singapore.

As an entry point for its mission, it concentrated first of all on animal welfare, and on the fur trade in particular. To do this, it prepared, since 2009 and with help from Australia, a training course for veterinary professionals in China, and it has been working with Chinese school authorities to champion, since 2012, concepts of empathy and compassion among children through Caring for Life Education, a curriculum covering all six years of primary school education. At the 8th China Urbanisation International Summit, ACTAsia was declared one of ten most influential organisations in China.

Unrelated to ACTAsia, on the 5th November 2016 *Channel 4* TV showed *China Between Clouds and Dreams*, in which children were being taught to care about the environment, birds and animals. Perhaps China is further ahead than we are in initiating issues of care in its education programmes. I remember how unfriendly China seemed when I first visited it. Now the people seem happy, and friendship is found everywhere except in its centre of government. If that should change over the decades, then China – like the brain's emotional centre, with a capacity to be Osler-like and with its newly inaugurated Osler Society – will have a place for global governance.

We discussed the organisation Skin Care for All: Community Dermatology, and spoke of the memo of understanding in China in 2002 which aimed to upgrade the training of one million village doctors. There has been training in the Dermatology Department at Oxford of Chinese military doctors, twelve of whom are now generals in charge of city burns hospitals. I have encouraged initiatives aimed at epidemics of diabetic foot ulcers and pressure ulcers in the elderly, as well as aims to promote better health care in western China beyond the cities and especially aimed at 56 ethnic minority groups.

Using animal welfare and the fur trade as entry points, I have created collaborations between ACTAsia and the London College of Fashion (LCF), at London University 'Better Lives' programme. Working together, they will hopefully be examining new ways to help with the disfigured, and the problems that follow the reduction of premature ageing. Both the LCF and ACTAsia use fashion shows to promote their mission.

Although lack of compassion has to be countered, there are many examples of exceptional kindness creating better lives. One to be especially recommended, that exists in the UK and in China, is that of the Paralympics. Doctors, nurses, occupational therapists and physiotherapists all encourage and create health and well-being of the severely disabled to an extent that they win international medals. I have argued that this cannot happen without compassion, as is illustrated by the role of Prince Harry. However, some experts who know the set-up suggest that only gold medals matter, and there is some bullying and anything less than gold can be rewarded by less kindness.

Dr Zhidao Xia, a Chinese traditional healer who came to learn from the Oxford International Wound Healing Foundation in Oxford's Dermatology Department, obtained a DPhil at Green College and became a leading expert in the field of stem cell research at Swansea University. He has always been helpful in forging links between me, Oxford and China. He obtained an appointment at Oxford Brookes University where he made links in rehabilitation and went on to explore the future management of the care of the elderly and where my emeritus professor status linked with nursing continues. This is now a global problem and one that Osler did not have to face. The end of life can be managed by the technologies of palliative care. In Sydney in 2016, I produced a DVD on the management of lymphoedema at the end of life. It is possible to suggest technologies but it is not easy to make the final years more happy. Indeed, the high technologies and safe homes aimed at the aged away from their homes and hopes are not aimed at happiness. It is books like *Being Mortal* that draw attention to this. It is difficult in the USA and the UK, and when giving advice to China, one meets in some places the highest technology and in other places an absence of care. ACTAsia's belief that one must aim at teaching children in China to care for the animal kingdom and the environment and then perhaps kindness to humans will follow, makes a lot of sense.

In choosing China rather than the UK to explore these concepts, it is because it has the largest population, and were it to become a compassionate country, in a decade or so it would have the greatest influence.

The UK created the grounds for 'Better Lives' so much earlier than anyone else, with its long and complex endeavour to survive a Civil War, its Industrial Revolution, and its fight against Hitler. To take the lead in solving global requirements for the best ethics needs more energy than it can recruit, and to change its establishment views built up over a decade or so.

Notes on Chapter 11

1) Price, E.W., Bailey D. (1984), 'Environmental factors in the aetiology of endemic elephantiasis of the lower legs in tropical Africa', in *Trop Geogr Med* 36: 1-5.

2) Fuller, L.C., Hay, R., Morrone, A., Naafs, B., Ryan, T.J. and Sethi, A, (2013) 52: 'Guidelines on the role of skin care in the management of mobile populations', in *International Journal of Dermatology* 52: 200-08.

3) Dreyer, G., Addiss, D., Dreyer, P., Noroes, J. (2002), *Basic Lymphoedema Management: The Treatment and Prevention of Problems*

Associated with Lymphatic Filariasis. New Hampshire, Hollis Publishing Co: 112.

Dreyer, G., Addiss, D., Gadelha, P. et al (2006), 'Interdigital skin lesions of the lower limbs among patients with lymphoedema in an area endemic for bancroftian filariasis', in *Trop Med Internat Health* 11: 1475-78.

4) Suma, T.K., Shenoy, R.K., Varghese, J. et al (1997), 'Estimation of ASO titre as an indicator of streptococcal infection precipitating acute adeno lymphangiitis in Brugian Lymphatic Filariasis', in *South East Asian J Trop Med Public Health* 1997.28: 826-30.

Shenoy, R.K., Kumaraswami, V., Suma, T.K. et al (1999), 'A double-blind, placebo-controlled study of the efficacy of oral penicillin, diethylcarbamazine or local treatment of the affected limb I'm preventing acute adenolymphangitis in lymphoedema caused by Brugian Filariasis', in *Ann Tropical Medicine Parasitol* 93: 367-77.

5) Vaqas, B. and Ryan, T.J., 'Lymphoedema: Pathophysiology and management in resource-poor settings – relevance for lymphatic control programmes', in *Filaria Journal* 2003, 2; 4: www.filariajournal.com/content/2/1/4

6) **Publications on CAM and Integrated Medicine**

Narahari, S.R., Ryan, T.J., Bose, K.S., Prasana, K.R., Aggithaya, M.G., (2011), 'Integrating Modern Dermatology and Ayurveda in the Treatment of Vitiligo and Lymphoedema in India', in *International Journal of Dermatology* 50: 310-34.

Ryan, T.J., Narahari, S.R. (2012), 'Reporting an Alliance Using an Integrative Approach to the Management of Lymphoedema in India', in *International Journal of Lower Extremity Wounds* 11: 5-9.

Ryan, T.J., (2013), 'Integrative Medicine Selects Best Practice from Public Health and Biomedicine', in *Indian Journal of Dermatology* 58: 63-72.

Narahari, S.R., Bose, K.S., Aggithaya, M.G., Swamy, G.K., Ryan, T.J., Unnikrishnan, B., Washington, R.G., Rao, B.P.S., Rajagopala, S., Manjula, K., Vandana, U., Thaivalath, T.A., Rojith. M., Shanappa, Y.. Shefuvan, S. and M. (2013), 'Community level morbidity control of lymphoedema using self-care and integrative treatment in two lymphatic filariasis endemic districts of South India: A non-randomised interventional study', in *Trans. R Soc Trop Med Hyg* 9: 566-77.

Narahari, S.R., Ryan, T.J., Aggithaya, M.G. (2013), 'How does yoga work in lymphoedema?, in *J Yoga Phys Ther* 3: 135.

Aggithaya, M.G., Narahari, S.R., Ryan, T.J. (2015), 'Yoga for correction of lymphoedema's impairment of gait as an adjunct to lymphatic drainage: A pilot observational study', in *International Journal of Yoga* 8: 54-61.

Narahari, S.R., Guruprasad, M., Therme, L., Bose, K.S., Ryan, T.J. (2016), 'Yoga protocol for treatment of breast cancer-related lymphoedema', in *International Journal of Yoga* 9: 145-55.

Arianayagam, S., Ryan, T.J. (2016), 'Disorders of pigmentation of the skin-hypotheses underlying interventions by multiple systems of medicine: Is there a role for integrated medicine?', in *Current Science* 111 Special Section: Integrative medicine.

Narahari, S.R., Aggithaya, M.G., Thermo, L., Bose, K.S., Ryan, T.J. (2016), Response to comment on the article, 'Yoga protocol for treatment of breast cancer-related lymphoedema', in *International Journal of Yoga* 2017.10: 52-54.

Bodeker, G., Ryan, T.J., Volk, A., Harris, J., Burford, G. (2017), 'Integrative skin care: dermatology and traditional and complimentary medicine', in *Journal of Alternative and Complementary Medicine* 04/2017; 23(6).

7) Ryan, T.J. (2016), 'Matts Hypothesis: How simple strategies can lead to better outcomes', in *J Lymphoedema* 11: 46-48.

Brooks, J., Ersser, S. (2017), 'Skin and wound care and effective water use in resource-poor countries', in *Community Dermatology Journal* 13-10.

8) Rawlings, A.V., Matts, P.J. (2005), 'Stratum corneum moisturisation at the molecular level: an update in relation to the dry skin cycle', in *J Invest Dermatol* 124(6): 1099-102.

9) Macdonald, J.M., Ryan, T.J. (2010), 'Global impact of the chronic wound and lymphoedema', in Macdonald, John M. and Geyer, Mary Jo (Eds.), *Wound and Lymphoedema Management*, World Health Organisation.

10) Moffatt, C.J., Franks, P.J., Doherty, D.C., et al. 'Lymphoedema: an underestimated health problem', in *QJM* 2003; 96: 731-38.

11) Ryan, T.J. (2011) 'The International Society of Dermatology's Task Force for Skin Care for All: Community Dermatology', in *International Journal of Dermatology* 50:548-51.

12) Kaur, V., Ryan, T.J. (1996), *Women in Dermatology: Joint Meeting of the International Society of Dermatology and the Dermatology and Venereology Society*, 8th June 1995 35: 68-71.

13) Clark, K. (1972), *The Nude*, Princetown University Press.

14) Anderson, L., Davis, M.P. 2017A 'Wake-Up call to dermatologists – Climate Change Affects the Skin', in *International Journal of Dermatology.*

15) Ryan T.J.(2017), 'Will China be a model for Health for all ?A view on both the technicalities of CARE as well as the attitude of CARE from the home of Sir William Osler in Oxford?', in *British-Chinese Medical Journal* 1:1-7.

16) Ryan, T.J. (2014), 'The *wow factor* as a determinant of funding for disorders of the skin', in *Military Medical Research* 2:14 – DOI: 10.1186/s40779-015-0040-7.

17) Aronson, J. (2016), "Collaborative care" is preferable to "patient centred care"', in *British Medical Journal* 2016;353: i 2926.

18) Golden, R. in Silverman, Mark E., Jock Murray, T., and Bryan, Charles S. (Eds.), *The Quotable Osler*. American College of Physicians, pp 283.

19) Francisco Kerdel Vegas (2016), *Medical Paradoxes: Contradictions in Modern Medicine*. London, Publications Violetta.

20) Gawande, Atul (2015), *Being Mortal: Illness, Medicine, and What Matters in the End*. London, Profile Books.

21) Wejuan Tao, Liangbiao Gu, Yanging Zhao, Kejian Li (2015), 'Humanism and medicine in China', in *The Lancet* (letter) 385: 9460.

22) Miller, T. (2017), *China's Asian Dream*. London, Zed Books.

Miller is Oxford-educated but has lived and travelled over many years in China. He describes the demise of Europe and the USA and the takeover by China. It is based much on China's investment of billions in the rest of the world, a gift that is asked for and needed but not greeted with love. It is my view that it will not be greeted with love until its care for technology is accompanied by promotion of an attitude of care based on Confucius, Buddha or

Jesus Christ – or even the caring parts of the Qur'an. Such preaching must be without fanaticism, and should be focused on kindness as a manifestation of friendliness rather than on 'dollars' as gifts.

23) David Cranston (2017), *William Osler*. Bicester, Words by Design.

12: Final Assessment

Frequent failure at the beginning of a career may sometimes be followed with success, but today few get given the second chances that I have been given. At least one of my university friends thought that not working hard enough was an explanation of my failing exams. In the Irish Republic, stationers have popular postcards providing the meaning of names. Terence, as mentioned in Chapter 2, is 'He is hard-working', but the truer meaning may be 'He never gives up'.

As a lonely and anxious child attending many different systems of education, it must be unusual for any child in the UK to have had such long stretches entirely alone. In my infancy, there were few playmates, while during the war at the age of eight in 1942, conversation was limited for a whole year in lodgings cared for by an elderly landlady speaking only at breakfast and supper. As the only boarder in a well-known prep school at the age of eleven, I was again alone. Reading about Boy Scouts was fun but my preference was to be a lone wolf and never to join a pack. There is a recognisable 'only child syndrome', but it does not quite fit the shy and anxious child avoiding adventure and his mother's noisy and often embarrassing humour.

All the recent generations of Ryans are reserved. Father and son together were an admiring, but not a friendly, pair. The same was true for Father and his father, brother and sister. My mother, with all her unusual features, after she came out of the WAAF, was a loving and devoted mother. During the war, she needed my companionship but only once was she more demanding of my attention than seemed reasonable.

It was probably a determining factor of my final career that my mother expected me to become a doctor from the age of four, but it was helpful to have a brief period with a religious step-grandmother. Saying prayers was cathartic and reduced my anxiety. Today, I have a scientific interest in spiritual influences on the mind with a major effect on the body but I am not persuaded by religions except for the initial spokesmen such as Buddha and Confucius, or spokespieces such as the 'Sermon on the Mount'.

Passing into Oxford University and qualifying as a doctor was not straightforward. What followed was not predicted. As something of a Cinderella meeting with Sir John Masterman, the Provost of Worcester, as a Dandini or Good Fairy, getting to and surviving Oxford, and one day to be Vice-Warden of a college, was a fairytale. Even in my final year as a student, there could be no expectation of getting the best jobs, or of discovery or travel. Suddenly, by being invited to take the best house job for the Regius Professor of Medicine, a career began that could not have been taken for granted, since each move was by invitation rather than through application.

Once qualified as a doctor, there was no expectation of doing research. The fact that I did make some fresh scientific observations and was awarded by an Oxford DM, a personal chair and several international achievement awards[1] was based on chance rather than intent. Much credit must go to the support provided by my wife Anne and to the team that made up the Dermatology Department. As a clinician, I could never claim to be much of a scientist (see Appendix 1), and eventually it was in the clinical fields of leg ulceration and lymphoedema that I was able to hold a position of some authority.

Marrying an Australian added new friends and experiences throughout my career from the age of 36. There was marvellous hospitality in Australia from Annes's parents, the family of her twin brother David and the family of her younger brother Paul and many of their friends. Their visits to us were always times of great enjoyment. My daughter Josephine took higher degrees at Monash University and Deakin University, and Melbourne became even better known when Rodney and Ellen Sinclair settled there. Knowing them well as tenants of our property in Oxfordshire and

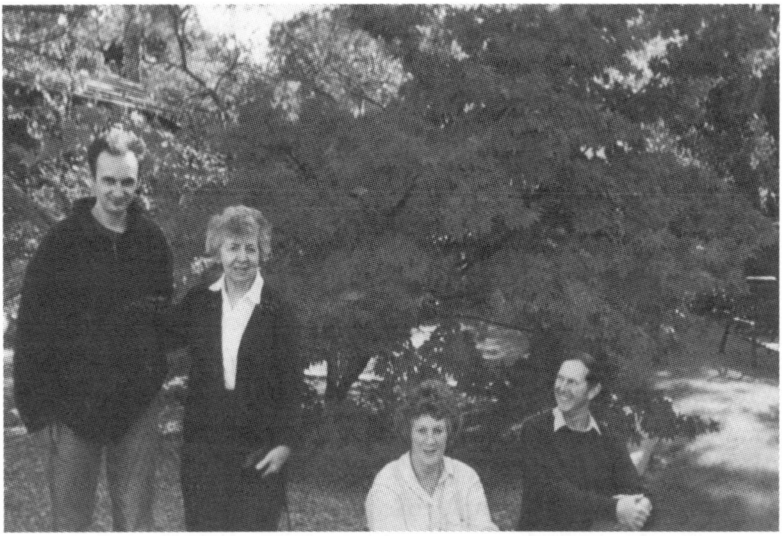

James Ryan, Judy Merry, Anne Ryan and David Merry in our show garden at Hill House, Iffley

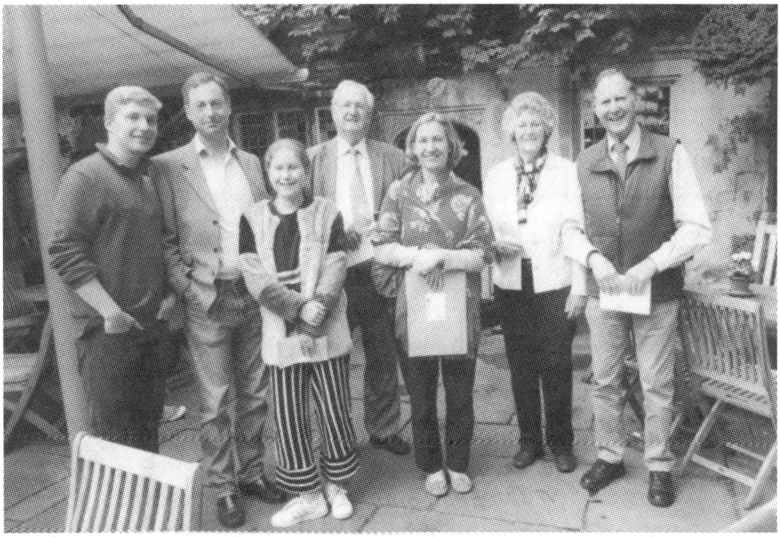

The twins Anne and David on far right. The Del Mars Cosmo, James and Adelaide far left, and myself with Josephine in the middle.

as a very promising junior in the Oxford Dermatology Department, it was no surprise that he has set up a very successful research base in Melbourne. All aspects of my career – dermatology, wound healing, St John Ambulance, lymphology and music – have been enriched, and a few of my watercolours grace homes and offices.

Moments of intense pleasure were often musical. There have been many high spots. Three best loves that have made a lasting impression have been Maria Callas in *Aida*, *La Traviata* and *Tosca*, Margot Fonteyn in many roles, though the feminine roles of Cleo or Juliet were preferred to the Firebird or Apollo. Marlene Dietrich who was the third love after a late night performance at the Edinburgh Festival. High on the list were Gré Brouwenstijn's Leonora in *Fidelio* in the Stuttgart and Glyndebourne productions. Hans Hotter's *Wotan*, Geraint Evans' *Falstaff* and *Beckmesser*, Welitsch's *Musetta*, Gobbi in *Don Carlos*, *Otello* or *Tosca*, Régine Crespin as the Feldmarschallin and Monserrat Caballé in the same role, both at Glyndebourne and Boris Chistoff as Boris Godunov several times. First night successes such as Gerda Lammers in *Electra*, the opening of the new Glyndebourne House with René Fleming as the Countess in *Figaro*, the *War and Peace* production which opened the Sydney Opera House and Richard Goodall's English Mastersingers and *Ring* were other favourites. Disappointments have been Dietrich Fischer Dieskau and Bryn Terfel in *Falstaff*. I have not always appreciated Joan Sutherland but saw her from her early priestess in *Aida* and first lady in *The Magic Flute*, a Gilda in *Rigoletto* which the Quartette was successfully encored at Oxford and her famous *Lucia*. Once when she had sung a Woodbird in Siegfried, I met her in the interval hailing a taxi and asked her who a substitute *Siegfried* had been. "I haven't a faintest," was the reply.

In late retirement, selling larger houses and moving into smaller ones as part of retirement plans and a way of boosting finances meant I had the pleasure of supporting Glyndebourne's superb *Meistersingers*, and getting more involved there. A neighbour in retirement was the Russian baritone Sergei Leiferkus, who gave recitals in our village and introduced young artists. At Glyndebourne, I took some Dutch opera-lovers to his dressing room. One of them asked him whether he sang at Bayreuth, and he responded, "They rang me and asked me to visit them and audition. Me audition!"

When the male nurse, Mr Haines, introduced me to a division of St John Ambulance, he was offering someone who was unable to lecture without reading from notes. My lectures were without merit. It was in St John Ambulance huts, sometimes talking to as few as two people, that I learned to talk with ease. Taking cadets to Turkey and Jerusalem, and tutoring some to win national prizes in First Aid, was one of the best things accomplished in my life: it got me onto the Community Health Council and overall introduced me to community rather than individual health. There were highlights like being in charge of First Aid for Churchill's funeral at Bladon, looking after an illegal pop festival, attending to transfusions of racehorses on air flights, and receiving from the Duke of Gloucester the Knighthood of The Order of St John. More bizarre was inspecting the underground offices to be shared with the Area Health Officer, Alex Gatherer with the idea of playing a key role in organising the people of Oxfordshire to survive an atomic war.

My love of opera introduced me to Josephine Whalley and her senior world of wine and top scientists whom she invited to see my notebooks.

Their glance at and corrections of my disorganised observations led to my being a founder-member of the British Microcirculation Society. Margaret Jennings, later the second Lady Florey, was asked to guide me to prepare for my DM. Eventually, the senior Oxford DM degree was acquired by publications. I became President of the largest and most successful World Microcirculation Conference, and acted as liaison officer for all national societies in the field. For a while, I was the only writer in the UK or USA focusing on blood supply of the skin.

However, all this was a sideline! My real job was dermatology. As a fortunate junior, there were invitations and sponsored national meetings where people were surprised by lectures containing what was then called 'lateral thinking'. Because of a lack of confidence, they were thoroughly rehearsed, and used skills learned from amateur dramatics.

It was extraordinary to have my own lab in London University with my own group of researchers from the USA, Lebanon and Japan, and to be at the famous Hammersmith Hospital was even more exceptional. No-one there had ever failed 'membership' as frequently. There are none who took it eleven times.

Never fully confident of my abilities, every now and then there would be a boost. For example, the dermatologist that led global dermatology advances at the end of the 1960s was the American Al Kligman, of the Department in Pennsylvania University. He surprised me by writing a letter in which he said:

> *You are disturbing the establishment. No better sign that you are finding an authentic path to greatness. Dowling agrees with me that you have the poetic touch; I hope you will continue to be a revolutionary, I did enjoy seeing you in England. Please come to the States. I appreciate your fervour, Don't let anyone dilute it. I hope I have a chance to be stimulated by you often. Onward! Go, man, go!*

My return to Oxford from London was partly in the expectation of the development of a research programme. Some of the work done with juniors and colleagues was of fairly high scientific calibre. With 650 or so publications at the age of 85, that job was done.

Throughout a career of interest in the field of microcirculation and lymphatics, my main role has been to interpret – when attending microcirculation or lymphatic societies, to tell people about the skin, and when visiting dermatology societies, to tell them about the blood supply and the lymphatic drainage. The value of the society meetings has been as a place for discussion and learning, and it has not been difficult to keep abreast of the field – and, for some reason, almost no-one else in the field of dermatology wanted to play a similar role. One thing, molecular biology, was to change this: the fact that the endothelial cell became recognised as a factory of important cytokines, and the mechanisms whereby the endothelial cell became involved in inflammation became linked with the behaviour of the surrounding tissues. These discoveries led many people to become much more interested in blood vessels. Peter Mortimer, while a registrar in Oxford, developed an interest in the lymphatics, and later became a distinguished authority in this field.

Foreign travel to the developing world became a major part of my career. The Venezuelan Ambassador, Kerdel Vegas, introduced me to the St Francis Leprosy Guild which opened up the possibility of visits to leprosy centres round the world. He and the tropical dermatology specialist, Orlando Canizares, introduced me to the International Society of Dermatology, Tropical, Ecologic and Geographic, to become its President, finally its Honorary President and, in late retirement, to chair their sub-committee on Skin Care for All: Community Dermatology.

Dr Colin McDougall, who secured Oxford's reputation as a leader in the field of leprosy research, retired in 1991 and died in 2006, the year in which WHO declared that leprosy had been eliminated as a public health problem, and in which Mikio Masuzawa hoped he might shortly inform me that he had grown the mycobacterium *in vitro* for the first time. But this extraordinary bacteria, probably originally derived from TB, had lost most of its genome, and needed to borrow very specifically from other living cells. These difficult bacteria continued to disappoint us.

Darrell Wilkinson introduced me to the International Committee of Dermatology, eventually to become the Chairman of the International Foundation for Dermatology, then paying attention to all five continents. It coincided with a change in the Department of Dermatology in Oxford, led by the American George Cherry. With his help, our philosophy led to becoming, not just a typical Dermatology Department with its thousands of named titles in Latin, to an organisation applying skincare to maintain skin function, in wound healing, lymphoedema and for tropical skin disease. It required a new purpose-built building on a new site at the Churchill Hospital, the development of a new kind of skin care nursing profession, and trainees from the developing world. Much was learned from successive members of the ISD, ICD and IFD.

Much thought had to go into the meaning and not just the technology of care. I favoured low technology of *care* at low cost available for all, and I was one of many repeatedly calling for such.[2] Being handed Osler's home, 13 Norham Gardens, to look after introduced me to new perspectives on best practice.

Being invited as mentor to the Institute of Applied Dermatology in Kerala, India, and being exposed to new ideas by several Indian colleagues, by cooperating with Professor Aldo Morrone on the topic of immigration in Rome, and cooperating with Dr Gerard Bodeker on Global Initiatives of Traditional Systems of Health, and with my Cousin Vanya on tribal needs in the Nilgiri Hills of South India, opened up important public health interests. Finally, entering discussions with the *Procter & Gamble* scientist, Paul Matts, on how the epidermis works, were all stimuli late in life that kept me active after retirement.

There have been close colleagues in the Department of Dermatology in Oxford who have advanced its reputation nationally and internationally: Rodney Dawber, Fenella Wojnarowska and George Cherry. My successor on the IFD, Rod Hay in London, has been a close colleague in international affairs and has forged links with major programmes of WHO, the CDC in Atlanta, while he has overseen new training schemes in Patagonia and Cambodia.

The arts played some part in my life, and the paint brush and piano have provided an important alternative interest. The use of flower shapes and colours to produce a picture, but not necessarily to identify a botanical specimen, began as a hobby when reaching the age of 50, as a response to an exhibition in Japan and learning the power of the black ink brush to heighten colour. By painting only about 6-10 paintings per annum, productivity is small. Dermatologists have purchased some but there are also several hung in the boardrooms and departments of Oxford and London hospitals, charitable foundations and the pharmaceutical industry.

To decorate the new dermatology building at the Churchill Hospital, paintings were collected from many dermatologists round the world. Sadly, my successors have not kept them.

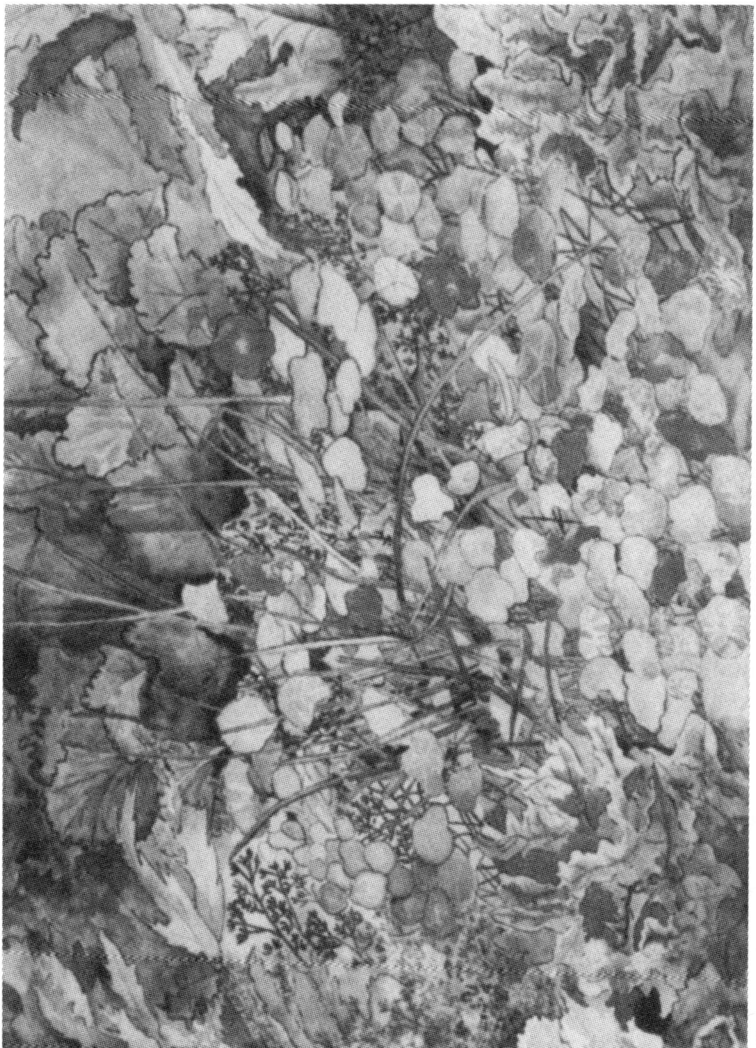

Above and overleaf: two watercolours which, with my piano playing, became a successful diversion

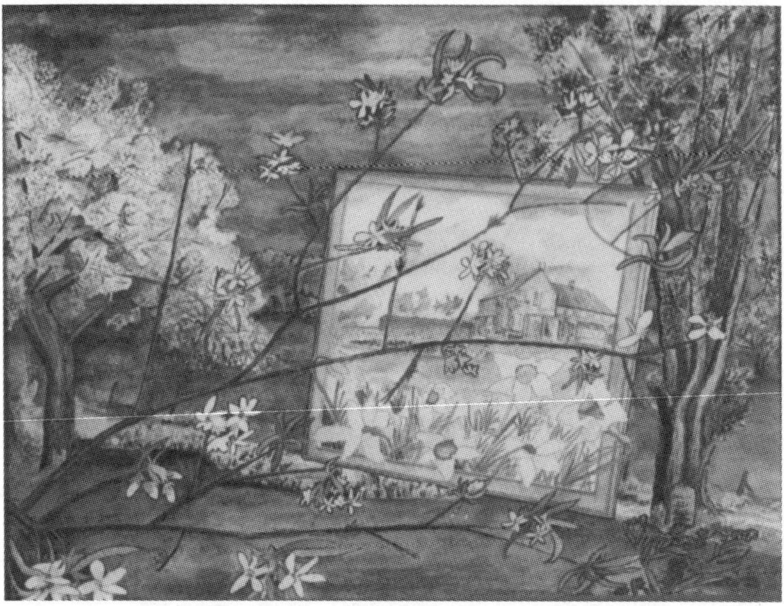

Watercolour of Abbey Willows in the Spring showing the house (inset) and the view of the garden

Work with a Hospital Art Committee had advisors from the Southern Arts Council. We bought a large mobile for the entrance roundabout at the John Radcliffe Hospital. It was disapproved of by the local press but became the site of many official photographs for many years. It was made up of three large sails which had a limited lifespan of three years. They were replaced three times and then it was decided to remove the mobile.

Flower paintings by the Rye artist, Leo Turpin, and by the daughter of Geoffrey Dowling, the doyen of dermatology, Jane Dowling, decorate our home. There was an occasion when the British Association of Dermatology received a query from the biographer of the painter Francis Bacon. It was unsurprisingly about a photograph of a nude young man wearing sun glasses. It was on the floor of his studio after his death and was clearly a dermatology textbook. I started trying to look for it in several libraries, and met other dermatologists such as Andrew Griffiths and Anthony Du Vivier doing the same thing, having also been

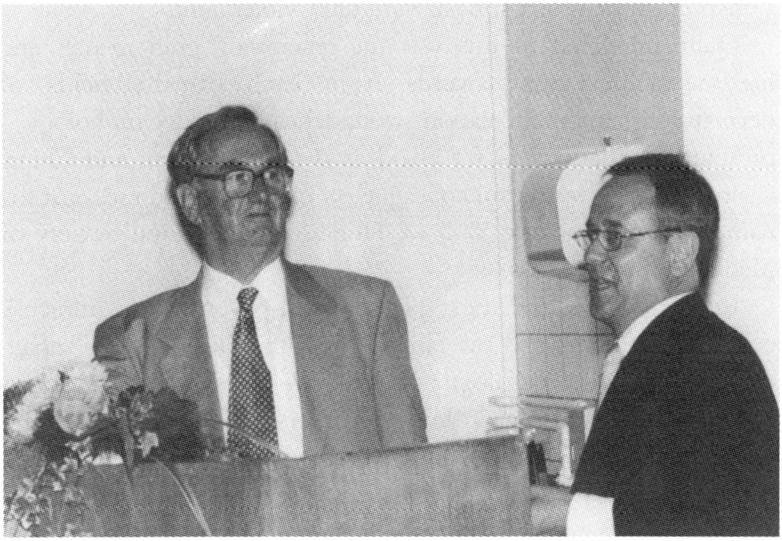

With Dr Wolfgang Marsch in Halle, South Germany, who was to arrange an Honorary Degree at Martin Luther University in 2007

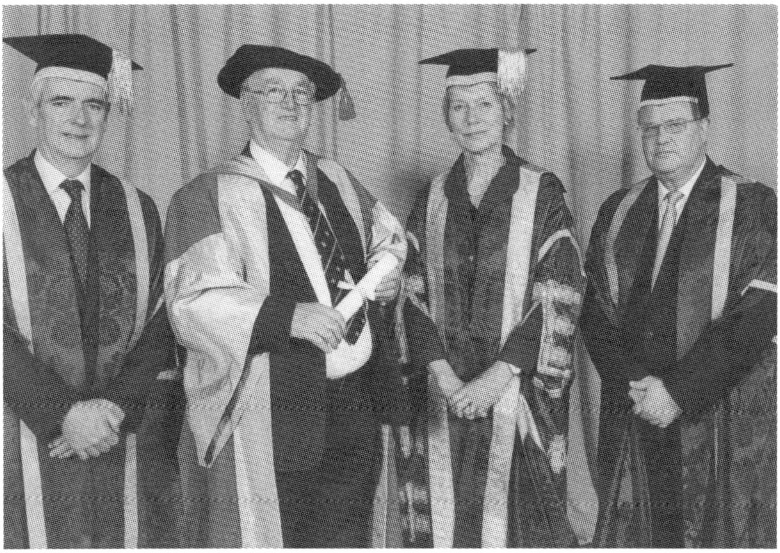

Receiving an Honorary Degree at Hull University in 2013

asked without success. Eventually, it was found in my own library in a chapter on treating psoriasis with ultra-violet light.

Quite unrelated to this was the receipt of gold medals and lifetime achievement awards from each of the fields of dermatology, microcirculation, wound healing and lymphology – presented in nations as far afield as the USA, Brazil and China. Claire Fuller, a wonderful colleague on many programmes, got my name engraved on the Wall of Honour at the Royal Society of Medicine.

In many ways, the most pleasure was given by an immense celebration for me and my family when, in Halle, Saxony-Anhalt, the German dermatologist Wolfgang Marsch organised an honorary degree at Martin Luther University. Also enjoyable were honorary degrees at Hull University, organised by Steve Ersser and while at Oxford Brookes University he organised there my appointment as a professor. I was surprised to get the Rotary's Paul Harris Award for relatively short-lived efforts in Tanzania and Guatemala. Lifetime achievement awards and honorary memberships abound (see the notes to this chapter).

Notes on Chapter 12

1)

Lifetime Achievement Awards

Sir Archibald Gray Medal of the British Association of Dermatologists for Outstanding Contributions to Dermatology 1997

European Tissue Repair Society 1995

Asian Union forMicrocirculation 1995

The Association for the Advancement of Wound Care: The John Boswick Memorial Award 2004

Ratschow Medal of the Curatorum Angiologica, Germany 2002

The International League of Dermatological Societies 2007

World Union of Wound Healing Societies Toronto 2008

International Lymphoedema Frame Work 2008

The International Society of Dermatology 1999

The Chinese Traumatology Society 2016

Honorary Memberships

Dermatology Societies of Sweden, Norway, Italy, Israel, France, Germany, Spain, America, Brasil, Argentina, Japan, Nepal, India.

The Sikhumba Club – Dermatology Registrars of South Africa

The Sky Club for Japanese Trainee Dermatologists

National Academy of Medicine – Venezuela

Honorary International Life Membership Indian Association of Dermatology Venereology and Leprosy 2011

British Microcirculation Society (Life) with named Annual Award for best research paper at Annual Meeting 1987

European Society for Microcirculation (Life)

2) *The World Health Forum, Vol 8,* p 305, published in 1987 the view of E.O. Attinger:

> *High technology has been vastly expanded and misused in the health care systems of many countries, There has been insufficient regard for the social and economic consequences. Health care systems should be restructured so as to strengthen the humane functions of doctors and others, Funds should be redirected towards technologies that can effectively improve the health status of the whole population.*

I wished to give greater emphasis on the attitude rather than the technology of care.

Appendix 1: Scientific Contributions

The following are scientific contributions advancing mechanisms which explain skin disease with examples from 650 publications.

1) The epidermis has a rough surface and this can be made smooth and non-reflective by putting a little oil on it. I had in my hand an instrument for mopping out the ear and dislodging wax. Pressing it on the skin covered in oil, it dislodged tissue fluid and increased the visibility of the superficial blood vessels, rather in the same way as a crinkled pillow produces red marks on the skin. The doyen USA dermatologist, Dr Sulzberger, on my first visit to the USA, pronounced it: 'Newtonian in its simplicity'. Four large notebooks were filled with observations. I presented this observation to the first meeting of the British Microcirculation Society at the Royal Microscopical Society.

Ryan, T.J. (1965), 'A new technique for studying the microcirculation of the skin', in *Journal of the Royal Microscopical Society* 84: 230.

Ryan, T.J. (1967), 'A new technique for studying the microcirculation of the skin', in *In Vivo Techniques in Histology.* Ed. G.H. Bourne), pp 192-202. London, Williams & Wilkins.

2) Over several years, descriptions of the superficial blood supply in different diseases and age groups followed. It was obvious that the different shapes of the capillaries close to the epidermis correlated with differences in the behaviour of the overlying epidermis. A rapidly growing epidermis in repair or in diseases such as psoriasis correlated with overgrown capillaries, while atrophic skin conditions, ageing skin or skin treated with steroids had a thin epidermis and reduced vasculature.

Ryan, T.J. (1967), '"Teach-in" on factors controlling the blood supply of the epidermis', in *British Journal of Dermatology* 79: 1-13.

This observation had to be explained, and it was postulated that the epidermis produced stimuli to its blood supply. Such a stimulus could be modified by other cells in the vicinity such as nerve endings, and white cells, as well as the amount and type of intervening connective tissue.

Ryan, T.J. (1970), 'Factors influencing the growth of vascular endothelium in the skin', in *British Journal of Dermatology* 82 (Suppl 5): 99-111.

3) It was the usual belief that the basal cells migrated away from the dermis, losing their nucleus as they reached the surface and were exfoliated. I stated that no cell habitually moves away from what it most needs, and this belief – that the epidermal cells move away from their blood supply – needed a rethink. I suggested that, when a basal cell divides to replicate itself, it loses its attachment to the dermis and is displaced by adjacent non-dividing cells, jostling it out of position outwards to its death away from its nutrition. This was published as a paper in the *British Journal of Dermatology*. I had given it as an oral presentation at an annual meeting, entitled 'The direction of growth of epidermis'. I was very junior and afterwards, standing by another registrar, later Miriam Stoppard, wife of the playwright, she spoke of the reaction as a stunned silence.

Ryan, T.J. (1970), 'Direction of epithelial growth', in *British Journal of Dermatology* 83: 701-02.

Not long after its publication, there was a paper in the *British Journal of Dermatology* by the USA's most senior pathologist, Herman Pinkus, giving reasons why Ryan's Hypothesis should be discounted. In a letter to the journal and in a later update I politely disagreed.

Ryan, T.J. (1975), 'The direction of epithelial growth is inwards' (Section on Dermatology, pp 1-3). *Proceedings of the Royal Society of Medicine* 68: 159-61.

A big fan mail followed and some well-known intellectuals, such as the South African George Findley, supported the concept. I returned to it in publications over the years and finally in 2014-15, when writing on how the pigment cell, the melanocyte, is exfoliated outwards or sometimes migrated inwards into the dermis, I restated my belief.

4) At a meeting in Gothenburg (1968), I learned how to test blood vessels for fibrinolysis, the property used to remove clots. At the Institute of Dermatology, visiting research workers were supplied, Bob Turner from the USA, Amal Kurban from Lebanon, and Kiyoshi Nishioka from Japan. Between us, we identified for the first time as a product of the epidermis, an inhibitor of fibrinolysis. We followed this by demonstrating in the skin, conditions of activation and the inhibition of fibrinolysis.

Kurban, A.K., Turner, R.H., Ryan, T.J. (1970), 'Fibrinolysis in relation to dermatology', in *British Journal of Dermatology* 82 (Suppl 5): 44-50.

5) With Kyoshi Nishioka, we examined how new blood vessel growth used a scaffold of fibrin which existed only when fibrinolysis was inhibited.

Nishioka, K., Ryan, T.J. (1972), 'The influence of the epidermis and other tissues on blood vessel growth in the hamster cheek pouch', in *Journal of Investigative Dermatology* 58: 33-37.

6) Once I was a consultant at Oxford, there was less time to innovate. There were clinical observations, and we tried out various treatments newly developed by others. There was much to write about, including half a book on blood vessels.

Ryan, T.J. (1973), 'Blood Vessels of the Skin', Vol 2, Chapters 16-21, in Jarrett, A. (Ed.), *Physiology and Pathophysiology of the Skin.* London, Academic Press.

A book on vasculitis, entitled *Microvascular Injury*, took the line that noxious agents did harm only if there were opportunities provided for them to localise. I described factors promoting localisation, such as gravitational stasis, cooling, absent fibrinolysis and the psychosomatic.

Ryan, T.J. (Ed.) (1976), *Microvascular Injury* (Vol 7, *Major Problems in Dermatology*). London, Lloyd Luke Medical, p 416.

7) With Wajdi Kanan and others in the Department, we showed that the septal mucosa of the anterior nose was an excellent model to study localisation.

Kanan, M.W., Ryan, T.J. (1974), 'Endonasal localisation of blood borne viable and non-viable particulate matter', in *British Journal of Dermatology* 92: 475-78.

Kanan, M.W., Ryan, T.J., Weddell, A.G.M. (1975), 'The behaviour of the nasal mucosa towards blood borne colloidal carbon in experimental animals', in *Pathology*, Europe 10: 264-76.

8) A new interest was the lymphatic of the skin, and I wrote the first review for dermatologists in the same major series, *Pathophysiology of the skin*, edited by Jarrett. In this, I drew attention to the elastic fibre that was found round the lymphatic in the skin. Later, this was to become a major interest and several publications from Oxford emphasised its importance.

Ryan, T.J. (1978), 'The lymphatics of the skin', in Jarrett, A. (Ed.), *The Physiology and Pathophysiology of the Skin*, Vol. 5. 2nd edition, pp 1755-80. London, Academic Press.

Ryan, T.J. (1978), 'Disorders affecting the lymphatic system', in Jarrett, A. (Ed.), *The Physiology and Pathophysiology of the Skin*, Vol. 5. 2nd edition, pp 1781-2808. Academic Press, London.

Ryan, T.J., Mortimer P.S., Jones R.L. (1986), 'Lymphatics of the skin: neglected but important', in *Jnl Dermatol* 10: 411-17.

Ryan, T.J. (1989), 'Structure and function of lymphatics', in *Invest Derm* 93: 18S-24S.

Mortimer, P.S., Simmonds, R., Rezvani, M., Robbins, M., Hopewell, J.W., Ryan, T.J. (1990), 'The measurement of skin lymph flow by isotope clearance – reliability, reproducibility, injection dynamics and the effect of massage', in *Invest Derm* 95: 677-82.

9) During the 1980s, quality of life became an issue specially led by Andrew Findley in Cardiff. I had discussed with Margaret Agerholm, who worked on polio rehabilitation, her classification of disabilities, and had emphasised the importance of appearance and body image. A paper had been published in which I had stated that everyone would like to be confident when nude! Andrew kindly told me that this had influenced him. The Department of Dermatology employed Sandra Jowett, a sociologist, to explore this theme and it added to a rapidly developing literature.

Ryan, T.J. (2003), 'Handicaps and the handicapped: a nomenclature and Classification of intrinsic handicaps', by M Agerholm, in *R, Soc Health J* 1975: 95 3-8. *Clinical and Experimental Dermatology* 28: 113-14.

Jowett, S., Ryan, T.J. (1985), 'Skin disease and handicap: An analysis of the impact of skin conditions', in *Social Science and Medicine* (Oxford) 20:425-29.

Jowett, S., Ryan, T.J. (1985), 'Dermatology patients and their doctors', in *Clinical and Experimental Dermatology* 10: 246-54.

Ryan, T.J. (1987), 'The confident nude or whither dermatology', in *Dermatology in Practice* 5: 8-12.

Finlay, A.Y., Ryan, T.J. (1996), 'Disability and handicap in dermatology', in *International Journal of Dermatology* 35: 305-11.

10) The influence of mechanical forces to tranduce biochemical signals became a major interest with colleagues such as Mikio Masuzawa, who used centrifugal forces to show that fibroblasts gripped their template and manufactured inhibitors of fibrinolysis. This was important as lysis prevented grip and stick.

Ryan, T.J. (1985), 'The Dowling Oration: Morphosis, occult forces and ectoplasm – the role of glues and proteolysis in skin disease', in *Clinical and Experimental Dermatology* 10: 507-22.

Ryan, T.J. (1989), 'Biochemical consequences of mechanical forces generated by distension and distortion', in *J American Acad Derm* 21: 115-30.

11) Sergio Curri was insisting that the blood supply of adipose tissue was of particular interest. It led me to read extensively about adipose tissue, and eventually we wrote a book together which was the first of its kind. It added fat cells to the supporting system of the skin that needed to be taken into account in all its disorders. When liposuction became a tool to treat lymphoedema, more thought to explain its effects resulted in more publications.

Ryan, T.J., Curri, S. (1989), *The Cutaneous Adipose Tissue* in the series *Clinics in Dermatology*. Philadelphia, J.B. Lippincott.

Ryan, T.J. (2007), 'What are subcutaneous adipocytes really good for?', in *Experimental Dermatology* 16: 45-70.

12) From my days as a medical student, listening to a lecture on India fakirs, I have been interested in those phenomena which science cannot explain. They include those religious ceremonies that do body-piercing without pain, bleeding or scarring. This can be contrasted with the Catholic stigmatists that have painful bleeding. It has some similarities to the painful bruising syndrome and psychosomatic purpura which I studied from time to time but for which I could find no explanations.

13) I did not have any new ideas after this time but helped others to massively develop the theme of skin care in the resource-poor developing world, first with the UNESCO collaboration on 'Healthy Skin for All', preparing UNIDERM for the International Committee of Dermatology, and then the task force with the International Society of Dermatology's Skin Care for All: Community Dermatology. Ryan, T.J. (1994), 'Healthy skin for all', in *International Journal of Dermatology* 33: 829-35.

Ryan, T.J. (1994), 'United Nations and Non-governmental Organisations 'Healthy Skin for All'. Contemporary Tropical Dermatology', in *Dermatology Clinics* 12: 611-19.

14) With a medical student, Babar Vaqas, I wrote an article on the morbidity control of lymphatic filariasis which stimulated Dr Narahari of Kerala to further develop yoga and Ayurveda for management of lymphoedema in South India. This has become one of the most successful and largest interventions for morbidity control of lymphoedema. There have been 3,000 patients treated for the massive oedema of lymphatic filariasis and fifty relevant publications.

Vaqas, B., Ryan, T.J., 'Lymphoedema: Pathophysiology and management in resource-poor settings-relevance for lymphatic control programmes', in *Filaria Journal* 2003, 2; 4 www.filariajournal.com/content/2/1/4

Podoconiosis, as discussed with Frederick Price when he visited my laboratory in 1970, is due to the effect of irritant soil on persons not wearing shoes. I have visited Ethiopia with Clare Fuller and Paul Matts to support studies by Gail Davey, and the initiation of footwear, washing and emollients. Rod Hay supervised a study by

Ferguson (*British Journal of Dermatology*) on trans-epidermal water loss (TEWL). The Paul Matts Hypothesis, which shows that the epidermis, when injured, allows increased transepidermal water loss and triggers the production of inflammatory mediators to the dermis, and that studies by Jill Brookes show that glycerine washes can reverse the process. Jill Brooks (2016) found that, in podoconiosis, the TEWL was severely compromised. What was gratifying was that an emollient 3% glycerine immediately reversed this. Glycerine/Glycerol has many ideal properties (Fluhr et al, 2010), and it holds moisture in the skin and is not expensive.

Ryan, T.J. (2016), 'The Matts Hypothesis: How simple strategies can lead to better outcomes', in *Lymphoedema* 11: 1-3.

Brooks, J., Ersser, S. (2017), 'Skin and wound care and effective water use in resource-poor countries', in *Community Dermatology Journal* 13 – 10.

With Sanju Arianayagam, I published three articles in Indian journals, suggesting that, as others had done, there was more to Melanin than light protection, and that one should look at Tyrosine metabolism millions of years earlier when it played a role in cell contact and synapse formation. At the beginning of my career, Professor J.D. Boyd, the Cambridge pathologist, suggested that mature melanocytes had lost the power to move and, in deeper locations, cannot be concerned with radiant energy in or near the wavelength of light. The emphasis in my later work with Arianayagam was on the role of lysis of grip, synapsis and stick in allowing movement.

Arianayagam, S., Ryan, T.J. (2014), 'Human pigmentation: A side effect adapted from a primitive organism's survival, acting through cell attachment with an affinity for the keratinocyte and for elastin: Part I', in *Indian Journal of Dermatology Online* 5: 201-13.

Arianayagam, S., Ryan, T.J. (2014), 'Human pigmentation: A side effect adapted from a primitive organism's survival: Part II The melanocyteas mentor of the keratinocyte', in *Indian Journal of Dermatology Online* 5: 328-33.

Arianayagam, S., Ryan, T.J. (2016), 'Disorders of pigmentation of the skin-hypotheses underlying interventions by multiple systems of medicine: is there a role for integrated medicine?', in *Current Science* 111, Special Section: Integrative medicine.

Appendix 2: Lay Participation in Medicine

In 1983 I had had experience of managing youth of one of the largest cadet forces. More children than adults belong to St John Ambulance, but it was very difficult to keep them as teenagers. I spoke to the senior officers of the Brigade at their Annual Conference saying that they should do more to advertise their role as a youth organisation and should copy Oxford's successful drive to enthuse teenagers. I went on to ask both Green College and the Oxfordshire Health Authority to read my paper 'Lay participation in medicine'.

Richard Doll wrote:

> *I found the paper very stimulating and indeed exciting. The role of and power of the professional vis–a-vis the patient (or pupils) are central matters of concern and I touched upon them in my inaugural lecture.*

John Walton wrote:

> *The organisation of a day's seminar on this topic would be well worthwhile and an important initiative for Green College.*

Muir Gray wrote:

> *I emphasise that community participation as one of the key elements of the much broader WHO concept of primary care.*

Alec Gatherer, as District Medical Officer, wrote:

> *Would it be possible to use your initiative in any way to highlight what could be done to get better overall participation between the 'lay' and the professional?*

John Rigby Secretary of Outward Bound wrote:

> *We could consider how Outward Bound can integrate some of the notions of healthcare into its programmes.*

At the time of the writing of these letters I had no experience of resource poor countries world-wide. Now in 2017 many of the concepts are more relevant than ever for helping a frail elderly population and victims of burns, land mines, the disfigured and disabled from disorders of the skin such as leprosy in a world-wide programme of collaboration between the professional and the 'lay' person to provide a social and family-orientated caring community, supporting health services, and having some training in care technology and attitudes.

China has the worst of problems. Communism led to the expectation that the state would provide all and abolished voluntary help. They also made it impossible for families to be the centre of voluntary help. In the rural areas even the one child will have moved to the cities. I am working with the charity Actasia to solve this problem.

Lay Participation in Medicine

(First given in 1983 as a lecture to Senior St John Ambulance officers at their Headquarters in London and upgraded for Green College in 2000 with further notes made in 2017.)

This document, concerning lay participation in medicine, for discussion by members and fellows of Green College, is an appropriate subject for development by the college.

Outlined first are the medical problems it is intended partly to solve, after which the role of the volunteer is then discussed. Emphasis is laid on the need for leadership by the medical and nursing professions and reasons are given why any such programmes should be aimed at youth.

Medicine in the year 2000

The problems are well-known. They have been outlined in many documents, including some for the World Health Organisation and in an Orations by our first Warden Sir Richard Doll. The greatest problem: 'The impending crisis of old age: a challenge to ingenuity.' I quote from Acheson (1982):

> *If current rates of disability and dependency were to continue to prevail, by the end of the century, at least half of the additional elderly over 85 might need help in taking a bath, one fifth of those living in their homes might be bed fast or house bound and a substantial proportion would be suffering from troublesome incontinence.*

Other increasing problems are the effects of alcohol, drugs, smoking, accidents, and sexually transmitted diseases. These have received much publicity even within the last few months because of 'football hooliganism', heroin addiction in London, and HIV/AIDS.

The World Health Organisation also emphasises pollution and food poisoning, and in this college Jeffrey Burley has drawn our attention to some direct consequences of the loss of the tree, which relate to pollution and to food poisoning.

We are all aware that the unemployment problem, linked with early retirement and a shorter working week are creating difficulties which the WHO claims will be a crisis for the next century. Richard Doll states, "What is a much greater social problem is the technological revolution which is altering our whole structure of remunerative employment."

I suspect that all of us in Green College will accept that these are significant difficulties which need to be solved. Most of us are doing little, however, to solve them.

Some of us will be anxious about Oxford's incapacity to influence events and to public reaction to our failure. There is criticism of high technology which does nothing to solve such problems but uses up all the resources. Oxford, in the next ten years, will see an enormous development in high technology costing many millions of pounds, none of which technology is aimed at alleviating any of the problems outlined above. It is my belief that we can both support this high technology in Oxford and also offset it by giving more attention within Green College to these other problems. High technology is needed to prevent genetic disease or to rid us of some of the major infections, but its prolongation of life and its preservation of the diseased creates as many problems as are solved. It creates tension between the humanist and technological traditions of medicine. Oxford University is doubtful about the value of humanism in medicine and Green College could do more to show its worth.

Lay participation is contemporary terminology replacing the Victorian voluntary help. It too is receiving a great deal of attention and study and so one might ask why? I am also suggesting that such study is receiving too little input from the health orientated professions and we medical and nursing professionals should study what can be done to make us better leaders of lay persons and of youth in particular.

The case for involving lay people is very well outlined by Maurice King in his chapter 'Medicine in an Unjust World' in the *Oxford Textbook of Medicine* (1983). Having first outlined the size of the problem and the distribution of ill-health and resources, he nicely indicates that the medical and nursing professions are incapable of carrying such a vast burden and none of the professions find the carrying of this burden the least bit attractive. The training we give our medical students and nurses in no way encourages problem-solving outside the confines of a well equipped surgery. Satisfaction in the practice of medicine, at least in middle age, requires computers, cleanliness and comfort, and takes us further away from the house-bound bedfast and the incontinent elderly or the young addict.

Maurice King gives us seven axioms which lead inevitably to the need for 'voluntary' help.

i) CARE for all humanity, which means care for those even when there are no doctors or nurses.

ii) CREATE, which means building a health service and therefore training people in all aspects of management and leadership, and the use of bricks and mortar rather than merely teaching only clinical acumen to only a professional few.

iii) TEACH, which means that 'Doctor' once again means teacher first and foremost.

iv) DELEGATE, which means that care for all humanity, creation and teaching can be effected by others and not just doctors and nurses.

v) APPLY the most cost effective technologies.

vi) GO widely rather than deeply, with higher technology and more specialisation.

vii) MAKE the community master – which means making the service sensitive to the wants of the community rather than to the wants of those who provide the service.

The word 'sensitive' is one that is linked to voluntary rather than to professional help. It is mentioned by Richard Crossman (1973) in his lecture to Oxford University, 'The Role of the Volunteer in Modern Social Service', and it was much used by those such as Rosemary Rue when Community Health Councils were first introduced to their new role as watchdog of the Health Service.

The synthesis of Maurice King's axioms is comprehensive primary health care delivered by community health workers.

Addendum 2017: High technology is desirable and so is the pharmaceutical industry and the advanced cosmetician's contribution to well-being. This does not stop an appeal for low technology care and attitudes of care such as kindness being even more desirable. I no longer focus on small populations such as the UK, but see countries such as India and China, with their enormous populations also suffering from the dominance of high technology but an increasingly frail and elderly population, with the added emphasis on dementia, as well as many who survive astonishingly severe injury, disease and transplantation. India and China will have to become better than anyone else at following King's axioms. They must seek lay participation and involvement of youth in their solutions. Axioms by William Osler are to be advertised in China from this year. Oxford is fortunate in being able to promulgate axioms from 13 Norham Gardens from leaders such as Osler, Pickering, Doll and Walton who once lived there.

Altruism

Richard Crossman in 1973 gave a remarkable lecture in which he referred to altruism. The lecture was dedicated to Richard Titmus who had written about blood transfusion. Given a modicum of leadership in a community, many derive much satisfaction from giving blood. Titmus believed that this satisfaction could be equated with a biological need to help. It was Crossman's view that the Health Service he had helped to create had suppressed this biological need and failed to provide the satisfaction which is inherent in voluntary work. He wrote,

> *It is my contention in this lecture that one of the main causes of social disintegration from which our community is now suffering is the frustration of the altruistic motive.*

Crossman discussed an Oxbridge product, The Workers Educational Movement, a two-way channel between university dons and working class men and women. He described on the one hand how public opinion was changed to sweep labour to victory in 1945, while at the same time as in Communist Russia and China, the do-good volunteer was replaced by professionals and trained administrators. He went on to describe the setting up of the professional establishment and the reaction to it by youth – known as anti establishment. The development of lay protest groups was a further consequence, so that today wherever we have lay groups, opposition to, rather than partnership with, the professions may arise.

What I want to see in a new Oxbridge product is a two-way channel between university dons and working people which seeks to reverse the trends: professionals joining the lay groups, establishment joining youth and the trained linking up with the 'do-good volunteers'. It is not new – see Hardy's novels such as *Jude the Obscure* or William Morris building the Natural History Museum.

Crossman, 1973, spoke of the alienation of youth, failure to abolish inequality and of inhuman and stupid decision making in the Health Service in particular. This was linked, in his view, to the administration by highly professional hands of the welfare state while abolishing "the amateurism of philanthropy". He wrote,

> *What I do maintain is that do-good volunteering is as essential to humane social services as highly trained professionalism and the professional who disregards this need for do-good volunteering is liable to make the most cruel mistakes.*

This would seem to be a somewhat right-wing view for a socialist, but Crossman gave an example of Oxford practice which many of our colleagues would regard as left wing.

> *The case for the big new district hospital is almost entirely a consultant's case. Certainly it saves time when he does not have to get in his car and drive, in the course of a week, to half-a-dozen small hospitals. Certainly it is an advantage when a rare case is suddenly presented in a hospital which needs four or five experts, that those four or five should be gathered round the patient's bedside in a single building.*

Crossman might have been talking about the GP health centre versus home visiting, Since he was illustrating an aspect of service of which lay people disapprove but of which the professional sees the advantages, it can be translated into terms of high technology versus primary care.

Like Crossman, I see high technology as possible in an environment in which the do-good volunteer provides the primary care. This will only happen if the professional joins the volunteer.

Addendum 2017: During my career I took on executive roles with Lay volunteers in the Psoriasis Association, the Eczema Society, St John Ambulance, The Red Cross and The Community Health

Council. My wife is currently a coordinator and driver of our Village and Neighbourhood Link Scheme, taking the disabled to wherever they have appointments for health reasons.

Crossman wrote further that the need for volunteers in primary care is because the professional is always going to be too few and too busy to give the time that is needed to solve the problem of the individual in primary care. The problems in primary care are chronic and time-consuming but not highly technical, as, for instance, giving the physically handicapped a bath.

Fifteen years have gone by since Titmus (1969) wrote about the voluntary worker in the social services describing how the professions create an opposition of frustrated pressure groups. Eleven years have gone by since Crossman called on governments to,

> *Link professional and volunteer in true co-operation to foster the care element in the care services and to recruit, train and organise volunteers for all the functions that are performed by them.*

Actually governments have continued to hope that all of this might happen and have made money available. It is because the medical and nursing professions as well as the attitudes of the Trade unions have not promoted this link between professions and volunteers that I am proposing Green College should take the initiative.

As Crossman (1973) indicated, the opposition to change is powerful since our professions demand that all jobs are done only by holding the necessary qualifications and no one should undercut an honest working-man's rate for the job – or reduce the number of jobs available for those in need.

Addendum 2017: Knowing that the number of elderly not able to cut their toenails was hugely increasing, I set up a minimal and safe service for Red Cross and St John Ambulance in Oxfordshire to provide, but had great opposition from the established chiropody services, even though they could not meet the demand, and there were many walking shoeless because shoes could not accommodate their long nails.

Existing Lay Practice

There are many hundreds of organisations concerned with health. Most of these are fund-raising or lobbyist. Few provide a service. Nearly every disease has its own association drawing attention to its need for more resources to identify its cause or to treat it. I have helped to form a few for skin diseases – the Psoriasis Association, the Eczema Society, the Dystrophic Epidermolysis Bullosa Association, and the Skin Disease Research Foundation. All of these have been critical at some time of the established dermatology services and some of the dermatologists have at times been strongly opposed to such organisations. On the whole co-operation is now excellent but any question of these organisation providing therapy or even detailed counselling is still opposed by some. Nevertheless, it must be true that a counsellor for parents of eczematous children trained by the professions would be welcomed by many parents.

Addendum 2017: the nursing profession has made great progress in providing a counselling service.

Some years ago, all dermatologists were written to by Renwick Vickers who asked them if they would support a volunteer based camouflage service – the use of cosmetic skin preparations by lay advisors to disguise birth marks and other disfigurements. Some dermatologists wrote that they would never use such a service and were opposed to it. Within one year the British Red Cross volunteers were providing an excellent service in many but not all Dermatology Departments. The Family Practitioner Peter Pritchard, who launched a lay participation scheme for Family Practitioner Health Centres, wrote that that there was much opposition to such involvement of patient participants, in spite of its obvious advantages.

The Community Health Councils were set up to provide a sensitive watch dog service, directing criticism towards improvement of the service rather than to financial gain through litigation as one important consequence. Much has been written about CHCs and especially about how the process of consultation will delay decision making because the CHCs work mainly in opposition to, rather than in participation with, the Health Service Management Teams. Recommended by the Red Cross and St John Ambulance, I was probably the only medically qualified academic to be elected to a CHC. The Oxford CHC was one of the most influential. I was on it for four years and I believe I provided factual advice based on experience, which is now lacking, since employees of the NHS are removed from its membership and there are no watch dogs with the necessary insider knowledge. Many of the discussions within the CHC needed better information. There was also a tendency for research within the CHC to be time wasting because it duplicated what was often already set up as an audit by the Health Authority.

The voluntary organisations providing a service like the Red Cross and St John Ambulance Brigade are few and mostly very much smaller. However, there is great difficulty in recruiting and providing a sustained service as we did sometimes for weeks at large pop festivals, national emergencies and ambulance strikes. They worked best when led by a medically or nursing qualified member of the British Red Cross or the St John Ambulance Brigade. Unfortunately such leadership is rare. Doctors and Nurses are far too busy to take off such a long time for a volunteer role and, as mentioned above, there is opposition by some professions for taking on a volunteer role such as bed making or toe nail cutting.

Richard Crossman (1973) suggested that transport was one area in which volunteers could be better used to support the health service. When a member of the CHC, I was put in charge of examining ways in which volunteers could get the frail elderly to appointments within the health service as bus services, village shops, chemists and health centres contracted. The professional Ambulance Service was not keen to solve such a need as their paramedics became expert in more and more high technology. We voluntary organisations were not enthusiastic when the Ambulance Services gave thought to creating its own cadet corps competing with and better funded than our own.

Home Defence is one professional organisation which is very well funded and which at threatening times is very keen to recruit lay people in massive numbers. Much of the teaching and leadership provided is concerned with survival and the use of widely based cheap and simple techniques to maintain the health of the population. Unfortunately, all the expertise thus propagated is linked to war and to nuclear attack in particular. Any suggestion that such expertise could be linked to peace time needs is opposed. I have some experience of this through courses at The Home Defence College and as Chairman of the Joint Emergency County Committee.

Finally, a look at the use of the paramedic in schemes for the Third World provides answers to problems even in Europe. Nevertheless, even this area lacks the co-operation and leadership of the professions. It has been imposed upon a few in China but in countries such as India, western biomedical practice is mostly more attractive to the professionals. When the role of the 'doctor' is given to lesser qualified persons there is opposition. The use of the 'headman' of a village or a traditional health practitioner to provide modern western medicine for snake bites or leprosy is criticised and yet it is economically viable to use those who are anyway first on call. Making available fully trained physicians and surgeons within easy reach of even a small proportion of 'all' is an impossibility.

During the last ten years I have joined in discussions with the Oxfordshire Health Authority on how best to use volunteers, especially for home nursing. It is an area of frequent failure. The volunteer cannot give a regular commitment and is frequently without the qualifications to manage all problems. The professional does not know how to use the volunteer and has little skill in thanking and rewarding those who help out.

One solution is to employ a Liaison Officer. Such person costs money but is neither professional nor volunteer. I have argued, without avail, that a professional should become a part-time volunteer. I could not have the trust of the St John Ambulance Brigade if I had not signed up to obey its rules, wear its uniform, and participate in its bureaucracy.

George Day of the Samaritans described in *The Lancet* how, as a doctor and a member of the Samaritans, he was actually more useful to depressed patients, but was unwelcome at meetings of local psychiatrists. He also describes how angry he felt when the backache of one his patients was cured by a back-street 'bone-setter'.

He raise the issue of co-operation and collaboration: "Can a doctor collaborate with 'unqualified' Samaritans?" The General Medical Council booklet, page 11, states: 'A doctor who improperly delegates to a person, who is not a registered medical practitioner, functions requiring the knowledge and skill of a medical practitioner is liable to disciplinary proceedings.'

In this section I am merely pointing out that there are many bodies with points of view which must be consulted if lay participation is to succeed. They include governments, trades unions, The Home Defence College, The General Nursing Council, The General Medical Council, and existing voluntary organisations. as well as 'the Church'. Only an independent body with considerable status is likely to get a hearing.

Should the Main Emphasis Be on Youth?

There is surely no chance of controlling teenage drug taking, alcoholism, smoking, motor bike accident and sexually transmitted diseases unless the emphasis is on youth. I would guess that problems of litter and pollution similarly require leadership at an early age. The problems of the aged can be shared with the young. It is stated that the old and the young tolerate each other better than many more closely aligned groups. Taken as a package, the problems for the year 2000, and onwards, are, in my view, especially a question of attitudes learned in childhood.

Young people in the 1980s – would they benefit from stronger leadership and if so of what kind? My own experience is limited to the St John Ambulance Brigade and to a small pilot study called 'The Enterprise Unit' which we set up initially in an attempt to keep the 14-22 age group interested in Brigade activities. Previously with some 600 or so 10-14 year olds of both sexes in the Brigade in Oxfordshire, one had the problem that few remained as members of the Brigade after the age of 14. This was largely due to poor leadership and dull programmes, with very little opportunity for the young to play adult roles. The Enterprise Unit provided fun as well as responsible role-playing which could be rewarded. Some 20 or so working class teenagers could combine service to the community, for example to the handicapped with night walks, camping at home and overseas, adventures in teaching first aid in the University of Istanbul or decorating a children's ward in the eye hospital in Jerusalem. It was successful but only because of the quality of leadership given by adults aged from 25-40 from medical, nursing and other relevant professions.

On a broader level, the whole question of what youth thinks or is capable of doing is described in a survey of 'Young People in the 80s' commissioned by the Review Group on the Youth Service for The Department of Education and Science. A study of 635 14-19 year old caucasians, West Indians and Asians of all social groups spread evenly over the UK .

The study shows that young people are friendly, responsible, happy and helpful. They are aspiring to be adults and this is achieved by employment, or experimenting with activities such as smoking, alcoholism drugs or sex. Enjoyment is a principle aim of leisure. They desire independence and freedom of choice but not responsibility of a kind which would restrict their independence. They see themselves as responsible people and want recognition by adults. Transport is one determinant of their independence. To take part in a programme of participation they need transport and minimal provisions. They aim for and have few ties which restrict their freedom of choice and they have therefore more time and can give a longer commitment to voluntary service. To be enjoyable this must provide fresh experience as well as some reward or recognition of their worth. If these are provided, smoking, alcoholism, drugs and sex become less consuming. The majority of the young in this study agreed that it was important for young people to be involved in some activities designed to improve the quality of life of the elderly or handicapped, to improve urban environments and to preserve those of rural locations. Involvement with the developing world and CND were rated highly but more important than for 'others' than themselves. Lack of access to such activities may be an explanation of lack of involvement.

Active involvement with social issues is in my view very much a question of access. For the St John Ambulance Enterprise group the opportunity to help any one is limited by the difficulty of making contact with those in need. Professionals are too busy to concern themselves with appointment making, transport and supervision of contact with the young volunteer and those in need, especially when one or the other does not turn up. Being busy is a question of priorities and hence attitude of mind.

A programme for youth aimed at smoking, alcoholism, drugs, pollution, accident prevention and caring for the infirm does not need to convince the young of its importance. It is not a question of information, since health education of this kind is constantly provided. The problem is active involvement of adults in the young's leisure time in a manner which solves their hopes for independence, meeting their aspiration of being adult and to gain fresh experience. Altruism, or the biological need to help, may be for the young much more the need to be recognised as both helpful and achieving like an adult.

Experience from the Scouts, Guides, Duke of Edinburgh Award and the St John Ambulance cadet movement suggests that awards in the form of medals, badges and certificates, publicly presented, are attractive to the young. Achievement is in each case a consequence of a programme that teaches proficiency. Even in the St John Ambulance Brigade there is little in the list of subjects which the cadets can study that is relevant to the major health problems outlined above. I have suggested elsewhere that proficiency in helping the handicap is as appropriate as is 'caring for animals', and a 'handyman's badge' could be replaced by proficiency in 'aids for the disabled' or 'the young gardener' could be more valuable as a 'planter of trees'. Sports medicine is similarly an uncharted area in youth programmes in this country, in spite of the enormous desire of the young to achieve in their sports..

Addendum 2017: Since writing the above the St John Ambulance Brigade, the St Andrews Association and the British Red Cross have produced a *Carers Handbook: A practical guide for looking after ill, disabled and elderly people.* London: Dorling Kindersley, 1997). The paralympics has also done much to promote rehabilitation of the wounded in armed conflict and from land mines.

One advantage of dealing with youth is that they are less clearly divided into social classes. It is a criticism of the medical profession is that it offers less information to the working class (Pendelton and Bochner, 1980) and relies on health visitors to give advice to this class on its lifestyle. Black and Strong (1982) state, "They will no longer be able to do so", but they do not say why! I believe that the young GP trainee is not class conscious and more could be done to give the trainee access to youth perhaps through sports medicine.

There is a need for the medical and nursing professions to involve themselves in the leisure time of youth through organisations such as the Scouts and Guides and St John Ambulance cadet movement. Programmes which are educational, exciting and meet the aspirations of the young for independence and adult role playing must be devised. Award systems with appropriate publicity are needed such as the Duke of Edinburgh Award Scheme. The professions can provide information and access to areas which at the moment are not often seen by the young, and even more rarely by working class young who most need education.

Casualty Union – an Example of the Value of Youth Theatre

Casualty Union is an organisation set up to provide casualties and patients with realistic acting and make up. Examples of their activities include: aircraft crash exercise, advanced trauma care for nurses, advanced trauma life support for doctors, bomb blast exercise, major traffic accident, car crash extrication for the emergency services, chemical spillage, and decontamination. They assist with training for first responders, major disasters, mortuary, paramedic, pharmacists, St John Ambulance, Red Cross and the armed forces. The list of activities they undertake is phenomenal. They also do occasional film work, a number of members going on to forge careers in the film and television industry. It is of immense value for teaching and it is fun for a group of young people. I have used acting and make up for the Enterprise Group teaching in the University of Istanbul and for many Oxfordshire village fete demonstrations, providing a role for the young in public education. I have shown that, provided there is a commentator, acting in this way can be effective even by the most incoherent of the young. It is successfully used by both African and Indian youth from orphanages to educate the public about HIV/AIDS. I have used it in public demonstrations about the management of confusion (dementia), drug addiction and football hooliganism.

The young are used to demonstrating, they are pleasing to watch, and they are happy to demonstrate all manner of subjects such as against the nuclear arms race, climate change and its hazards, and the needs of the frail elderly, at pop festivals and other events. I believe they could play a greater role in education in the market place, as strolling players, folk groups, or morality players, but they must have professionals as one or more of their team.

What role for the Medical and Nursing Professions?

> *Even so, the impact on the health of the population served was disappointing. It became clear that doctors and nurses were trained for the part they were required to play.*

So stated Webb at the Green College lecture entitled Medicine in the third world.

> *They (doctors) had no administration nor management skills, no preparation for the supervision and support of health auxiliaries and no experience which would help them to work with rural communities and their leaders.*

Elsewhere Webb states, "and often it is the village worker and not the doctor who comes up with the answers." Still better if it is both working together.

Faced with the massive problem of health needs in the year 2000 it is an enormous indictment of the professions that they are doing so little to mobilise the large resources of the volunteer. They are not trained to do so, and there is nothing in the curriculum of the medical student nor nurse which would draw attention to the need to support auxiliaries and to lead lay people.

Rudolph Klein (2001) suggests that the dominant role of the medical profession will survive in western health care systems only if it shows that medicine is more than applied technology, because it manages to show consumers that doctors are their best allies in coping with the organisational complexities of the health care systems. The theme is thus a a recurring one – participation is a two way phenomenon. Being an ally is more than being a liason officer, it is joining the ranks.

References

Acheson, E.D.(1982). 'The impending Crisis of old age: a challenge to ingenuity', *Lancet*, 592-594.

Brister, J. (1984). 'Healthy changes for medical practice', *Development Forum* March, 13.

Crossman, R.H.S. (1973). Sidney Ball Memorial Lecture. *The Role of of the Volunteer in the Modern Social Science.* Oxford: Clarendon Press.

Day, G.H. (1983). 'The Samaritans and the medical profession', *Lancet*, 1477-1479.

Young People in the 80s: A Survey. Her Majesty's Stationary Office:Department of Education and Science, 66.

King, M.H (1983). 'Medicine in an Unjust World' in D,J, Weatherall, D.J., Ledingham, J.G.G. & Warrell, D.A. (Eds.), *Oxford Textbook of Medicine.* Oxford University Press.

Klein, R. (1982). 'Health care in the age of disillusionment', *British Medical Association*, 285:2.

Lapwood, R. (1982. 'Chaplain to casualty', *British Medical Journal* 285, 194-195.

Pritchard, P. (1981). 'Patient participation in general practice', London: Royal College of General Practitioners: Occasional paper No 17.

Smail, S.A. (1982). 'Helping agencies', *British Medical Journal* 285, 121-1674.

Titmus, R. (1970). *The Gift Relationship.* London: George Unwin, 198.

Webb, J.K.G. (1984). 'Medicine in the Third World', Green College Lectures 1984, *British Medical Journal* 288, 1141-1144.

Index